Monographs on Endocrinology

Volume 28

Philip L. Ballard

Hormones and Lung Maturation

With a Contribution by Roberta A. Ballard

With 85 Figures and 80 Tables

Springer-Verlag
Berlin Heidelberg New York Tokyo

Philip L. Ballard, M.D., Ph.D.

Professor of Pediatrics
Department of Pediatrics and
Cardiovascular Research Institute
University of California Medical Center
San Francisco, CA 94143/U.S.A.

Roberta A. Ballard, M.D.

Chief of Pediatrics and
Director of the Intensive Care Nursery
Mt. Zion Hospital and Medical Center
San Francisco, CA 94120/U.S.A.

ISBN-13:978-3-642-82485-2 e-ISBN-13:978-3-642-82483-8
DOI: 10.1007/978-3-642-82483-8

Library of Congress Cataloging in Publication Data
Ballard, Philip L. Hormones and lung maturation.
(Monographs on endocrinology; v. 28) Includes bibliographies and index.
1. Lungs – Growth. 2. Fetus – Physiology. 3. Thyroid hormones – Physiological effect. 4. Sympathomimetic agents – Physiological effect. I. Ballard, Roberta A. II. Title. III. Series [DNLM: 1. Hormones – physiology. 2. Lung – embryology. 3. Lung – physiology. W1 M057 v. 28 / WF 600 B189h]
QP121.B23 1985 599'.012 85-17266
ISBN-13:978-3-642-82485-2 (U.S.)

Softcover reprint of the hardcover 1st edition 1986

2127/3020-543210

Preface

As I reflect on the evolution of this book, I am struck by the differences between my early conceptions and the final product. When I was first approached by Springer-Verlag regarding a monograph on my interests in the area of fetal lung development, I imagined that it would be relatively easy to summarize my contributions, plus the work of other investigators as needed for proper perspective. This rather naive idea was abandoned as I prepared my initial outlines for the monograph. I quickly realized that contributions from my laboratory are not sufficient for telling the story of "hormones and lung maturation". The result of this decision is a longer and more heavily-referenced book than I originally envisioned.

Although I have attempted to discuss in considerable detail most aspects of hormones and the fetal lung, I know with certainty that I have not included all relevant references in each area. In most of these instances this reflects my impatience or lack of diligence, and I offer my apologies to those investigators whose work has been so omitted. In some situations published work has not been cited in a deliberate decision to limit the breadth of discussion or, rarely, due to my judgment of major shortcomings in experimental design or execution.

Thus, this book has evolved into an overview of hormones and pulmonary development, with a major emphasis on research with which I have been involved. I have attempted to discuss the biochemical mechanisms of hormone action with particular emphasis on receptor systems in the lung. It will be evident on reading several of the following chapters that we know considerably more about receptor mediation of hormone action than about other details of biochemical effects in lung cells.

A major challenge of future research in this area, in my opinion, is the definition of specific gene products influenced by hormones and the role of the induced proteins in cellular metabolism and lung physiology. Investigation at this level will no doubt involve many years of future effort to provide a detailed understanding of hormonal influence. The chore ahead of us is made both more complex and interesting since lung development is under the influence of several hormones which interact in both negative and positive fashion. The rewards of research in this field include insights into basic themes and mechanisms of differentiation, the role and mechanism of hormone action in modulating developmental processes, and the application and hopefully improving efficacy of therapeutic intervention with hormones to improve the outcome for infants delivered prematurely.

I have focused my discussion in this book on three classes of hormones: glucocorticoids, thyroid hormones, and β-adrenergic agonists. This represents not only my bias, based on my personal research experiences, but also hopefully objective assessment of information in the literature. The effects of treatment with each of these hormones are extensively documented, and there is considerable reason to believe that endogenous hormones of each class influence lung differentiation during normal and/or abnormal gestations. Accordingly, the bulk of the chapters relate to various aspects of these three hormones in the lung.

Glucocorticoids are discussed in Chaps. 2 through 6 and in Chap. 10. Chapter 2 reviews the various effects of in vivo corticosteroid treatment on development of the fetal lung. In Chap. 4 I have collected and discussed various lines of evidence relating to the influence of endogenous corticoids in modulating the rate of fetal lung maturation. Chapter 3 describes various properties of glucocorticoid receptors in lung, and summarizes the evidence that effects of glucocorticoids are mediated by the receptor system. Two chapters are devoted to the use of glucocorticoids for prevention of respiratory distress syndrome and other diseases of premature infants. Roberta Ballard, my wife and frequent collaborator, has contributed Chap. 5 which reviews clinical aspects of corticosteroid therapy. Chapter 6 describes the pharmacokinetics of administered corticosteroid as well as effects of treatment on various endogenous hormones. Finally, in Chap. 10 I discuss interactions between glucocorticoids and other hormones in lung maturation.

There is considerably less information on thyroid hormones in lung differentiation. I discuss in Chap. 7 various effects of thyroid hormones both in vivo and in culture systems, thyroid hormone receptors of the lung, and the evidence that receptors mediate thyroid hormone effects. A relatively recent area of investigation is the interaction between thyroid hormones and glucocorticoids, which in many cases is synergistic, and this topic is included in Chap. 10.

Adrenergic agonists are discussed in Chap. 8 which reviews the effects of these hormones and information on the receptor-adenylate cyclase system of the lung. The limited data regarding interactions between β-agonists and other hormones are included in the final chapter.

Although this book focuses primarily on three hormones, I discuss in Chap. 9 various other hormones which also affect the fetal lung. In general, there is less information about the effects and mechanism of the other hormones and their possible role during normal development is not established. I have not included a discussion of all agents and hormones which have been examined with regard to the fetal lung. It is highly likely that research of the future will add to the list of hormones deserving discussion. In particular, preliminary data indicate that prostaglandins and endorphins will fall into this category.

I have not approached the subject matter of this book from a historical viewpoint, but I touch on this aspect in Chap. 2. Certainly my own view of this field is strongly influenced by the perspective of time. I have been fortunate to be a participant in this area of research since its modern beginnings, which date to 1969 and the first of many contributions by G. C. Liggins. In that year I was working in the laboratory of Gordon Tomkins at the NIH as a postdoctoral research fellow. Those were exciting times in the study of hormone action, and Tomkins' laboratory provided a particulary stimulating scientific atmosphere. At that time the first information on steroid receptors was becoming available and I was both intrigued and excited by these first glimpses at how hormones acted within cells. My interest in endocrinology from a biochemical point of view had been initially stimulated by H. G. Williams-Ashman during my M. D./Ph. D. training years at the University of Chicago.

Although I was not aware of the work of Liggins in 1969, an interest in neonatology began during my internship at Stanford in 1968 and was nurtured by frequent discussions with my wife, who was a neonatal fellow during our two years in Washington, D.C. Thus, appropriately primed in both research and clinical interests, I arrived at the University of California, San Francisco in 1970. Clearly the highlight of the following year of pediatric residency was becoming aware of the relationship between glucocorticoids and fetal lung maturation. It occurred precisely between 9:00 and 10:00 a.m. on a Saturday morning. At the urging of my wife, a fellow in the Cardiovascular Research Institute, I attended a Saturday morning seminar directed by Julius Comroe. As I listened to Arnold Platzker describe the effects of administering dexamethasone to fetal lambs, I pondered questions about steroid receptors and other details of the glucocorticoid effect. My questions led to further discussions and with the help and encouragement of William Tooley and John Clements, I prepared a supplemental application to their SCOR grant, received funding, and began studies of glucocorticoid receptors in fetal rabbit lung. I received advice from John Baxter, by then already a local authority in receptorology, bench space and encouragement from Gordon Tomkins, who was then a member of the Department of Biochemistry and Biophysics at San Francisco, and collaboration from Roberta Ballard. In 1972 we published a paper describing the presence of glucocorticoid receptors in the lung. My interest in the lung and hormone action has persisted these past 14 years. In part, the following chapters chronicle my interests and accomplishments over this time.

This book has required a lot of time and help. For the past two years or so I have been absent from the laboratory on Wednesdays to work on "The Book". I thank my colleagues in the laboratory during this time for their understanding and patience; these include Linda Gonzales, Robert Ertsey, Madeleine Huey, Ta-Mund Chou, Leslie Hovey, and Raimund Hümmelink. I have had help from many sources. I thank the following people for reading and reviewing various chapters: James Roberts, Ian Gross, Linda Gonzales, Joseph Kitterman, and Roberta Ballard. The initial typing of the manuscript, and most of the organizational effort were provided by Marilyn Biagini. I am sure that we share equally the satisfaction and relief of completing the project, and I extend my special thanks to her. I also thank Carol Dahlstrom for her many hours of help in word processing, including several revisions of each chapter. My thanks also to Mary Helen Briscoe for the art work on many of the figures which I used. I am grateful to the NIH for continuing support of my research and writing. This undertaking has been supported in part by Grants HL-24075, HL-24056, and HL/HD-30541. I also thank Melvin Grumbach for his encouragement in this project and J. Wieczorek and other editors at Springer-Verlag for their patience as I missed more than one projected completion date. Finally, I particularly acknowledge the help and encouragement of my wife, Roberta Ballard, who is Chief of Pediatrics and Director of the Intensive Care Nursery at Mt. Zion Hospital, San Francisco. She has contributed a detailed and provocative discussion of clinical topics (Chap. 5) and is a highly-valued and loved colleague in both this and other undertakings.

San Francisco, October 1985 Philip L. Ballard

Contents

1 Lung Development

1.1 Introduction

At birth, the major transition for the newborn infant is switching from a passive to an active role in gas exchange. Success in this process is the major determinant of the well-being and survival of newly-born infants. When delivery occurs at term the transition is normally accomplished with ease. With premature delivery, however, the ability of the lung to exchange gas is often inadequate.

The importance of the lungs in the transition to extrauterine life has long been recognized. However, only in recent times have we begun to understand the physiologic and biochemical processes underlying lung development. The process of preparing the lung for birth may be considered to include four areas: 1) morphologic development of the terminal airspaces (saccules and alveoli) to allow gas exchange from airways to capillaries; 2) biochemical differentiation of alveolar cells to provide for reabsorption of lung fluid and production of surfactant; 3) development of the respiratory musculature through in utero breathing movements; and 4) development of the extrathoracic components such as the various chemoreceptors and medullary control center that regulate ventilatory activity.

The most recent phase in the study of lung development relates to the regulation of the maturational processes. During the last decade and a half, the importance of hormones in lung maturation has become apparent. In particular, hormonal effects on the first two areas mentioned above have received considerable attention. The goal of this book is to bring together current information on the effects and mechanisms of various hormones in preparing the lung for birth. The discussion is restricted almost entirely to hormonal influence on changes occurring relatively late in pulmonary development rather than during embryogenesis and early fetal development.

To date, most descriptions of hormone action in the lung have been concerned with either lung structure or the surfactant system of type II alveolar cells. An additional area of increasing interest is the process of lung fluid secretion and reabsorption. Background information on this topic is included in Chap. 8, along with a discussion of beta-adrenergic influence. There has been relatively little research regarding hormone effects on interstitial cells, endothelial cells and macrophages, and these areas are mentioned only in passing in subsequent chapters.

This review of lung development, as well as the following discussion of hormonal effects, focuses almost entirely on the respiratory function of the lung. As detailed in Chaps. 2, 7, 8, 9 and 10, investigations of effects of glucocorticoids and other hormones have been restricted almost entirely to lung morphology and the physiologic and biochemical aspects related to respiratory function and the surfactant system. Nevertheless, it is well recognized that the lung performs a number of metabolic activities unrelated to gas exchange. Capillary endothelial cells produce biologically active substances as well as modifying and inactivating a variety of compounds presented by the pulmonary circulation. A recent review of lung metabolic activities has appeared in the series of Ciba Foundation Symposia (1980). Many of the metabolic activities of the lung are no doubt important in the process of birth and air breathing. These include, for example, the kallikrein-kinin system, the renin-angiotensin system, inactivation of monamines, and, in particular, the production and metabolism of prostaglandins. In some instances, hormones are known to influence metabolic processes of adult lung (e.g., glucocorticoids and prostaglandin synthesis). Future research will no doubt more clearly define the influence of various hormones in non-respiratory functions of the developing lung.

This chapter provides an overview of lung development during fetal and neonatal life, concentrating on morphologic aspects and the surfactant system. When possible, data for the human lung are presented; comparisons between species are included, since a variety of animal models have been used in studies of hormone action. For more detailed discussions and reviews of lung development, the reader is referred to other publications on this topic (Sorokin 1959; Kikkawa et al. 1968; Kikkawa et al. 1971; Williams 1977a; Kauffman 1980; Inselman and Mellins 1981; Meyrick and Reid 1977, 1982; Grant et al. 1983; Fukuda et al. 1983; Gail and Lenfant 1983; and Burri 1984) and several chapters in books edited by DeReuck and Porter (1967), Hodson (1977), and Farrell (1982).

1.2 Structural Development

1.2.1 Architecture and Pattern of Growth

The anatomy of the mature respiratory system may be considered as containing three regions: 1) the upper airways, which are primarily extrathoracic, and consist of the nose and mouth, pharynx, and trachea as the portals of gas entrance and exit; 2) the lower conducting airways, which start with the mainstem bronchi and continue to the terminal bronchioles, and constitute the main gas distributing system within the lung; 3) the acinar region which is composed of respiratory bronchioles, alveolar ducts, and alveoli in the mature lung. The latter area accounts for 80–90 % of the tissue volume of the lung and is the region in which exchange of oxygen and carbon dioxide occurs. Most of the hormonal effects which have been described during fetal life occur in the acinar region.

The majority of the conducting airways are lined by ciliated epithelium and characterized by the presence of cartilage. The bronchioles, the most peripheral of the conducting airways, are distal to the last plates of cartilage which diminish progressively as the airways proceed peripherally. The terminal bronchioles are clustered with their associated acini in groups of three to five per lobule. The acini are thin-walled structures lined by nonciliated cells which have a high ratio of airspace to tissue in the mature, inflated lung.

The pulmonary vasculature has the dual role of carrying out gas exchange and providing the metabolic needs of pulmonary cells. Two vascular systems exist in the lung. Branches of the pulmonary artery and veins provide the blood supply to the terminal respiratory units and most of the pleura. The bronchial arteris and veins, which originate from the aorta, provide branches to the airway walls and hilar region of the lung. Consistent with the large volume of acinar tissue, the pulmonary artery system accounts for more than 90 % of the total pulmonary blood flow. Effective functioning of the lungs depends upon appropriate blood flow from pulmonary arteries to those regions of the lung that are inflated.

The overall pattern of development of the respiratory system is worth outlining before the specific details are discussed. The general concepts of the process for the human situation have been formalized by Reid (1967). First, division of the bronchial tree is fully developed by the 16th week of gestation. At this time, there are 15–25 sequential segments of conducting airway from trachea through the terminal bronchioles. Formation and differentiation of the airway structure occur in a centrifugal manner from hilum to lung periphery. In experimental animals, at least, there are lobar differences in the formation of lung structure. The upper lobes mature at a somewhat faster rate than the lower lobes of the lung (Brumley et al. 1967; Kikkawa 1971; Kotas et al. 1977). Second, development of the pre-acinar blood vessels follows temporally airway formation, while the acinar arteries and veins develop concurrently with the alveoli. By 16 weeks gestation, nearly all the pre-acinar vessels are formed. Subsequently, these vessels grow in diameter and length, while new vessels continue to be formed in the intra-acinar region. During the canalicular phase of lung development (defined below) acini are slowly invaded by developing capillaries. This process occurs in a centripetal direction and concludes with extension of capillaries to respiratory bronchioles. Third, alveolar development occurs primarily after birth in the human.The alveoli develop in a centripetal fashion, appearing first on saccules, and then on alveolar ducts and respiratory bronchioles. The size and number of alveoli increases throughout childhood until thoracic growth ceases.

1.2.2 Stages of Growth

Formation of the lung from the earliest stage to the mature structure has been divided into five chronological periods. These phases describe the morphology of the developing airways and airspaces, and the actual delineations of different stages are accordingly somewhat arbitrary. The stages of lung development are summarized for six species in Table 1.1. Differences in the timing of differentiation are apparent, with maturation (formation of canaliculi or saccules) occurring relatively early in the human and later in rodents where the lung is still relatively immature at birth.

The photomicrographs in Fig. 1.1 illustrate the canalicular, saccular, and early alveolar stages of lung development in the human fetus. These specimens are from human fetuses of 22–36 weeks gestation, spanning the age

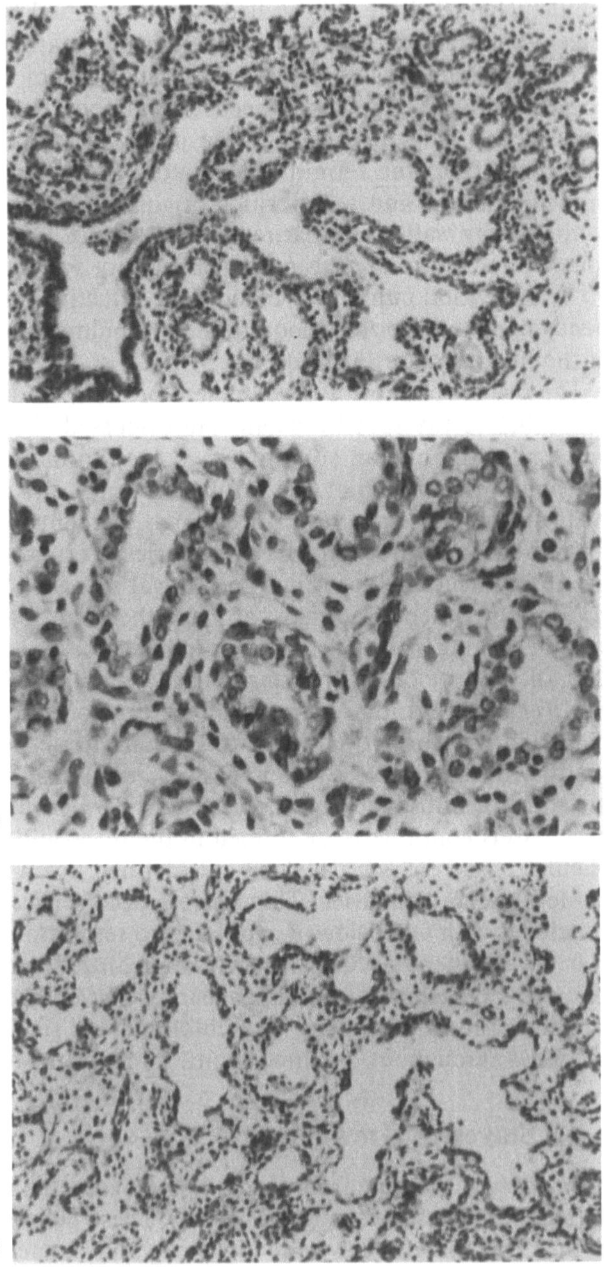

a

b

c

Fig. 1.1. **a** Section of lung from a 22-week human fetus showing the smooth-walled respiratory channels characteristic of the canalicular stage (×200). **b** Higher magnification (×500) of lung from the canalicular period. The potential airspaces are lined by a uniform cuboidal epithelium separated by abundant interstitium containing randomly dispersed blood vessels. **c** Lung of a 23-week fetus showing development of the wavy internal configuration of the respiratory channels. The epithelial cells remain cuboidal and the interstitium is abundant (×200). **d** Lung of a 29-week infant illustrating the saccular stage. The interstitium is thinner and epithelial cells have flattened, particularly in areas where blood vessels adjoin the epithelium. The *arrows* illustrate

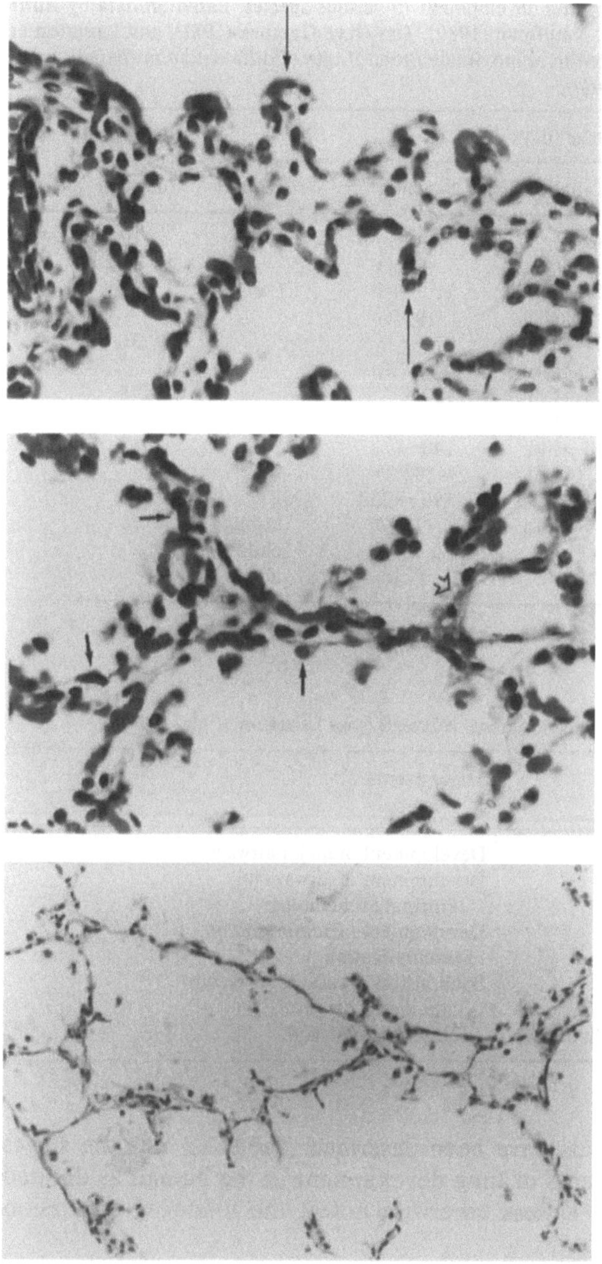

d

e

f

secondary crests which subdivide the saccules (×500). **e** Section of a lung from an infant at 36 weeks gestation illustrating development of septae containing both double capillary networks *(single arrows)* and thinner areas containing a single capillary network *(double arrows)* (×500). **f** Well-developed alveoli in lung from an infant at 36 weeks gestation (×200). Reprinted from Langston et al. (1984), by permission

Table 1.1. Stages of morphologic lung development in various species. Based on data by Burri (1974), Meyrick and Reid (1977), Kauffman (1980), Ten Have-Opbroek (1981), and Langston et al. (1984). The species are arranged in approximate order of rate of differentiation (based on development of canalicular structure)

Species	Development stage (days of gestation)				Length of gestation (days)
	Glandular	Canalicular	Saccular	Alveolar	
Mouse	14→16	16.5→17.4 (87 %)	17.4→+5 (91 %)	+5→	19
Rat	13→18	19→20 (86 %)	21→+7 (95 %)	+7→21	22
Rabbit	19→24	24→27 (77 %)	27→ (87 %)	–	31
Sheep	→95	95→120 (64 %)	120→ (81 %)	–	148
Monkey (Rhesus)	50→80	80→140 (48 %)	140→ (83 %)	–	168
Human	42→112	112→196 (40 %)	196→252 (70 %)	252 through childhood	280

Table 1.2. Phases of human lung development. Adapted from Langston et al. (1984)

Phase	Gestational age (weeks)	Major events
Embryonic	3½–6	Development of major airways
Glandular	6–16	Development of airways to terminal bronchioles
Canalicular	16–28	Development of acinus and its vascularization
Saccular	28–36	Subdivision of saccule by secondary crests
Alveolar	36 through childhood	Acquisition of alveoli

range when hormonal effects have been described. Table 1.2 lists the stages and major morphologic events of lung development in the human as defined by Langston et al. (1984). Unless otherwise noted, the following discussion refers to the human situation.

1.2.2.1 Embryonic

Following formation of the primitive gut, the lung first appears as a ventral bud off the prospective esophagus near the end of the fourth week of gestation. Epithelial components of the lung are derived from the endoderm, and the connective tissue arises from the mesodermal germ layer. Through successive dichotomous divisions, the lung bud separates distally from the gut and grows into the surrounding mesenchyme. The branching determines the pattern for the corresponding conductive airways which develop later. By the end of the sixth week, the lobar and segmental sections of the airway tree are established as tubes lined by high columnar epithelial cells. The undifferentiated epithelial cell is a rapidly dividing stem cell which is felt to give rise to at least 12 different types of differentiated epithelial cells in the mature lung. The internal organization of the undifferentiated cell is unremarkable; the cytoplasm contains ribosomes, glycogen granules, and only small quantities of endoplasmic reticulum and Golgi apparatus.

During this stage the pulmonary arteries bud off from the sixth pair of aortic arches, growing into the mesenchyme where they surround the developing tubules. This vascular plexis is first connected only to systemic veins draining the gut and trachea, but subsequently they connect to the pulmonary veins which grow out of the atrial portion of the heart. The embryonic period extends from approximately 26 to 42 days gestation.

1.2.2.2 Glandular

This stage, also referred to as the pseudoglandular stage, is characterized by the complete formation of prospective airways (15–25 orders of branching depending on the segment) and by the first appearance of the acinar outlines. This process occurs through continuous growth and branching at the periphery of the epithelial tubes. The rate of cell proliferation in both the mesenchyme and epithelium is higher during the glandular stage than at any subsequent time. During this stage vascular branching also occurs but the vessels remain small with little blood flow.

Interactions between mesenchymal and epithelial cells appear to influence the rate and type of branching pattern. Intimate contacts between these cell types occur (Bluemink et al. 1976), and in animals the mesenchyme regulates budding of the epithelial tubes (Alescio and Cassini 1962; Wessells 1970). Removal of mesenchyme from the tip of a developing tube prevents further branching, whereas transplantation of mesenchymal tissue next to a lower order tube or the trachea induces new outgrowth. The mesenchymal requirement is organ but not species-specific; mediators and mode of action of this effect are not yet defined.

At the beginning of the glandular stage the lining cells are a homogeneous population of high columnar epithelial cells. In the proximal airways, cells differentiate into ciliated, non-ciliated, goblet and basal types, and both cartilage and smooth muscle appear in the trachea. By about the twelfth week mucous glands appear in the trachea and these develop secretory activity two weeks later. By the end of the glandular stage, the peripheral tubules, lined by columnar or cuboidal epithelial cells, represent the future acini of the lung parenchyma.

1.2.2.3 Canalicular

Between about 112 and 196 days gestation, the framework for future acini are laid down and vascularization occurs. Formation of acini proceeds by further peripheral branching and lengthening of terminal tubules, and eventually there is a marked widening of the airspaces at the expense of interstitial tissue. These new airspaces resemble small, blind-ending channels separated by mesenchymal tissue of relatively sparse cellularity. The channels assume an irregular wavy configuration as further subdivisions of the acinus are developed. During this stage the capillaries progress from a loose network within the mesenchyme to a close arrangement around the potential airspaces. Where close contact occurs, the first thin air-blood barriers are formed.

Initially during this period the respiratory channels are lined uniformly by cuboidal epithelium. As subdivisions of acini are formed, the lining epithelium begins to thin, particularly in the proximal portions, representing differentiation into type I alveolar cells. In the human lung, type II cells containing recognizable lamellar bodies are first detected at 20–24 weeks gestation (Campiche et al. 1963; Hage 1973). Maturation of type II cells (as studied in the rat) occurs at a time when proliferation of epithelial cells is low, consistent with the notion that withdrawal from the cell cycle is necessary for differentiation. Thus, surfactant synthesis and storage occur relatively early during fetal development, long before mature alveolar structure and substantial secretion of surfactant normally occur (see Fig. 1.3). If sufficient surfactant is present in air spaces during late canalicular stage, however, structural development is often adequate to support normal gas exchange and allow survival.

The inter-relationship between type II cells and type I cells during differentiation is not fully defined. Nevertheless, there is considerable evidence suggesting that type I cells arise from cuboidal epithelial cells containing lamellar bodies, apparently mimicking the process for regeneration of type I cells from type II cells in adult lung following both injury (Evans and Bils 1969; Adamson and Bowden 1974; Kauffman 1974) and pneumonectomy (Brody et al. 1978).

At term, in both the rabbit (Wang et al. 1971) and rat (Kauffman 1977), air spaces are lined with approximately 45 % differentiated type II cells and 55 % type I cells; the proportion of epithelial cells containing lamellar bodies does not exceed 50 % at any point during fetal life. Early in the third trimester most cells are cuboidal without lamellar inclusions; as maturation proceeds, the percentage of differentiated type II cells exceeds the percentage of flattened, type I cells. This pattern is consistent with differentiation of type I cells from surfactant containing cuboidal cells. A similar sequence of cell appearance apparently occurs in developing human lung, although this question has not been studied in detail (Hage 1973; Campiche et al 1963).

There are other more direct data supporting the proposal that the type II cell is the progenitor of the type I epithelial cell. Adamson and Bowden (1975) examined fetal rat lung near term by both microscopy and radioautography after labeling with [^{3}H]thymidine. DNA synthesis and cell division were maximal when terminal airways were lined exclusively by type II cells and undifferentiated cuboidal cells, and mitosis was not observed in differentiated type I cells. Furthermore, intermediate cell forms were observed prior to appearance of type I cells, consistent with differentiation of type I cells from type II cells. Well-differentiated type II cells undergo mitosis in fetal lung (Williams 1977a) and occasional type I cells are found to contain remnants of lamellar bodies (Williams 1977a; Balis and Conen 1964; Suzuki 1966; Mecurio and Rhodin 1977). In an electron microscopic study of fetal cat lung, Mercurio and Rhodin (1977) concluded that forthcoming differentiation of type I cells was heralded by cytoplasmic attenuation and not by an absence of lamellar bodies. The greatest proliferative activity of type II cells in the postnatal rat (day 7) coincides with development of septal crests and increasing accumulation of both type I and type II cells; labeling with [^{3}H]thymidine is not observed in type I cells at this time (Kauffman et al. 1974).

It has been postulated that a physical interaction between developing capillaries and neighboring type II cells is involved in differentiation of type I cells (Adamson and Bowden 1975). Cytodifferentiation during normal development is an asynchronous process with mature cell types present in increasing porportion during the canalicular and saccular stages. Exposure to exogenous glucocorticoids both in vivo (Chap. 2) and particularly in culture (Chap. 4) produces an accelerated and more synchronized process of cytodifferentiation.

1.2.2.4 Saccular

Between about 28 and 36 weeks gestation there is continued expansion of potential airspaces which is characterized morphologically by a marked decrease in interstitial tissue and development of narrower and more compact layers of lining cells. Cellular proliferation, as assessed by labeling experiments in the rat, is several times greater in fibroblasts and endothelial cells than in the epithelium at this time. Secondary crests appear in the distal airspaces, producing the progenitors of future alveolar ducts and sacs. However, the saccular walls retain their double capillary structure as distinct from the single capillary epithelial layer in mature alveoli. During this stage there is increasing deposition of elastin within the interstitial space as the volume of that area decreases. The type I and type II epithelial cells are well-differentiated at this time and secretion of surfactant into the fluid-filled saccules begins.

1.2.2.5 Alveolar

Although the appearance of alveoli in the human lung prior to birth is still controversial, recent observations by Langston et al. (1984) found alveoli in all lungs examined at 36 weeks gestation. They defined an alveolus as a "thin-walled, flask-shaped or multi-faceted polygonal structure with a single capillary network." It has been assumed that the continuing process of capillary apposition in the condensing interstitial space results in the fusion of the two septal capillary networks into a single vessel. There is agreement that alveolarization is a continuing process which lasts throughout much of childhood. Estimates of alveolar number at term range between 20 and 70 $\times$ 10^6. Since many infants at 36 weeks gestation have no respiratory difficulty, it is clear that adequate gas exchange occurs in the absence of significant alveolarization. The data of Table 1.3 illustrate the continued growth of the human lung after birth. Lung weight and volume increase by approximately 10- and 25-fold, respectively, during childhood. There is a similar increase in respiratory bronchioles, alveolar ducts, number of alveoli and total alveolar surface area. Thus, growth is a continuing process, whereas cytodifferentiation is completed before birth.

Table 1.3. Growth of human lung after birth. Compiled from data of Burri and Weibel (1977) and Meyrick and Reid (1977)

	At birth	Adult
Number respiratory bronchioles and alveolar ducts	1.5×10^6	14×10^6
Acinar length (mm)	1	1 000
Distance from terminal bronchiole to pleura (mm)	1.1	4
Number of alveoli	20×10^6	300×10^6
Alveolar size (μ)	40–120	250–300
Alveolar surface area (m^2)	2.8	75
Lung volume (ml)	200	5 500
Lung weight (g)	60	700

1.2.3 Cells of the Acinus

The mature lung is an extremely heterogeneous organ containing about 40 different cell types (Sorokin 1970). The parenchymal area is less complex, however, being comprised primarily of type I and type II cells, interstitial cells, endothelial cells and macrophages. The relative distribution of these cell types for adult rat lung is shown in Table 1.4. Capillary endothelial cells and interstitial cells are the most numerous types. The numbers of type I and type II epithelial cells are similar; however, type I cells have a greater area and occupy approximately 98 % of the alveolar surface. In the human, it has been estimated each alveolus contains 113 type I cells and 170 type II cells, with type I cells occupying approximately 95 % of the surface area (Meyrick and Reid 1977).

1.2.3.1 Type I Cells

These cells have a centrally-located oval nucleus from which extend thin sheets of cytoplasm of 0.1–0.3 μm thickness. The cytoplasm of the type I cell can extend through pores of Kohn and thus provide the epithelial lining for neighboring alveoli. Alveolar capillaries lie immediately below type I cells separated only by a single basement membrane. Thus, the diffusion barrier between blood and the airspace consists only of the endothelial cells, base-

Table 1.4. Cell types in lung parenchyma (adult rat). Data from Weibel and Gil (1977)

	Relative distribution (%)	Alveolar surface area (%)
Type I epithelial cells	10	98
Type II epithelial cells	12	2
Endothelial cells	40	
Alveolar macrophages	5	
Interstitial cells	33	

ment membrane, and the thin cytoplasmic extension of type I cells. There are relatively few mitochondria, ribosomes, and pinocytic vesicles in both endothelial and type I epithelial cells, further facilitating gas diffusion. Type I cells are relatively susceptible to injury due in part to their large surface area and limited metabolic capacity for repair processes. Following acute injury, new type I cells differentiate from type II cells which undergo division and differentiation (Evans and Bils 1969; Evans et al. 1973).

1.2.3.2 Type II Cells

These cells appear morphologically as cuboidal cells which are often located in the corners of alveoli. They form tight junctions with type I cells and their apical surface is often partially covered by cytoplasm of the type I cell. The luminal surface of type II cells are characterized by microvilli. In the mature animal, lamellar bodies are present in the cell cytoplasm, particularly near the luminal surface. The cytoplasm of the type II cell is also rich in mitochondria, golgi bodies and rough endoplasmic reticulum. In late fetal and early postnatal life most type II cells were found to have foot processes penetrating discontinuities in the basement membrane (Grant et al. 1983). These extensions may interact with underlying interstitial cells, perhaps reflecting cell-cell influences on structural differentiation or surfactant synthesis.

The major known function of these cells is the synthesis and secretion of surfactant (described in the following section). Type II cells undergo hyperplasia in response to injury, and serve as the progenitor of type I cells. Finally, these cells in postnatal lung have an active ion transport system which promotes movement of water from the alveolar lumen into the pulmonary circulation and lymphatics.

1.2.3.3 Fibroblasts

Interstitial fibroblasts are located in alveolar septae and are the sites for synthesis and secretion of collagen, elastin, proteoglycans, and other proteins of the interstitial space. There are at least two classes of interstitial cells in the lung during late fetal life as distinguished by the absence or presence of neutral lipid inclusions. On the basis of their location and morphology, it has been assumed that both cell types are fibroblasts.

Various properties of the lipid interstitial cells have been determined in morphologic studies (Brody and Kaplan 1983; Vaccaro and Brody 1979; Brody and Vaccaro 1979; Maksvytis et al. 1981; Tordet et al. 1981). In the rat, the cells are first detected at about 19 days gestation. The number and volume of lipid vacuoles per cell increases both before and especially just after birth; there is a 2-fold increase between days 4 and 7 after birth, a time of rapid alveolar proliferation. The labeling index with [^{3}H]thymidine is relatively high at 4 days of age and quite low a week later. After this time, the cells gradually decrease in number and are infrequently observed in adult lung. It has been reported that lipid interstitial cells are also present in lung of the fetal primate. Lipid-containing cells are often found adjacent to the more typical and abundant non-lipid containing fibroblasts and in contact with type II cells.

The lipid interstitial cells contain the enzyme lipoprotein lipase, probably explaining in part their accumulation of intracellular lipid. Studies of cAMP generation suggest that the cells contain receptors for glucagon, β-adrenergic agonists and PGE_2. Based on the thymidine labeling experiments, it has been concluded that lipid interstitial cells are not derived from non-lipid containing cells or vice versa. These and other morphologic studies support the concept that more than one type of fibroblast is present in the alveolar interstitium during fetal and early postnatal life. The possible specialized functions of the lipid-containing fibroblasts are not yet known, although it has been speculated that they might provide substrate for phospholipid synthesis in type II cells or have a role in alveolar formation.

Heterogeneity of interstitial fibroblasts has also been described in adult lung. As first reported by Kapanci et al. (1974), adult lung contains a population of interstitial cells with abundant microfilaments which stain for both actin and myosin. These interstitial cells are observed during septal formation (day 5–15 in the rat), produce elastin, and are commonly situated at the junction of intra-alveolar septae with cytoplasmic processes extending along the air-blood barrier (Brody and Vaccaro 1979). It has been suggested that the contractile interstitial cells (which occasionally contain lipid droplets) may arise from the lipid-containing fibroblasts (which have some cytoplasmic filaments). Myofibroblasts are felt to be contractile and to have a role in determining alveolar shape during respiration (Kapanci et al. 1983).

1.2.3.4 Endothelial Cells

Capillary endothelial cells are a major cell type in lung acini. These cells comprise the final portion of the barrier for gas exchange from alveolus to the circulation. As in other capillaries, pulmonary endothelial cells contain vesicles which participate in transport of fluid and macromolecules across the cells. As mentioned previously, these cells possess numerous metabolic activities involved primarily in the generation and metabolism of vasoactive and other biologically active compounds (Ciba Foundation Symposium 1980; Gail and Lenfant 1983). The close apposition of capillaries with the potential air spaces in fetal lung represents a critical event in lung maturation.

1.2.3.5 Macrophages

Another cell of the acinar area is the alveolar macrophage. In adult lung, these cells are found in the alveolar airspace where they perform a phagocytic function. They contain a number of enzymes and are the last line of defense in the lung against foreign particles and microorganisms. They also ingest and metabolize surfactant as discussed in the following section. Most if not all macrophages arise from blood monocytes.

The ontogeny of macrophage alveolar influx and function has been documented in the rabbit lung (Zeligs et al. 1977a, b; Nerurkar et al. 1977). Macrophages are first detected during late gestation and their numbers increase many-fold postnatally. It is conceivable that the paucity of macrophages in the fetal lung results in differences in the metabolism and recycling of surfactant between the fetus and the adult animal.

1.3 The Surfactant System

Pulmonary surfactant may be defined as a complex mixture of lipids and protein, characterized by high surface activity, which is absorbed as a monolayer at the alveolar air-liquid interface to promote alveolar stability on deflation. Surfactant may also have a role in fluid movement and pulmonary defense mechanisms, but these functions are not yet well defined. There have been numerous review articles on surfactant and its discovery, synthesis and secretion, isolation, composition, physiologic function, and clinical importance. These include, among others, contributions by King (1974), Goerke (1974), Clements and Tooley (1977), Clements and King (1976), Sanders (1982a, b, c), King (1982), and articles by several authors in Robertson et al. (1984). The following discussion is limited to an overview of the surfactant system.

1.3.1 Discovery/Physiologic Function

Awareness of pulmonary surfactant in modern times is generally credited to the report by Von Neergaard in 1929. He appreciated the unique situation in lung where gas exchange must occur through an air-liquid interface within a spherical structure of relatively small radius. The high surface tension in this structure predisposes to eventual collapse of alveoli unless the surface tension can be reduced. It is now well-documented and generally accepted that pulmonary surfactant, through adsorption to the air-liquid interface, progressively reduces surface tension during expiration (compression of the lipid layer) and prevents alveolar collapse. Subsequent studies by Clements (1957), Pattel (1958), Clements et al. (1958) and Clements and Tierney (1965) demonstrated that lung fluid produces stable bubbles, and, when placed on a surface balance apparatus, lowers the surface tension at the interface in a manner dependent on surface area.

In 1959, Avery and Mead published the first information relating to surface active material in lung of the human infant. In this important study, minces of lung were agitated in saline and the filtered extract was tested for surface activity on a Langmuir-Wilhelmy surface balance. Data for the lowest surface tension obtained on the films is plotted vs. the birthweight of the infant in Fig. 1.2. A low surface tension (5–10 dynes/cm) was found with lung extracts of most infants over 1,200 g dying from causes other than hyaline membrane disease. By contrast, lung extracts from 9 infants dying of hyaline membrane disease did not produce a low surface tension. Extract from one infant of a diabetic mother had little surface activity, consistent with delayed lung maturation as subsequently established (Chap. 9). The findings of Avery and Mead (1959) and subsequent investigators have established that hyaline membrane disease, or respiratory distress syndrome (RDS), of premature infants is primarily a disease of surfactant deficiency. In such infants, progressive atelectasis occurs due to the high surface tension within alveoli, and the infants develop a clinical syndrome characterized by progressive respiratory distress (Chap. 5).

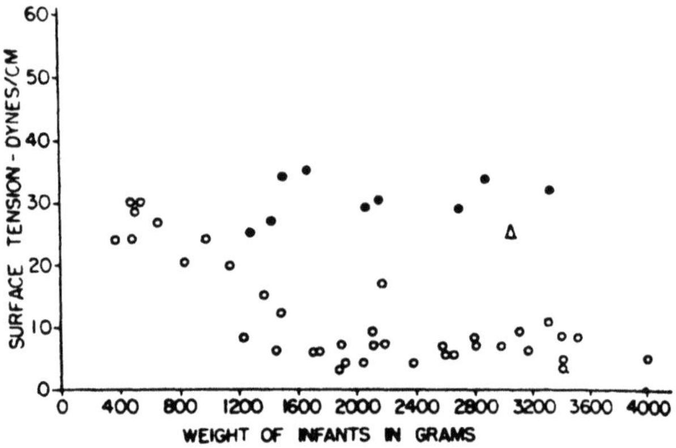

Fig. 1.2. Lowest surface tension obtained with lung extracts in the study by Avery and Mead (1959). Data are shown for infants dying from causes other than hyaline membrane disease *(open circles)*, infants dying with hyaline membrane disease *(closed circles)*, and one stillborn infant of a diabetic mother *(triangle)*. Reproduced from Avery and Mead (1959), by permission

1.3.2 Ontogeny

In the human, the concentration of saturated phosphatidylcholine (PC) in lung tissue increases around 20 weeks gestation during the canalicular stage (see Fig. 4.7). This timing is in agreement with morphologic studies examining epithelial cell cytodifferentiation in general and the appearance of intracellular lamellar bodies in type II cells in particular. The period of time required for differentiation of most alveolar epithelial cells in the human is

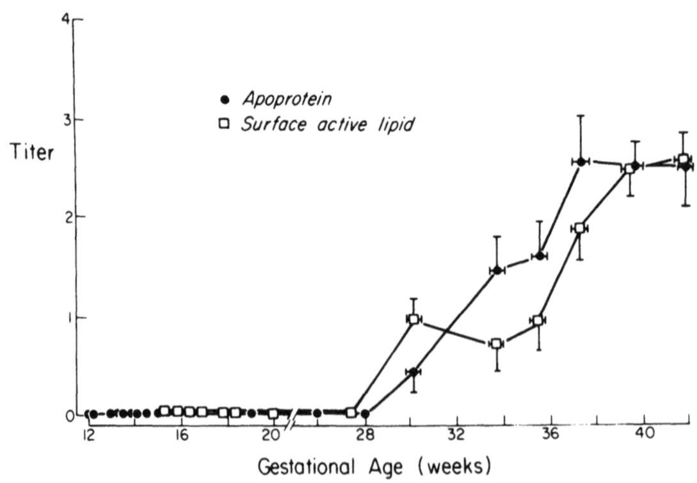

Fig. 1.3. Ontogeny of surface activity and surfactant apoprotein during human gestation. Surface activity was estimated by foam stability and apoprotein concentration was determined by a latex agglutination assay in amniotic fluid samples. Data are mean ± SE for 14–32 samples at each point. Reproduced from King et al. (1975), by permission

unclear, but it appears that this may occur over a period of only a few weeks. In the fetal rabbit, for example, surfactant is present by 27 days gestation, and most of the accumulation of lamellar bodies occurs over a period of a few days during the saccular stage of development. Surfactant is detected in mouse, rat and sheep lung at about 18, 19 and 120 days gestation, respectively (Meyrick and Reid 1977).

Although intracellular surfactant is present in human lung at relatively high concentrations soon after mid-gestation, surfactant does not normally appear in amniotic fluid (reflecting secretion into alveolar spaces) until about 30 weeks gestation (Fig. 1.3). The occurrence of RDS reflects in part the timing of surfactant accumulation in alveoli. RDS is almost uniformly present in infants at 26 weeks gestation, and the incidence of the disease falls to about 50 % by approximately 31 weeks. The temporal discrepancy between amniotic fluid tests of lung maturity and the actual incidence of RDS no doubt relates to several factors of which labor (promoting secretion of surfactant) is particularly important (see Chap. 8).

1.3.3 Composition

The chemical composition has been studied in surfactant isolated from a variety of starting materials and from numerous species. The most common procedure has been isolation of surface-active material from bronchoalveolar lavage of adult animals. Numerous preparative procedures have been utilized for purification with most involving density gradient sedimentation.

Table 1.5 compares the phospholipid composition in whole rat lung, two cell populations, and isolated surfactant. The enrichment for PC (most of which is saturated) and phosphatidylglycerol in type II cells and, to a greater extent, in lavage surfactant is demonstrated. There is also relatively less of the common phospholipids of membranes in these two sources. This type of distribution pattern is seen in adult lung of several species which have been studied. Although saturated PC is present in all tissues, the concentration (in both

Table 1.5. Phospholipid composition in adult rat lung (% of total phospholipids). Data from Mason and Williams (1977)

Phospholipid	Lung tissue	Lavage surfactant	Type II cells	Macrophages
Phosphatidylserine + lyso PC	4.8	0.2	1.4	6.0
Phosphatidylinositol	8.5	1.8	2.0	3.4
Sphingomyelin	9.8	0.3	1.6	16.3
PC	45.9	83.3	75.0	49.2
Phosphatidylglycerol	3.3	9.3	6.1	1.5
Phosphatidylethanolamine	19.1	1.9	10.7	17.0
Diphosphatidylglycerol lyso (bis) phosphatidic acid	4.0	1.8	1.4	3.7
Unidentified	4.1	0.9	1.8	2.8

absolute amount and as a percent of total PC) is highest in lung tissue (Mason 1973).

The composition of surfactant is shown in greater detail in Table 1.6 which shows representative data for material isolated from dog lavage fluid. Surfactant purified from lavage, at least, is clearly a complex mixture of lipid and protein. On a weight basis, phospholipids are the major constituents, with smaller amounts of neutral lipids and proteins. The major component is saturated PC, in particular dipalmitoyl PC, which is primarily responsible for the property of surfactant to reduce the surface tension at an air-aqueous interface to nearly zero. Saturated fatty acids also predominate in the other phospholipids of surfactant; the amount of saturated fatty acids in total surfactant phospholipids ranges from 65–80 % in various species. Although there is variability between species, the fatty acid composition of surfactant phospholipids is as follows: 16:0 accounts for 55–85 % of the fatty acids; other fatty acids are 18:1 > 18:0 ~ 18:2 ~ 16:1 > 14:0 ~ 18:3 (reviewed by Sanders 1982b).

The physiologic role of the other phospholipids and neutral lipids is not certain. Particular attention has been focused on phosphatidylglycerol which is the second-most abundant phospholipid of surfactant. This lipid is present in only trace amounts in most tissues other than the lung, apparently located in mitochondria where it serves as an intermediate in cardiolipin synthesis. Relative to the whole lung, surfactant is more enriched in phosphatidylglycerol (approximately 4-fold) than with saturated PC. For these reasons, phosphatidylglycerol has been considered as a rather specific biochemical marker for surfactant. Furthermore, the presence of phosphatidylglycerol is a reliable indicator of fetal lung maturity; the presence of phosphatidylglycerol in amniotic fluid correlates closely with lung maturity, and phosphatidylglycerol is not

Table 1.6. Composition of pulmonary surfactant isolated from bronchoalveolar lavage fluid of dog. Data from King and Clements (1972) and Metcalfe et al. (1980)

	%	by dry weight
Phospholipid	75.2	
Saturated PC		36.2
Other PCs		19
Phosphatidylglycerol		7
Phosphatidylethanolamine		4.5
Phosphatidylinositol		4.5
Other		4
Neutral lipids	12.7	
Monoglyceride		0.2
Diglyceride		0.5
Triglyceride		2.8
Cholesterol		7.4
Cholesterol ester		0.4
Free fatty acids		0.9
Unidentified		0.5
Protein	11.1	
Hexose and hexosamine	≦1.0	

detected in lungs of infants with RDS (Hallman et al. 1976; Hallman et al. 1977). Based on these observations, it has been suggested that phosphatidylglycerol has an important functional role in pulmonary surfactant (Hallman and Gluck 1976). However, studies by Beppu et al. (1983) and Hallman et al. (1985) found that the properties of surfactant from rabbit lung were not affected by nearly complete substitution of phosphatidylinositol for phosphatidylglycerol, obtained by feeding the animals myoinositol. While these and other data clearly indicate that the presence of phosphatidylglycerol is not necessary for normal properties of surfactant both in vitro and in vivo, it remains likely that phosphatidylglycerol has either a direct or indirect influence on surfactant function in the newborn infant.

Approximately 10 % of isolated surfactant is protein. The total amount and numbers of proteins associated with surfactant has varied considerably between investigators and preparative procedures. All surfactant preparations contain serum protein in varying amounts. It is still not clear whether these proteins are an integral part of secreted surfactant or rather represent non-specific contaminants which are either normally present in alveoli or are produced by the lavage procedure.

The major proteins of surfactant are specific lipid-associated proteins with molecular weights of about 35,000 and 10,000 daltons (reviewed by Clements and King 1976, and King 1974, 1982). The ontogeny of apoprotein in human amniotic fluid has been determined by radioimmunoassay (King et al. 1975). As shown in Fig. 1.3, apoprotein and surfactant rise in parallel during gestation. In rat lung, the 35K protein has been localized by immunocytochemistry to the endoplasmic reticulum and Golgi apparatus of type II cells and to phagocytic inclusions of both macrophages and type I cells (Williams and Benson 1981), and was first detected in fetal lung on day 19 of gestation (Katyal and Singh 1983).

The structure and function of the apoproteins has been extensively investigated. It now appears that the 35K protein is the major species of a series of isoforms ranging from approximately 32,000–36,000 daltons and differing primarily in the amount of glycosylation (Katyal and Singh 1984, Whitsett et al. 1985); the primary translation products have molecular weights of 29,000–31,000 daltons (Floros et al. 1985). Quite recently, the amino acid sequence of the protein has been determined (Benson et al. 1985; White et al. 1985). Dog apoprotein contains 231 amino acids and the human protein has 228 amino acids. The primary structure of each is characterized by repeat sequences of glycine-X-Y (where X and Y represent other amino acids and Y is often hydroxyproline); this structure is typical of collagen. The presence of the collagen-like runs, along with disulfide bridges, suggests the possibility that the native molecule could be a triple helix with a molecular weight of 180,000 daltons or greater. Despite these major advances in determining the structure, the role of the apoprotein in surfactant is not yet established. Apoprotein may be important for surfactant structure and/or absorption of the material to the air-aqueous interface (Hawgood et al. 1985). It is certain that surfactant apoprotein will continue to receive considerable attention in the future with regard to its function and as a specific marker for hormonal effects on surfactant production.

1.3.4 Life Cycle

Surfactant is a product of the alveolar type II cell. Within these cells surfactant is packaged and stored as characteristic lamellar bodies which are eventually discharged at the cell surface into the alveolar space. An electron micro-

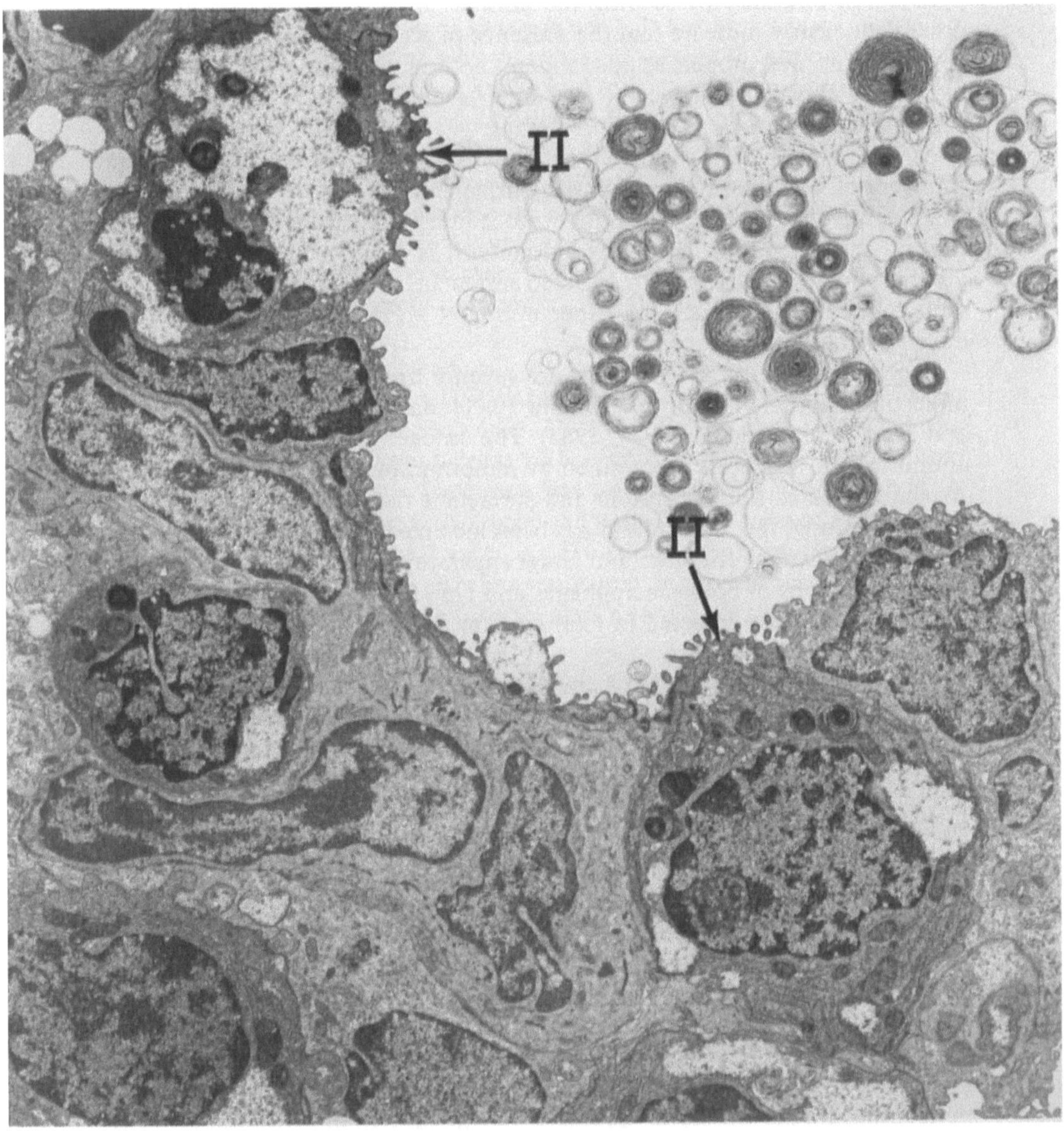

Fig. 1.4. Electron micrograph of fetal rat lung at 21 days gestation. Two type II cells containing lamellar bodies and glycogen are designated by the *arrows*. The two cells are separated by a type I cell. The potential airspace is filled with secreted surfactant in the forms of intact but swollen lamellar bodies, lamellated vesicles, and tubular myelin (×4000). The micrograph is courtesy of Mary C. Williams

graph of type II cells from the near-term fetus (Fig. 1.4) shows both intracellular lamellar bodies and surfactant secreted into the alveolar space. Surface-active material has been found in numerous vertebrate animals and the amount correlates well with alveolar surface area (Clements et al. 1970). Lamellar bodies have also been demonstrated in type II cells from lungs of many species with some apparent minor differences in ultrastructural appearance (Kikkawa and Spitzer 1969).

Figure 1.5 outlines the major steps in the life cycle of pulmonary surfactant as proposed by Clements et al. (1984). The intracellular events in this scheme are based on considerable data from autoradiographic, cytochemical and immunocytochemical studies, whereas the extracellular pathways are primarily speculative. Synthesis of surfactant occurs in the endoplasmic reticulum utilizing substrates derived from the circulation. The biochemical pathways for phospholipid synthesis in the lung are discussed in Chap. 2. The newly-synthesized surfactant passes into the Golgi apparatus where modifications (e.g.,

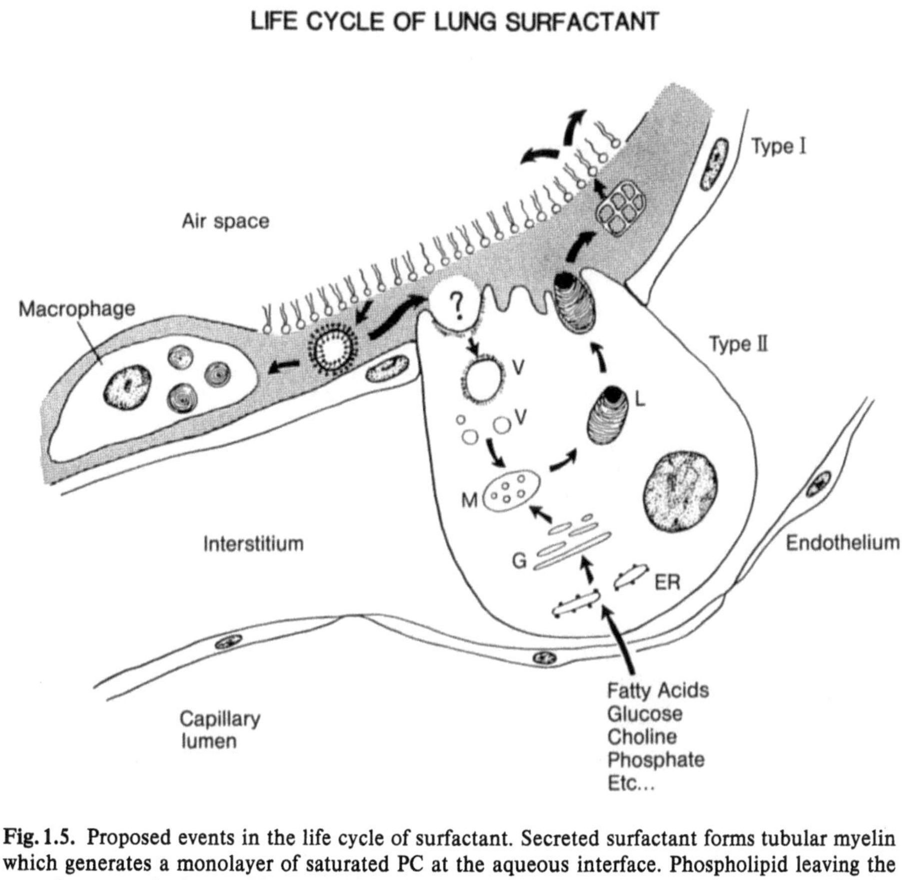

Fig. 1.5. Proposed events in the life cycle of surfactant. Secreted surfactant forms tubular myelin which generates a monolayer of saturated PC at the aqueous interface. Phospholipid leaving the monolayer may be ingested by macrophages or recycled into the type II cell as vesicles. Abbreviations are: *ER*, endoplasmic reticulum; *G*, golgi apparatus; *M*, multivesicular body; *L*, lamellar bodies; and *V*, vesicles. Reprinted from Clements et al. (1984), by permission

glycosylation of protein) may occur. The earliest recognizable precursor of the lamellar body has been termed a multivesicular body, and this structure is felt to evolve into mature lamellar bodies characterized by the lamellated layers of lipid and dense core at one end. Secretion occurs by fusion of the limiting membrane of the lamellar body with the cell membrane and subsequent expulsion of the lamellar body contents into the aqueous subphase of the alveolar space. Surfactant has been detected in alveoli in multiple forms, including intact lamellar bodies, loosely packed multi-lamellar membranes, vesicles, and the unique tubular myelin characterized by its square tube-like lattice structure. The inter-relationship of these different forms of surfactant is unclear, but it has been postulated that lamellar bodies unwind into tubular myelin which is an immediate precursor of the active monolayer of surfactant at the air-aqueous interface (Goerke 1974; Williams 1977b). Recent evidence indicates that formation of tubular myelin is dependent on calcium ions (Benson et al. 1984). It is further postulated that compression of the monolayer film on expiration forces out all surfactant components other than dipalmitoyl PC. Removal of surfactant from the airspace occurs by at least three mechanisms: 1) migration up the airway on the mucocilliary blanket; 2) uptake by macrophages and degradation within lysosomes; and 3) uptake by type II cells with possible re-utilization at the level of multivesicular bodies. The latter step in the proposed uptake process is supported by the recent observation that type II cells can take up substances from alveoli by absorptive endocytosis and deposit the ingested material in multivesicular and lamellar bodies (Williams 1984a, b).

References

Adamson IYR, Bowden DH (1974) The type 2 cell as progenitor of alveolar epithelial regeneration. A cytodynamic study in mice after exposure to oxygen. Lab Invest 30:35

Adamson IYR, Bowden DH (1975) Derivation of type 1 epithelium from type 2 cells in the developing rat lung. Lab Invest 32:736

Alescio T, Cassini A (1962) Induction in vitro of tracheal buds by pulmonary mesenchyme grafted on tracheal epithelium. J Exp Zool 150:83

Avery ME, Mead J (1959) Surface properties in relation to atelectasis and hyaline membrane disease. Am J Dis Child 97:517

Balis JU, Conen PE (1964) The role of alveolar inclusion bodies in developing lung. Lab Invest 13:1215

Benson BJ, Williams MC, Sueishi K, Goerke J, Sargeant T (1984) Role of calcium ions in the structure and function of pulmonary surfactant. Biochim Biophys Acta 793:18

Benson B, Hawgood S, Schilling T, Clements T, Damm D, Cordell B, White RT (1985) Structure of canine pulmonary surfactant apoprotein: cDNA and complete amino acid sequence. Proc Natl Acad Sci USA 82:6379

Beppu OS, Clements JA, Goerke J (1983) Phosphatidylglycerol-deficient lung surfactant has normal properties. J Appl Physiol: Respirat Environ Exercise Physiol 55:496

Bluemink JG, vanMaurik P, Lawson KA (1976) Intimate cell contacts at the epithelial/mesenchymal interface in embryonic mouse lung. J Ultrastr Res 55:257

Brody JS, Burki R, Kaplan N (1978) Deoxyribonucleic acid synthesis in lung cells during compensatory lung growth after pneumonectomy. Am Rev Resp Dis 117:307

Brody JS, Vaccaro C (1979) Postnatal formation of alveoli: interstitial events and physiologic consequences. Fed Proc 38:215

Brody JS, Kaplan NB (1983) Proliferation of alveolar interstitial cells during postnatal lung growth. Evidence for two distinct populations of pulmonary fibroblasts. Am Rev Respir Dis 127:763

Brumley GW, Chernick V, Hodson WA, Normand C, Fenner A, Avery ME (1967) Correlations of mechanical stability, morphology, pulmonary surfactant, and phospholipid content in the developing lamb lung. J Clin Invest 46:863

Burri PH (1974) The postnatal growth of the rat lung. III. Morphology. Anat Rec 180:77

Burri PH, Weibel ER (1977) Ultrastructure and morphometry of the developing lung. In: Hodson WA (ed) Lung Biology in Health and Disease, Vol 6, Development of the Lung, Marcel Dekker, New York, pp 215–268

Burri PH (1984) Fetal and postnatal development of the lung. Ann Rev Physiol 46:617

Campiche MA, Gautier A, Hernandez EI, Reymond A (1963) An electron microscope study of the fetal development of human lung. Pediatrics 32:976

Ciba Foundation Symposium 78 (1980) Metabolic Activities of the Lung, Excerpta Medica, New York

Clements JA (1957) Surface tension of lung extracts. Soc Exp Biol Med Proc 95:170

Clements JA, Brown ES, Johnson RP (1958) Pulmonary surface tension and the mucus lining of the lung: some theoretical considerations. J Appl Physiol 12:262

Clements JA, Tierney DF (1965) Alveolar instability associated with altered surface tension. In: Handbook of Physiology, Vol 2, Fenn WO, Rahn H (eds), American Physiological Society, Washington, D.C., pp 1565–1583

Clements JA, Nellenbogen J, Trahan HJ (1970) Pulmonary surfactant and evolution of the lungs. Science 169:603

Clements JA, King RJ (1976) Composition of the surface active material. In: The Biochemical Basis of Pulmonary Function, Vol 2, Lung Biology in Health and Disease, Part 4, The Surfactant System of the Lung, Crystal RG (ed), Marcel Dekker, New York, pp 363–387

Clements JA, Tooley WH (1977) Kinetics of surface-active material in the fetal lung. In: Lung Biology in Health and Disease, Vol 6, Development of the Lung, Marcel Dekker, New York, pp 349–366

Clements JA, Goerke J, Wright JR, Beppo O (1984) Turnover of lung surfactant. Prog Resp Res 18:133

De Reuck AVS, Porter R (eds) (1967) Ciba Foundation Symposium: Development of the Lung, Little, Brown & Company, Boston

Evans MJ, Bils RF (1969) Identification of cells labeled with tritiated thymidine in the pulmonary alveolar walls of the mouse. Am Rev Resp Dis 100:372

Evans MJ, Cabral LJ, Stephens RJ, Freeman G (1973) Renewal of alveolar epithelium in the rat following exposure to NO_2. Am J Pathol 64:559

Farrell PM (ed) (1982) Lung Development: Biological and Clinical Perspectives, Vol 1, Biochemistry and Physiology, Academic Press, New York

Floros J, Phelps DS, Taeusch HW (1985) Biosynthesis and in vitro translation of the major surfactant-associated protein from human lung. J Biol Chem 260:495

Fukuda Y, Ferrans VJ, Crystal RG (1983) The development of alveolar septa in fetal sheep lung. An ultrastructural and immunohistochemical study. Am J Anat 167:405

Gail DB, Lenfant CJM (1983) Cells of the lung: Biology and clinical implications. Am Rev Resp Dis 127:366

Goerke J (1974) Lung surfactant. Biochim Biophys Acta 344:241

Grant MM, Cutts NR, Brody JS (1983) Alterations in lung basement membrane during fetal growth and type 2 cell development. Develop Biol 97:173

Hage E (1973) The morphological development of the pulmonary epithelium of human foetuses studied by light- and electron microscopy. Z Anat Entwickl-Gesch 140:271

Hallman M, Kulovich M, Kirkpatrick E, Sugarman GR, Gluck L (1976) Phosphatidylinositol and phosphatidylglycerol in amniotic fluid: indices of lung maturity. Am J Obstet Gynecol 125:613

Hallman M, Gluck L (1976) Phosphatidylglycerol in lung surfactant. III. Possible modifier of surfactant function. J Lipid Res 17:257

Hallman M, Feldman HB, Kirkpatrick E, Gluck L (1977) Absence of phosphatidylglycerol (PG) in respiratory distress syndrome in the newborn. Pediatr Res 11:714

Hallman M, Enhorning G, Possmayer F (1985) Composition and surface activity of normal and phosphatidylglycerol-deficient lung surfactant. Pediatr Res 19:286

Hawgood S, Benson BJ, Hamilton RL Jr (1985) The effects of a surfactant associated protein and calcium ions on the structure and surface activity of lung surfactant lipids. Biochemistry 24:184
Hodson WA (ed) (1977) Lung Biology in Health and Disease, Vol 6, Development of the Lung, Marcel Dekker, New York
Inselman LS, Mellins RB (1981) Growth and development of the lung. J Pediatr 98:1
Kapanci Y, Assimacopoulos A, Irle C, Zwahlen A, Gabbiani G (1974) "Contractile interstitial cells" in pulmonary alveolar septa: A possible regulator of ventilation/perfusion ratio? J Cell Biol 60:375
Kapanci Y, Baud M, Mo Costabella P (1983) Alveolar contractile interstitial cells. Their morphology and reactions to hypoxia and to epinephrine stimulation. In: Current problems in Clinical Biochemistry: 13. The Cells of the Alveolar Unit, Favez G, Junod A, Leuenberger P (eds), Hans Huber, Bern, pp 134–141
Katyal SL, Singh G (1983) An enzyme-linked immunoassay of surfactant apoproteins. Its application to the study of fetal lung development in the rat. Pediatr Res 17:439
Katyal SL, Singh G (1984) Analysis of pulmonary surfactant apoproteins by isoelectric focusing. Brochim Biophys Acta 194:411
Kauffman SL (1974) Kinetics of alveolar epithelial hyperplasia in lungs of mice exposed to urethane. I. Quantitative analysis of cell populations. Lab Invest 30:170
Kauffman SL, Burri PH, Weibel ER (1974) The postnatal growth of the rat lung II. Autoradiography. Anat Rec 180:63
Kauffman SL (1977) Acceleration of canalicular development in lungs of fetal mice exposed transplacentally to dexamethasone. Lab Invest 36:395
Kauffman SL (1980) Cell proliferation in the mammalian lung. Int Rev Exp Pathol 22:131
Kikkawa Y, Motoyama EK, Gluck L (1968) Study of the lungs of fetal and newborn rabbits. Ann J Path 52:177
Kikkawa Y, Spitzer R (1969) Inclusion bodies of type II alveolar cells: Species differences and morphogenesis. Anat Rec 163:525
Kikkawa Y, Kaibara M, Motoyama EK, Orzalesi MM, Cook CD (1971) Morphologic development of fetal rabbit lung and its acceleration with cortisol. Am J Pathol 64:423
King R, Clements JA (1972) Surface active materials from dog lung. II. Composition and physiological correlations. Am J Pathol 223:715
King RJ (1974) The surfactant system of the lung. Fed Proc 33:2238
King RJ, Ruch J, Gikas EG, Platzker ACG, Creasy RK (1975) Appearance of apoproteins of pulmonary surfactant in human amniotic fluid. J Appl Physiol 39:735
King RJ (1982) Pulmonary surfactant. J Appl Physiol: Respirat Environ Exercise Physiol 53:1
Kotas RV, Farrell PM, Ulane RE, Chez RA (1977) Fetal rhesus monkey lung development: lobar differences and discordances between stability and distensibility. J Appl Physiol: Respirat Environ Exercise Physiol 43:92
Langston C, Kida K, Reed M, Thurlbeck WM (1984) Human lung growth in late gestation and in the neonate. Am Rev Respir Dis 129:607
Maksvytis HJ, Vaccaro C, Brody JS (1981) Isolation and characterization of a lipid-containing interstitial cell from the developing lung. Lab Invest 45:248
Mason RJ (1973) Disaturated lecithin concentration of rabbit tissues. Am Rev Respirat Dis 107:678
Mason RJ,Williams MC (1977) Type II alveolar cell. Defender of the alveolus. Am Rev Respirat Dis 115 (Suppl):81
Mercurio AR, Rhodin JAG (1977) An electron microscopic study of the type I pneumocyte in the cat: Differentiation. Am J Anat 146:255
Metcalfe IL, Enhorning G, Possmayer F (1980) Pulmonary surfactant-associated proteins: their role in the expression of surface activity. J Appl Physiol: Respirat Environ Exercise Physiol 49:34
Meyrick B,Reid L (1982) Pulmonary arterial and alveolar development in normal postnatal rat lung. Am Rev Respir Dis 125:468
Meyrick B, Reid L (1977) Ultrastructure of alveolar lining and its development. In: Development of the Lung, Hodson WA (ed), Marcel Dekker, New York, pp 135–214
Nerurkar LS, Zeligs BJ, Bellanti JA (1977) Maturation of the rabbit alveolar macrophage during animal development. II. Biochemical and enzymatic studies. Pediatr Res 11:1202
Pattle RE (1958) Properties, function and origin of the alveolar lining layer. Proc Roy Soc London, Ser. B 148:217

Reid L (1967) The embryology of the lung. In: Development of the Lung, deReuck AVS, Porter R (eds), Little, Brown and Company, Boston, pp 109–124

Robertson B, van Golde LMG, Batenburg JJ (eds) (1984) Pulmonary Surfactant, Elsevier, Amsterdam

Sanders RL (1982a) The chemical composition of the lung. In: Lung Development: Biological and Clinical Perspectives, Vol 1, Biochemistry and Physiology, Academic Press, New York, pp 179–192

Sanders RL (1982b) The composition of pulmonary surfactant. In: Lung Development: Biological and Clinical Perspectives, Vol 1, Biochemistry and Physiology, Academic Press, New York, pp 193–210

Sanders RL (1982c) Major phospholipids in pulmonary surfactant. In: Lung Development: Biological and Clinical Perspectives, Vol 1, Biochemistry and Physiology, Academic Press, New York, pp 211–238

Sorokin S, Padykula HA, Herman E (1959) Comparative histochemical patterns in developing mammalian lungs. Dev Biol 1:125

Sorokin SP (1970) The cells of the lungs. In: Morphology of Experimental Respiratory Carcinogenesis, Nettesheim P, Hanna MG, Deatherage JW Jr (eds), U.S. Atomic Energy Commission Division of Technical Information, pp 3–43

Suzuki Y (1966) The structural differentiation of the alveolar lining cells: I. Electron microscopic studies on the prospective alveolar epithelium in the lung tissue of rat embryos. Okaj Fol Anat Jap 42:119

Ten Have-Opbroek AAW (1981) The development of the lung in mammals: An analysis of concepts and findings. Am J Anat 162:201

Tordet C, Marin L, Dameron F (1981) Pulmonary di- and tri-acylglycerols during the perinatal development of the rat. Experimentia 37:333

Vaccaro C, Brody JS (1979) Ultrastructure of developing alveoli. I. Role of the interstitial fibroblast. Anat Rec 192:467

Von Neergaard K (1929) Neue Auffassungen über einen Grundbegriff der Atemmechanik. Z Ges Exptl Med 66:373

Wang NS,Kotas PV, Avery ME, Thurlbeck WM (1971) Accelerated appearance of osmiophilic bodies in fetal lungs following steroid injection. J Appl Physiol 30:362

Weibel ER, Gil J (1977) Structure-function relationships at the alveolar level. In: Bioengineering Aspects of the Lung, West JB (ed), Marcel Dekker, New York, pp 1–81

Wessells NK (1970) Mammalian lung development: Interactions in formation and morphogenesis of tracheal buds. J Exp Zool 175:455

White RT, Damm D, Miller J, Spratt K, Schilling J, Hawgood S, Benson B, Cordell B (1985) Isolation and characterization of the human pulmonary surfactant apoprotein gene. Nature 317:361

Whitsett TA, Hull W, Ross G, Weaver T (1985) characteristics of human surfactant-associated glycoproteins A. Pediatr Res 19:501

Williams MC (1977a) Development of the alveolar structure of the fetal rat in late gestation. Fed Proc 36:2653

Williams MC (1977b) Conversion of lamellar body membranes into tubular myelin in the alveolar spaces of late fetal rat lung: TEM and HUEM observations. J Cell Biol 72:260

Williams MC, Benson BJ (1981) Immunocytochemical localization and identification of the major surfactant protein in adult rat lung. J Histochem Cytochem 29:291

Williams MC (1984a) Endocytosis in alveolar type II cells: Effect of charge and size of tracers. Proc Natl Acad Sci USA 81:6054

Williams MC (1984b) Uptake of lectins by pulmonary alveolar type II cells: Subsequent deposition into lamellar bodies. Proc Natl Acad Sci USA 81:6383

Zeligs BJ, Nerurkar LS, Bellanti JA (1977a) Maturation of the rabbit alveolar macrophage during animal development. I. Perinatal influx into alveoli and ultrastructural differentiation. Pediatr Res 11:197

Zeligs BJ, Nerurkar LS, Bellanti JA (1977b) Maturation of the rabbit alveolar macrophage during animal development. III. Phagocytic and bacterial functions. Pediatr Res 11:1208

2 Glucocorticoid Effects in Vivo

With the material of Chap. 1 as background, this chapter discusses the effects of in vivo glucocorticoid treatment on lung maturation. This topic has been the subject of numerous reviews over the past 15 years. These include articles and chapters by Avery (1975), Taeusch and Avery (1977), Gross (1977), Hallman and Gluck (1977), Brown et al. (1978), Farrell and Hamosh (1978), Ballard (1979), Rooney (1979), Batenburg and Van Golde (1979), Olson (1979), Smith and Bogues (1979), Hitchcock (1980), Ballard (1982), Possmayer (1982), Ballard (1983), Rooney (1983) and Smith (1984). Rather than providing a detailed accounting of all of the numerous contributions in the literature on this topic, this chapter summarizes the different types of experimental approaches and the various effects observed with in vivo corticosteroid treatment. Other aspects of corticosteroids and lung maturation are discussed in subsequent chapters. Responses of lung tissue in culture are included in Chap. 3, 4, 9, and 10. Chapter 4 is devoted to the role of endogenous corticosteroids in lung maturation, and includes experiments employing ablation and replacement therapy. Thus, this chapter is restricted to a summary of in vivo glucocorticoid treatment of the intact fetus with only occasional references to in vitro systems for comparison.

2.1 Historical Perspective

The area of glucocorticoids and lung maturation is a recent one. Although the scientific foundations for this area encompass much earlier research in the areas of pulmonary physiology, surface tension, and developmental endocrinology, the first work specific to fetal lung dates from the report by Liggins in 1969. For an extremely interesting and insightful historical review of this topic, I recommend the series of articles by Comroe (1977a,b,c). He describes many of the scientists in this field and their contributions during the past century, including the circumstances leading to the important discovery by Liggins.

During the 1960s, Liggins was concerned with the question of whether fetal hormones influence the timing of delivery. One of the experimental approaches was treatment of the fetus with adrenocortical hormones. He administered dexamethasone by continuous infusion into lamb fetuses and found that indeed premature delivery occurred. When he reported these results, he included the following astute observations (Liggins 1969):

"Gross examination of the lungs of 10 lambs delivered spontaneously at 117–123 days after dexamethasone infusions showed that in six, none of which had been artificially ventilated, there was partial aeration. In most instances the aeration consisted of patchy expansion in the uper lobes, but in one lamb delivered at 123 days the lower lobes were also partly expanded. This lamb was found alive at least an hour after being born and survived for a further hour until killed. The body weight of 2349 g, the general appearance and the bone age determined by X-ray of the limbs corresponded with the duration of pregnancy calculated from the date of mating. During the period of observation, the lamb bleated and showed some signs of respiratory distress. Histological examination of the lungs removed 4 h after death confirmed that alveolar expansion had been maintained ... According to Howatt, Avery, Humphreys, Normand, Reid and Strang (1965), and Reynolds, Jacobsen, Motoyama, Kikkawa, Craig, Orzalesi and Cook (1965), maintenance of alveolar expansion in the lung is dependent on adequate surfactant activity. These authors and also Brumley, Chernick, Hodson, Normand, Fenner and Avery (1967), found that alveoli collapse and the lungs become airless at maturities of less than 125–127 days. Persistence of partial expansion of the lungs in the corticosteroid-treated lambs in the present series at 117–123 days strongly suggests accelerated appearance of surfactant, possibly as a result of premature activity of enzymes involved in a biosynthetic pathway."

Although the report by Liggins (1969) was the first demonstration of accelerated lung maturation, this possibility was suggested earlier by Buckingham et al. (1968). In their abstract, they proposed that the lung, as an analog of the developing intestine, might undergo accelerated differentiation with glucocorticoid treatment. Apparently Liggins was not aware of this proposal at the time of his study, since he does not cite the abstract by Buckingham. Over the past 16 years, both the observations and predictions of Liggins have been confirmed by the work of many investigators. The initial confirmatory studies were carried out by Avery and her colleagues (DeLemos, Germeta, Knelson, Kotas, Taeusch, Heitner, Bater, Robert, Carson and others) in a series of studies with lambs and rabbits. Other early reports included studies by Kikkawa et al. (1971), Platzker et al. (1972), and Sundell et al. (1973).

An influence of glucocorticoids on lung maturation is perhaps not unexpected in view of the well described effects in other developing tissues (reviewed in Ballard, 1979). Glucocorticoids are known to accelerate developmental processes and induce specific proteins or enzymes in at least 12 different differentiating tissues. In many organs, corticosteroids act during late fetal life, while in other tissues the effects are observed during postnatal development (e.g., the suckling period). A common theme of these effects is precocious appearance of normal developmental events. The same theme applies to glucocorticoid action in fetal lung.

In 1972, Liggins and Howie published the results of their clinical trial with prepartum betamethasone treatment to prevent RDS. These exciting findings, combined with the early studies in animals, produced a nearly exponential increase in interest and research in hormonal acceleration of pulmonary development. The following sections summarize the different experimental approaches, the types of responses observed, and some of the factors influencing glucocorticoid responsiveness in vivo.

Table 2.1. Effects of in vivo glucocorticoid treatment on lung maturation[a]

Effect	Sheep	Rabbit	Rat	Mouse	Monkey
Increased aeration	Liggins 1969	Motoyama et al. 1971			
Increased survival time	Liggins 1969	Motoyama et al. 1971 Taeusch et al. 1972	Frank et al. 1985		
Less severe respiratory distress	Sundell et al. 1973				Kessler et al. 1982
Morphologic maturation	Platzker et al. 1975 Brumley et al. 1977 Vilos et al. 1983	Wang et al 1971 Kikkawa et al. 1971 Motoyama et al. 1971		Kauffman et al. 1977a	Bunton & Plopper 1984
Increased surface activity of tissue extracts	Delemos et al. 1970 Knelson et al. 1971	Kotas & Avery 1971 Russell et al. 1974			
Increased surfactant in tracheal fluid or lung lavage	Platzker et al. 1975 Vilos et al. 1983	Motoyama et al. 1971 Rooney et al. 1976 Ballard et al. 1980 Freeze & Hallman 1983			Kessler et al. 1982
Increased maximum lung volume and/or deflation stability	Delemos et al 1970 Brumley et al. 1977 Thiebeault et al. 1978 Vilos et al. 1983	Kotas & Avery 1971 Robert et al. 1975			Johnson et al. 1978 Kessler et al. 1982
Increased rate choline incorporation into PC		Farrell & Zachman 1973 Brehier et al. 1977 Possmayer et al. 1979 Rooney et al. 1979	Farrell et al. 1977 Gross et al. 1984	Brehier & Rooney 1981	
Increased tissue content of saturated PC or PC	Platzker et al. 1975	Farrell & Zachman 1973	Nelson et al. 1976 Gross et al. 1984		

[a] Initial and representative confirming references are given for each category and species.

2.2 Experimental Approaches

Table 2.1 lists the types of studies that have been performed with in vivo glucocorticoid administration in the sheep, rabbit, rat, mouse and monkey. In these species, glucocorticoids have been shown to accelerate lung maturation as judged by morphologic, physiologic and biochemical criteria.

A variety of corticosteroids as well as ACTH have been utilized, and the route of administration has included intravenous infusion into the fetus (sheep), intramuscular injection into both the fetus (rabbit and rat) and into the mother (rabbit, rat, mouse and monkey). Dexamethasone and betamethasone are more appropriate than cortisol (or corticosterone) for maternal treatment since the synthetic corticosteroids are not inactivated by placental 11β-hydroxysteroid dehydrogenase (discussed in Chap. 4). Pharmacologic doses of corticosteroid have been used in many studies, but lower doses are also effective. Only a few dose-response studies have been carried out in vivo. Using mice, Kauffman (1977a) found a maximal response for increasing potential airspace at a dose of ~ 2 μg maternal dexamethasone/g (Fig. 2.1). In another study with mice, maximal stimulation of choline incorporation by fetal lung occurred at a daily maternal dose of about 3.5 μg/g (Brehier and Rooney 1981). The optimal dose of betamethasone in rats for choline incorporation was 1 μg/g (Gross et al. 1984), and in rabbits 0.1 μg/g is maximal (Ballard, unpublished data). In each of these studies a dose-response relationship was es-

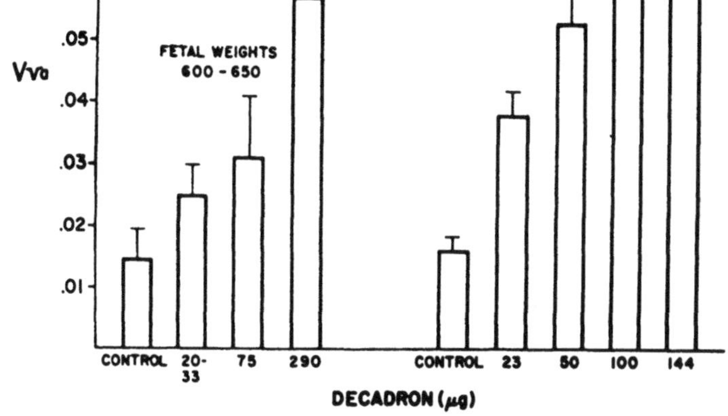

Fig. 2.1. Dose-response study with dexamethasone in fetal mice. Increasing doses of steroid were administered to pregnant mice (~50 g) on day 16 of gestation and the volume density of air space (Vva) in fetal lungs were determined after 24 h exposure. Dexamethasone dose dependency of Vva is best illustrated in the group of heavier fetuses. From Kauffman (1977a), with permission

tablished. Production of cortisol levels equivalent to those at term are effective in the premature sheep fetus (discussed in Chap. 4), and in both the rabbit and monkey betamethasone has been used at doses similar to those for human prenatal therapy (0.2 μg/g).

Several of the experimental models offer unique advantages. The in utero fetal sheep preparation has been particularly useful for studies of glucocorticoid action on surfactant flux in tracheal fluid. As originally described by Platzker et al. (1972, 1975), in this preparation the fetal trachea is cannulated and lung fluid is diverted to an intra-amniotic reservoir which may be sampled at desired intervals. If twin pregnancies are utilized, an intra-uterine control is available. This approach has allowed quantitative determination of surfactant flux over time. Because of the relatively large size of the lamb fetus, pressure-volume studies are also easily carried out. The long gestation in the sheep has been convenient for studies of endocrine ablation and hormone replacement therapy during the third trimester. Because placental passage of steroids is very restricted in the sheep, hormones must be infused directly into the fetus.

The rabbit has been a popular experimental model because of the relatively short gestation, large litter number, and fetuses of sufficient size for both tracheal lavage and pressure-volume determinations. In contrast with the sheep, the rabbit fetus may be treated either directly or through maternal administration. This species has also been used for a number of developmental studies of lung physiology and biochemistry, and accordingly normal developmental patterns are available. PC synthesis (Fig. 2.6) and alveolar content of surfactant (Table 2.2) begin to increase at approximately day 27 and 28, respectively; glucocorticoid treatment has usually been given for 1 or 2 days prior to these points in gestation.

The rat has been utilized primarily for investigation of lung biochemistry and morphology. Tracheal lavage to assess secreted levels of surfactant is not feasible in this species. Some investigators have attempted to assess surface active material in alveolar and airway spaces by collecting the incubation medium from minces of lung tissue. However, this approach is not as satisfactory

Table 2.2. Developmental changes in PC content of lung lavage and tissue in the rabbit. Data from Rooney et al. (1976b) and Rooney and Gobran (1977)

Gestational age (days)	Lung lavage			Lung tissue	
	L/S ratio	Total PC[a]	Saturated PC[a]	Total PC[a]	Saturated PC[a]
27	0.8	2.6	1.3 (50%)	1300	350 (27%)
28	1.9	5.4	3.0 (56%)	1700	580 (34%)
29	5.1	7.4	3.4 (46%)	1700	580 (34%)
30	4.1	8.4	4.2 (50%)	1800	630 (35%)
31	9.9	25.4	13.4 (53%)	2200	920 (42%)
+1	31.1	274	161 (59%)	2400	1090 (45%)
Adult	> 50	264	143 (54%)	2500	720 (29%)

[a] g PC phosphorus/g lung dry weight

as collection of tracheal fluid or lung lavage. The relatively short gestation of the rat facilitates data acquisition, but by the same token the timing of pregnancies is critical. Major increases in surfactant content and synthetic rate, for example, occur over the last 2 days of gestation (Maniscalco et al. 1978, Fig. 2.6). The same situation holds for the mouse, which has been used both for biochemical and morphologic studies.

There have been a limited number of studies in the monkey. The main advantage of this model, of course, is the general similarity to the human. Disadvantages include the difficulty of performing chronic determinations as in the sheep, and the inherent expense of a monkey colony.

2.3 Morphology

The effects of in vivo glucocorticoid treatment on lung structure have been described by both light and electron microscopy and are illustrated by the micrographs in Fig. 2.2. In this study, Kikkawa et al. (1971) injected fetal rabbits with 1 mg of cortisol at various times in gestation and examined the fetal lungs 2 days later. Accelerated development in response to treatment was observed at each gestational age examined. At the earliest age examined (21 days), treatment resulted in more airway branching, enlargement of the glands, and some shortening of lining epithelial cells. At 24 days, further flattening of epithelial cells was observed along with increased volume of potential air space. By 26 days gestation, treatment produced complete precocious maturation of type II cells with loss of glucogen and appearance of lamellar bodies; type I cells exhibited extension of their cytoplasm resulting in relatively thin septae. The authors state that all of the changes noted with cortisol treatment represented normal developmental events and they estimate that cytodifferentiation in the lung was accelerated by approximately 1½ days of gestation compared with saline-injected littermates.

The effects of glucocorticoid treatment by light microscopy can be quite striking. After dexamethasone infusion into fetal lambs, the lungs show greatly increased potential airspaces and reduced interstitial volume (DeLemos et al. 1970; Platzker et al. 1975). In monkeys, 3 days exposure to betamethasone increased the average size of airspaces about 25 % on morphometric analysis (Beck et al. 1981).

These and subsequent findings indicate that glucocorticoid treatment causes precocious maturation of type I and type II cells, and possibly other pulmonary cell types. It seems likely, for example, that glucocorticoids stimulate proliferation of pulmonary capillaries and alter fibroblast production of matrix proteins, although these aspects have not been carefully evaluated. The question of precisely which cell types are directly influenced by glucocorticoids has not been fully defined. Autoradiographic studies of dexamethasone binding in adult lung suggest that most but not all cell types are potential targets for glucocorticoid action (see discussion in Chap. 3).

Kauffman (1977a) performed a quantitative study of morphologic changes in fetal mouse lung. As shown in Fig. 2.1, there was a dose dependent increase in total airspace volume (canal formation) as estimated by morphometrics; a

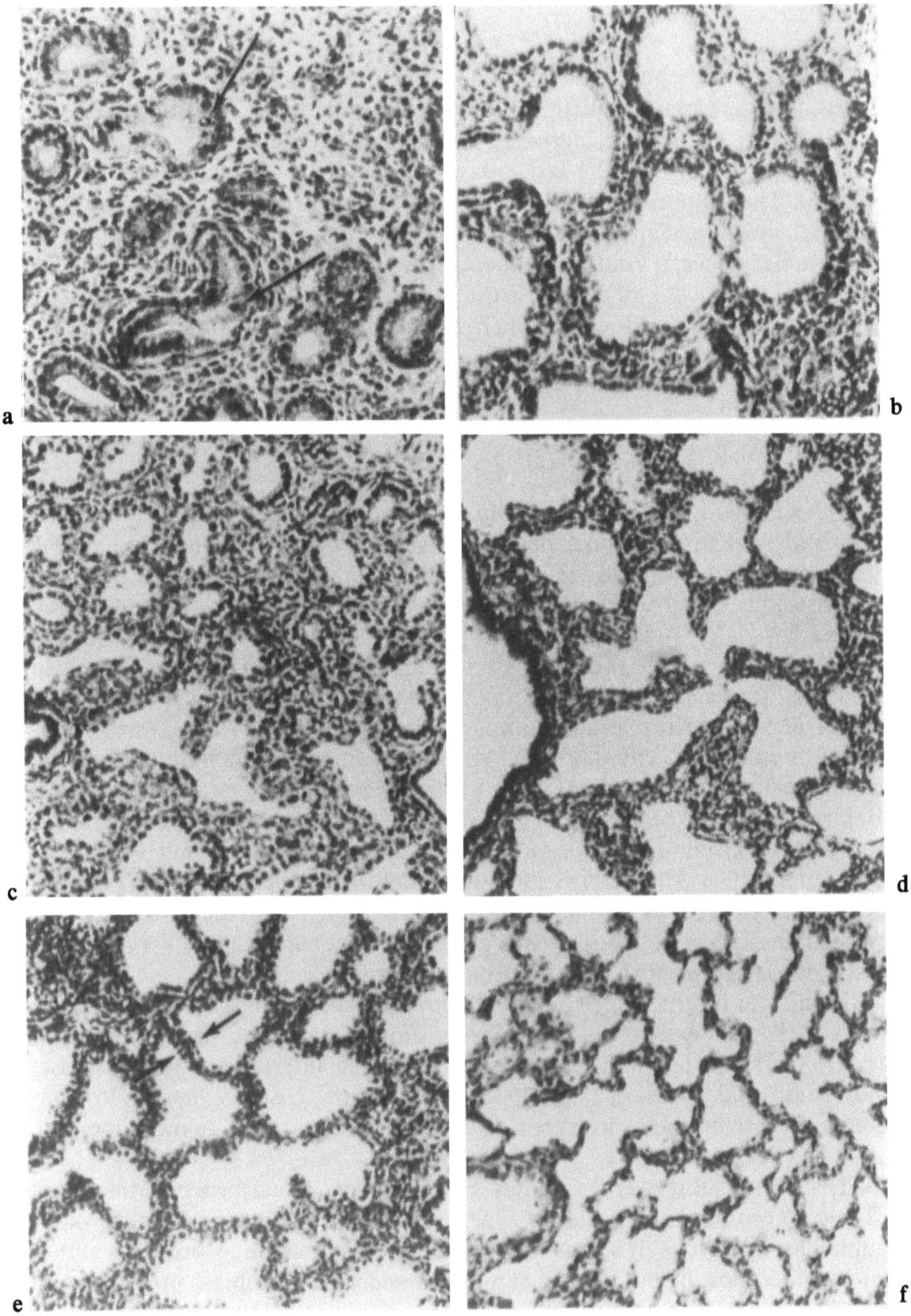

Fig. 2.2a–f. Light micrographs of fetal rabbit lung (×160). **a** 21-day control showing abundant interstitial tissue and glandular-like ducts lined by columnar epithelial cells in active mitosis *(arrows)*. **b** fetus treated with cortisol for 2 days and delivered on day 21 showing decreased mesenchyme, dilated and more tortuous ducts, and low columnar or cuboidal epithelial cells. **c** Control animal at day 24 showing mixture of glandular and more tortuous ducts with low columnar or cuboidal epithelial cells. **d** Cortisol-treated fetus at day 24 exhibiting thinner septae and larger ducts lined by cuboidal cells. **e** Control fetus at day 26 with relatively thin septae and cuboidal epithelium. **f** Cortisol-treated animal on day 26 showing mature appearing structure with thin septae and abundant potential air spaces. From Kikkawa et al. (1971), with permission

response was first observed 14 h after treatment. In control animals the proportion of epithelial cells containing granules increased from 18.3 to 41.9 % between 17 and 18 days. Fetuses treated with dexamethasone for 24 h had granules in 36.2 % of their epithelial cells on day 17. In contrast with results for volume of air space (Fig. 2.1), the increase in granules required 2 μg dexamethasone/g for 24 h. It was concluded that glucocorticoid-induced changes in lung structure occur more rapidly and with lower doses of steroid than for appearance of lamellar bodies in type II cells. This proposal, which appears to be supported by data in the monkey (discussed below), suggests a difference in the rate or timing of expression of glucocorticoid action in different cell types. It is unlikely that mesenchymal cells are more *sensitive* to corticosteroid than epithelial cells, since receptor number and affinity are similar in different pulmonary cell types (Chap. 3); also, differences in steroid metabolism should not be a factor using dexamethasone. The apparent dose-response difference could arise if the formation of mature lamellar bodies was a reversible process and occurred at a considerably slower rate than the structural changes. Under these conditions, dexamethasone at the lower doses might be sufficiently cleared before 24 h, preventing a detectable response. Additional quantitative data on this question would be useful.

If glucocorticoid effects occur at different rates in various pulmonary cell types, this could influence the type and degree of lung maturity produced after various times of treatment in the human infant. However, the type and rate of response to treatment in the clinical situation is certainly influenced by many factors of which gestational age is of major importance. This point is illustrated by findings reported for structural effects of triamcinolone in the lung of the fetal Rhesus monkey (Bunton and Plopper 1984). They treated pregnant monkeys with triamcinolone acetonide (1 or 10 mg/kg) at the end of either the first or second trimester, and the lungs were examined several weeks later. The nature and degree of response was dependent on the gestational age of the fetus. When treatment occurred during the glandular phase, growth of alveolar septae was retarded, but treatment later in gestation accelerated alveolarization. Perhaps the most striking finding of this study was the persistence of the structural changes for an extended time during gestation. In fact, accelerated alveolarization was still evident late in the third trimester, 40 days after administration of triamcinolone. It is not clear whether this finding represents irreversibility of the corticosteroid effect on structural development, or persistence of triamcinolone acetonide in the fetus. The response of the surfactant system under these conditions was not determined. It should be noted that the doses of triamcinolone in this study were equivalent to 5 to 50 times the dose of betamethasone used clinically; also, lung of the Rhesus monkey is essentially mature at birth, whereas this is not true for the human (Bunton and Plopper 1984).

The mechanisms of glucocorticoid effects on morphogenesis are largely unexplored. They may be related in part to inhibition of division of fibroblasts and stimulation of elastogenesis by these cells. The subsequent condensation and alteration of interstitial matrix could conceivably promote alveolarization. Similarly, arrested division of epithelial cells may promote maturational changes in structure as well as function (see Sect. 2.6.4); prolonged exposure to glucocorticoids conceivably could reduce the number of alveoli formed through inhibition of septation. Although exogenous corticosteroids apparently act through the same mechanisms utilized during normal development, it does appear that either prolonged exposure or excessive levels of glucocorticoids early in gestation can result in altered lung structure.

2.4 Alveolar Surfactant

As noted in Table 2.1, glucocorticoids increase the amount of airway surfactant in several species. Experimentally, various investigators have assessed surface activity, PC or saturated PC content, the L/S ratio, or the phosphatidylglycerol:phosphatidylinositol ratio in tracheal fluid or lung lavage. Changes in amniotic fluid phospholipids also occur after glucocorticoid treatment, but this measurement is less sensitive than assays in tracheal fluid and lung lavage due to the dilution factor.

The phospholipid content of the airways correlates well with surface activity and as such probably represents the best biochemical assessment of lung compliance. Table 2.2 presents data for the normal developmental increase of lavage PC, saturated PC, and L/S ratio in the rabbit. In this species there is a 10-fold increase in these parameters during late gestation. The magnitude of the changes provides relatively sensitive indices for evaluating hormonal effects; it also can introduce considerable biologic variability, especially if dating of pregnancy is not well controlled. Treatment of the rabbit fetus with corticosteroid for 2 days increases lavage L/S ratio, total phospholipid, and PC content by 50–100% (Rooney et al. 1979, Ballard et al. 1980, Fig. 7.4). By contrast, there is only a small increase in tissue phospholipid levels detected after treatment (see Sect. 2.6.1), consistent with the relatively modest (percentage-wise) change during normal development (Table 2.2).

Figure 2.3 shows the effect of dexamethasone infusion on surface activity in tracheal fluid of the fetal sheep (Platzker et al. 1975). Forty-eight to 72 h of treatment increased surfactant content at each gestational age studied. In the younger fetuses, surfactant was low but detectable in treated fetuses, whereas no activity was found in the untreated twin. With increasing gestational age, the response increased. A response to dexamethasone was noted within 36 h of starting the infusion, and the flux continued to increase over the experimental period. In tracheal fluid of the sheep, at least, there is a close correlation between the amount of surface activity and the content of saturated PC (Kitterman et al. 1981).

In the fetal monkey (135 days gestation), Kessler et al. (1982) found that the content of saturated PC in lavage fluid more than doubled after 3 days treatment with maternal dexamethasone. Results were equivalent whether the data were expressed per g dry lung weight or tissue saturated PC. The amount of tissue saturated PC was not significantly increased; this is not surprising in view of the relatively large pool of PC in lung. Johnson et al. (1978) estimated alveolar surfactant by measuring the minimum surface tension obtained with the saline extract of minced lung from a group of fetuses ranging from 124–143 days gestation. The minimum surface tension in saline vs. betameth-

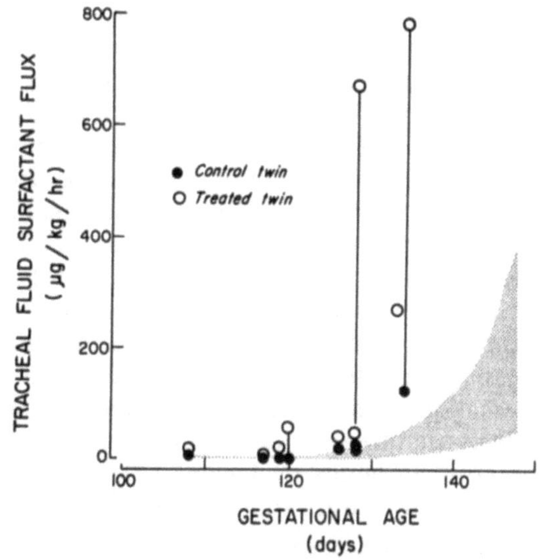

Fig. 2.3. Surfactant flux in tracheal fluid of fetal lambs. Twin fetuses received continuous peritoneal infusion of either diluent (control) or dexamethasone (400 µg/day, treated) for 1.5 to 4 days prior to delivery by cesarean section at the gestational ages shown. Data points represent surfactant collected during the last 12 h prior to delivery, and the *stippled area* shows mean ± 1 SD for flux in other control animals. Treatment increased surfactant in 8 of 9 experiments, with more pronounced stimulation later in gestation. From Platzker et al. (1975), with permission

asone-treated fetuses in this study was not different. However, this experimental approach does not quantitate the content of alveolar surfactant, and the complexities involved in surface balance measurements of this type have been noted (Kotas 1982).

The major mechanism for glucocorticoid-induced accumulation of surfactant in airways is probably stimulation of surfactant synthesis. The time course of response in both sheep (Platzker et al. 1975), and in rabbits (Corbet et al. 1978) indicates that corticosteroids do not have an immediate effect on surfactant release such as seen with beta-adrenergic agonists. However, the glucocorticoid effect may be mediated in part through induction of beta-adrenergic receptors and subsequent increased sensitivity to endogenous catecholamines (discussed in Chap. 8). There is little relevant information on the reversibility of the glucocorticoid stimulation of alveolar surfactant in vivo; data from culture studies indicate that stimulation of PC synthesis is reversible (Chap. 3). The reversibility aspect relates directly to the question of whether retreatment is required in the clinical situation (Chap. 5).

2.5 Pulmonary Function and Viability

Glucocorticoids enhance both maximal lung volume and the stability of the lung on deflation. The effect in fetal rabbits is illustrated by the data of Kotas and Avery (1971). Fetuses were injected with saline or 9-fluoroprednisolone acetate (0.05 mg) at day 24 of gestation, and pressure-volume studies were performed 2 and 3 days later. Maximal lung volume (ml/gm lung at 35–40 cm H_2O pressure) was approximately doubled in treated fetuses vs. controls, obtaining values equivalent to those normally seen at 30–31 days (2.8–3.5 ml/gm). This increase probably reflects a combination of both accelerated acinar development (formation of saccules and decreased connective tissue) and recruitment of air spaces due to increased surfactant. As shown in Fig. 2.4, treatment also produced more stable lungs on deflation at both ages. The stability of treated lungs was advanced by about 2½ days of gestation. The enhanced ability of alveoli to remain expanded as the distending pressure decreases is primarily a result of surfactant lowering surface tension in the air spaces. It is possible that deflation stability also is influenced by corticosteroid-induced formation of more spherical terminal respiratory units. These pressure-volume effects are often evident on gross inspection of ventilated lungs as originally observed in lambs by Liggins (1969) and are typically greater in the upper lobes which mature somewhat faster than the lower lobes.

In monkeys, 3 days treatment with betamethasone or dexamethasone increases maximal lung volume on air inflation (ml/kg) by about 50 % (Johnson et al 1979; Mitzner et al 1979, 1982; Kessler et al 1982). Lungs were also inflated with saline to assess maximal volume in the absence of an influence of surfactant. Distensibility with saline filling was also greater in the treated group than the controls, although the possibility of variable leaks complicates interpretation of these results. In contrast to findings in other species, glucocorticoid treatment produced relatively minor changes in deflation stability

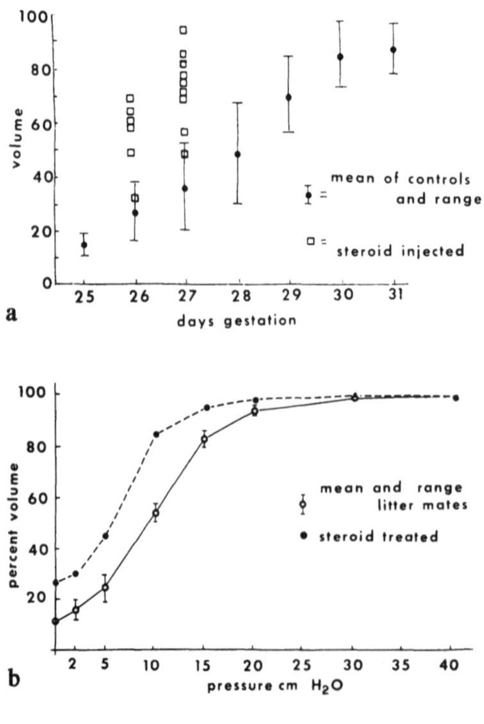

Fig. 2.4a, b. Effect of 9-fluoroprednisolone acetate on deflation stability in rabbit fetuses. Fetuses were injected with steroid or saline on day 24 and pressure-volume studies were performed on day 27. **a** Volume of air retained on deflation of lungs to 10 cm water pressure. **b** Results of deflation study in one litter. From Kotas and Avery (1971), by permission

after air filling. The apparently greater effect of corticosteroids on distensibility than deflation stability is unexpected in view of the normal pattern of pulmonary development in the monkey (see Table 4.3). Thus, data from two groups provide evidence that corticosteroids enhance lung volume at least in part by mechanisms independent of changes in surfactant production.

The findings in the pressure-volume studies led to the proposal that a major effect of glucocorticoids, in the fetal monkey at least, is on pulmonary connective tissue producing increased distensibility. The possible nature of changes induced in the mesenchyme are largely unexplored. Beck et al. (1981), reported a somewhat increased ratio of collagen: elastin after betamethasone treatment. In cultured human lung, cortisol increased incorporation of $^{35}SO_4$ into heparin, heparin sulphate and sulfated glycoproteins, and decreased [^{3}H]mannose uptake into glycoproteins (Heifetz and Snyder 1981).

Glucocorticoid treatment diminishes respiratory distress and increases survival of prematurely-delivered animals. In fetal sheep, Liggins (1969) noted survival of treated lambs at a gestational age when animals were normally previable. In rabbits, glucocorticoid treatment is associated with an increased viability score (Motoyama et al. 1971), and longer survival times (Taeusch et al. 1972; Barrett et al. 1978) compared with control littermates. Survival time correlated with deflation stability of lungs, suggesting the importance of lung maturity in outcome. It has been difficult to document that glucocorticoids increase long-term survival in animals such as the rabbit because of the narrow window of time which normally occurs between pulmonary immaturity (with non-survival) and adequate maturity for survival. In monkeys, dexamethasone treatment at 135 days gestation was associated with a lower incidence and severity of respiratory distress (Kessler et al. 1982). Based on the human experience, there seems little doubt that glucocorticoid therapy is associated with improved viability.

2.6 Biochemical Effects

2.6.1 Phospholipid Synthesis

The major focus of studies on glucocorticoid action has been the synthesis of surfactant. Since the surface active properties of surfactant are primarily determined by its major component, dipalmitoylphosphatidylcholine, considerable attention has been directed toward the synthesis of this phospholipid. The pathways for synthesis of PC and three other phospholipids are outlined in Fig. 2.5. The first phospholipid in each of the pathways is 1-acylglycerol-3-phosphate which is formed through acylation of either dihydroxyacetone phosphate or glycerol-3-phosphate. In adult type II cells, at least, these two pathways are of approximately equal importance in PC synthesis. Glucose, which is converted to dihydroxyacetone phosphate through glycolysis, is the major precursor of the glycerol backbone of phospholipids. Glucose also contributes to lipogenesis through conversion to acetate and synthesis of fatty acylCoA. Glycerol is also readily incorporated into the backbone of phospholipids in cultured lung (e.g., Fig. 10.1). In vivo, however, this may be an rela-

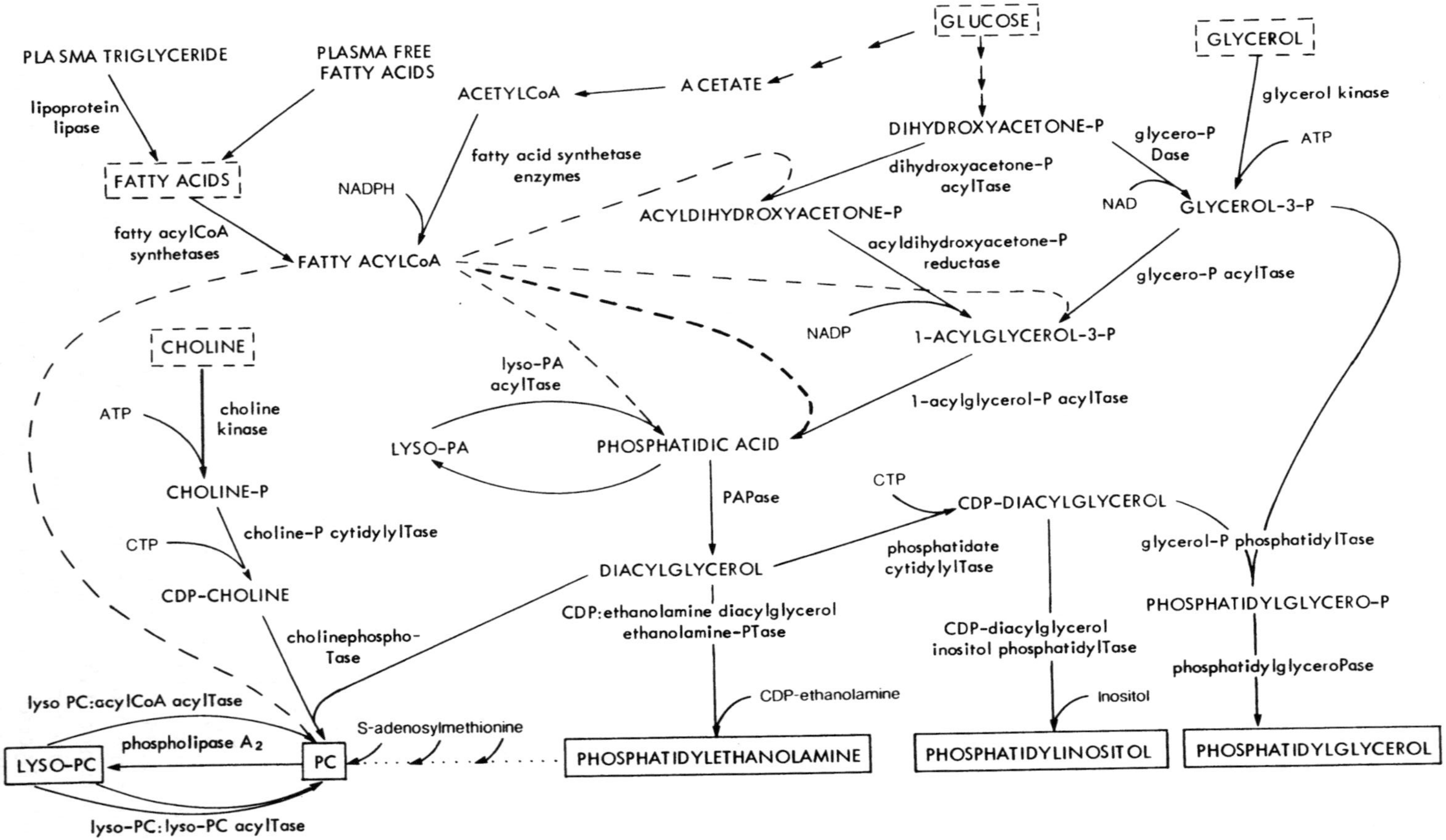

Fig. 2.5. Pathways of phospholipid synthesis in the lung. Abbreviations: *P*, phosphate; *PC*, phosphatidylcholine; *PAPase*, phosphatidic acid phosphatase; *Pase*, phosphatase; *Tase*, transferase; *Dase*, dehydrogenase. Phospholipid precursors are shown in *dashed boxes* and products in *solid boxes*. Methylation of phosphatidylethanolamine (-o-o-) is a minor pathway for PC synthesis in lung

tively unimportant pathway since circulating glycerol levels are low and uptake into lung is much less than for glucose. Glycerol-3-phosphate, formed primarily from dihydroxyacetone phosphate, also is incorporated into phosphatidylglycerol through esterification to the phosphate moiety of the C-3 position.

The fatty acids arise from three sources: hydrolysis of plasma triglycerides (lipoprotein lipase), uptake of circulating free fatty acids, and de novo synthesis from acetylCoA catalyzed by the group of fatty acid synthetase enzymes. The contribution of triglycerides in vivo is probably limited, whereas both uptake of fatty acids and lipogenesis within lung cells are important pathways. As shown in Fig. 2.5, fatty acyl groups are incorporated into phospholipids at multiple sites in the synthetic pathways.

Phosphatidic acid is formed from l-acylglycerol-phosphate by a second acylation step; at this point, synthesis of PC and phosphatidylglycerol diverge. Phosphatidic acid is dephosphorylated in a reaction catalyzed by phosphatidate phosphatase (phosphatidic acid phosphatase, PAPase), forming diacylglycerol which is an immediate precursor of PC. Three enzymes are involved in formation of PC from choline; choline kinase, cholinephosphate cytidylyltransferase, and cholinephosphotransferase. Considerable evidence in recent years indicates that the rate limiting step in this pathway is formation of CDPcholine catalyzed by cholinephosphate cytidylyltransferase. In vivo, most choline in the lung is probably derived by uptake from the circulation.

Little saturated PC is formed de novo in the lung; rather, the major product is 1-saturated-2-unsaturated PC. This compound is converted to disaturated PC through lysoPC and reacylation by two possible reactions. The predominant reaction in adult lung and type II cells in deacylation through phospholipase A_2 and reacylation via acylCoA in a reaction catalyzed by lysoPC acylCoA acyltransferase; in lung, this enzyme preferentially incorporates palmitate into the 2-position. PC may be also synthesized by sequential N-methylation of phosphatidylethanolamine, but this pathway is of minor importance in the lung.

Another important phospholipid of surfactant is phosphatidylglycerol. This compound is synthesized from phosphatidic acid in a reaction catalyzed by phosphatidate cytidylyltransferase. Subsequently, glycerophosphate is added to CDP-diacylglycerol to form phosphatidylglycerophosphate which is dephosphorylated to produce phosphatidylglycerol. CDP-diacylglycerol is also an intermediate in the pathway for synthesis of phosphatidylinositol. As the concentration of inositol increases, phosphatidylinositol synthesis is enhanced at the expense of phosphatidylglycerol production. It is worth noting that synthesis of both PC and phosphatidylglycerol is dependent on CTP. CMP is produced in the pathways for synthesis of PC, phosphatidylglycerol, and phosphatidylinositol. It has been proposed that increasing CMP levels in fetal lung (due to increasing PC synthesis during gestation) plus decreasing concentrations of inositol promote the reverse reaction catalyzed by CDP-diacylglycerol; inositol phosphatidyltransferase, thus enhancing phosphatidylglycerol synthesis at the expense of phosphatidylinositol (Hallman and Epstein, 1980; Quirk et al. 1980).

For detailed information and references on the pathways and enzymes of

tween the glycerol and fatty acid moieties of PC was not altered. By contrast, Freese and Hallman (1983) found a substantially *decreased* rate of glucose incorporation into saturated PC in treated pups. In these experiments, incorporation into the glycerol moiety of PC was not altered, whereas incorporation via de novo fatty acid synthesis was markedly reduced. These workers also found no stimulation of [^{14}C]pyruvate incorporation into saturated PC, consistent with other data indicating that the glycerol moiety of surfactant PC is primarily derived from glucose and glycogen rather than by gluconeogenesis.

In organ culture studies with fetal rabbit lung, glucocorticoids stimulate incorporation of glucose, glycerol, and acetate into PC, although not to the same extent as seen with choline (see Fig. 10.1). With cultures of human lung, dexamethasone stimulates incorporation of glycerol, choline, and acetate into PC by about 80 %, 120 % and 800 %, respectively (Gonzales et al. 1985). The apparent differences between in vivo and in vitro results for precursor incorporation may reflect the different substrate milieu. Additional studies on precursor incorporation, particularly with culture systems, may help to pinpoint the biochemical site of glucocorticoid action.

2.6.1.2 Tissue Phospholipid Content

The tissue concentration of both total PC and saturated PC increases during fetal development. Since there is a correlation between tissue saturated PC and total number of lamellar bodies per lung as estimated by electron microscopy (Faridy et al. 1981), most of the increase in saturated PC represents accumulation of surfactant. In some species glucocorticoid treatment produces a precocious rise in saturated PC, and to a lesser extent, total PC content. In the rabbit corticosteroid treatment of neither the fetus (Russell et al. 1974; Rooney et al. 1976a) nor the mother for 2 days (Gilden et al. 1977; Brehier et al. 1977; Rooney et al. 1979) affected the content or composition of lung phospholipid, whereas Farrell (1973) reported a 37 % increase in lung PC 3 days after fluoroprednisolone. Corticosteroid treatment of the rat for 2 days (representing a relatively greater proportion of total gestation than in the rabbit), increases saturated PC content by 30–45 % (Gross et al. 1984; Frank et al. 1985). Lung saturated PC was greater in treated vs. control twin lambs in the study by Platzker et al. (1975), with less effect noted in the older animals. In hypophysectomized fetal sheep, ACTH infusion for 3 days increased tissue phospholipid and saturated PC about 50 % whereas lavage saturated PC increased several-fold (Liggins et al. 1981; see Table 4.4). Finally Kessler et al. (1982) found a substantial increase in lavage but not lung tissue saturated PC of fetal monkeys after dexamethasone.

The limited hormonal response, particularly for total PC, is due to the relatively large pool of phospholipids in lung tissue, from both surfactant and membrane sources, the relatively short treatment times, and the modest increase in tissue PC content (compared with synthetic rate or lavage content) during normal development (e.g., see Fig. 2.6 and Table 2.2). The specificity of this determination for surfactant could be enhanced by assaying saturated PC in isolated type II cells or lamellar body preparations.

2.6.1.3 Enzymes

Since the corticosteroid induced increase in PC synthesis is mediated by receptor requiring de novo protein synthesis (Chap. 3), it has been assumed that this effect occurs via induction of one or more enzymes which are involved in the biosynthesis of phospholipids. Despite considerable research on this topic, the identity of induced enzymes remains uncertain. For many of the enzymes that have been examined, controversy exists in the literature regarding changes in specific activity after glucocorticoid treatment. Furthermore, to date only one study has attempted to measure either amount of enzyme or rate of synthesis after hormone treatment. The slow progress in the field of lung enzymology has severely limited our understanding of the details of glucocorticoid action in fetal lung.

It has been assumed that target enzymes for glucocorticoid would catalyze rate-limiting reactions in phospholipid synthesis and show a spontaneous developmental increase (discussed by Farrell 1973, and Rooney 1983). In liver, lung and isolated type II cells from adult rat, the reaction catalyzed by cholinephosphate cytidylyltransferase appears to be the rate-limiting step in the choline incorporation pathway (Rooney and Brehier 1982; Post et al. 1984a,b; Rooney 1983). Less is known about the relative rates for reactions leading to production of diacylglycerol in fetal lung. The developmental pattern for activities of many of the enzymes of both PC and phosphatidylglycerol synthesis have been determined in rabbit, rat and mouse lung. The ontogenic profiles are generally similar between species although some pronounced differences have been reported between laboratories. As recently reviewed by Rooney (1983), most experimental data indicate a developmental rise for PAPase, cholinephosphate cytidylyltransferase, phosphatidate cytidylyltransferase, lipoprotein lipase, and the acyltransferases involved in remodeling PC. By contrast, most studies have found little or no developmental change in the activity of choline kinase and choline phosphotransferase, while the pattern for glycerophosphate phosphatidyltransferase plus phosphatidylglycerophosphatase shows apparent species differences.

Table 2.3 summarizes studies of in vivo corticosteroid treatment on enzymes of phospholipid biosynthesis in fetal lung. There is considerable disagreement between different reports for many of the enzymes listed. These differences may arise from biologic differences between species, differences in the treatment protocol (choice of corticosteroid, dose and route of administration, duration of hormone exposure, and time of treatment during gestation), and differences in enzyme assay systems. Relatively few of the studies have characterized the enzyme response and included appropriate determinations to document corticoid responsiveness with the treatment protocol used. To be convincing, a study of in vivo induction of an enzyme(s) should include all of the following: 1) demonstration that treatment increases the rate of PC synthesis or saturated PC content of tissue or lavage fluid in the same animals where enzyme induction occurs, 2) a fully characterized and optimal assay system for enzymes evaluated, 3) assay of several enzymes to evaluate the specificity of hormone response, 4) characterization of both enzyme induction and another parameter of surfactant synthesis with regard to both time course and dose response. Few if any of the studies in Table 2.3 meet all of these criteria. Several studies of enzyme activities did not evaluate the effect of treatment on surfactant synthesis or content (Das et al. 1981; Mostello et al. 1981; Oldenborg and Van Golde 1977; Rooney et al. 1975), and other studies report the effect of hormone on only a single enzyme (Mostello et al. 1981; Farrell 1973; Farrell et al. 1977). Similarly, only a few of the reports include information on the time course of effect (Mostello et al. 1981; Brehier et al. 1977; Brehier and Rooney, 1981; Farrell 1973) or response at various doses of steroid (Gross et al. 1984; Brehier et al. 1977; Brehier and Rooney 1981). When the literature on enzyme induction is viewed from this perspective, the disagreement between investigators for many enzymes is perhaps not surprising. Nevertheless, some tentative conclusions are possible. With regard to inducibility by glucocorticoids, the enzymes of Table 2.3 may be listed in three categories.

a) No response detected. Three or more groups failed to detect a response for choline kinase, glycerophosphate phosphatidyltransferase, phosphatidylglycerophosphatase, and CDP-diacylglycerol:inositol phosphatidyltransferase. Although there is some disagreement with regard to the two enzymes for phosphatidylglycerol synthesis, the unexpected time course data (Rooney et al. 1975, 1976a) and the modest stimulation seen by Possmayer et al. (1979) argue against a major effect of corticosteroids on these enzymes. In addition, there are single reports in the literature regarding lysophosphatidic acid acyltransferase, CDP-ethanolamine:diacylglycerol ethanolaminephosphotransferase, and phospholipase A_2.

b) Confirmed increase in activity. There is substantial evidence that the activity of cholinephosphate cytidylyltransferase is increased after glucocorticoid treatment. This effect was first described in fetal rabbit by Rooney et al. (1976a), and subsequent studies have confirmed the finding in rat and mouse. The activity of this enzyme in vitro is greatly enhanced by the presence of acidic phospholipid cofactor. As noted in Table 2.3, there is little, if any, stimulation of activity by corticosteroid when cytidylyltransferase is assayed in the presence of cofactor. It seems likely that glucocorticoids, as well as other hormones (Chap. 7 and 9), increase the activity of cholinephosphate cytidylyltransferase primarily through production of endogenous acidic phospholipids which serve as cofactor. Additional studies are required to determine whether the rate of enzyme synthesis is also enhanced.

Two studies failed to observe an increase in cytidylyltransferase activity. In the study of Oldenborg and Van Golde (1977) pregnant mice received one intravenous dose of 30 μg dexamethasone and enzyme activities were assayed in fetal lung 3 and 4 days later. Based on the dose-response data of Brehier and Rooney (1981) and Kauffman (1977a), and the expected clearance rate of dexamethasone, it is unlikely that this treatment schedule would be an effective stimulus to the fetal lung; synthesis or content of surfactant was not assessed. In the studies by Freese and Hallman (1983) and Hallman (1984) the treatment protocol was similar to that of Rooney et al. (1979) except that lungs were examined at 27 rather than 26 days gestation. Also, the levels of enzyme activity found by Freese and Hallman (1983) and Hallman (1984) were lower than in the studies by Rooney and colleagues, suggesting differences in the assay system.

If acidic phospholipids have the same stimulatory effect on cytidylyltransferase activity within intact cells as seen in vitro, this could provide a mechanism to amplify the hormonal response to corticosteroids. Treatment would increase the rate of phospholipid biosynthesis through a primary effect on other enzymes, and then PC synthesis would be further enhanced as phospholipid cofactor for cholinephosphate cytidylyltransferase accumulated. This possibility is supported by the recent data of Gilfillan et al. (1984) showing that exogenous phosphatidylglycerol stimulated choline incorporation into PC in type II cells. Alternatively, it is conceivable that stimulation of cytidylyltransferase is a major site of action of glucocorticoids on phospholipid synthesis in type II cells. In this scenario, glucocorticoids acting through receptors would stimulate de novo production of fibroblast-pneumonocyte factor (FPF) in fibroblasts. Within type II cells, FPF would activate cytidylyltransferase activity by a mechanism (possibly via adenylate cyclase) not involving de novo protein synthesis. This possibility is supported by a preliminary report that FPF acts rapidly in isolated type II cells to accelerate disappearance of radioactivity (from choline) from cholinephosphate and into PC (Post and Smith, 1984). Since glucocorticoids apparently induce specific proteins within type II cells (as discussed in Sect. 2.6.2), it is unlikely that this proposed scheme involving FPF would be the only mechanism for glucocorticoid action in these cells.

A second enzyme in this category is PAPase. Increased activity of this enzyme in rabbit lung after corticosteroid treatment has been confirmed by four separate laboratories. By contrast, PAPase activity is not affected by 17β-estradiol in this species, although estrogen increases choline incorporation (Khosla et al. 1980, Chap. 9). Specific activity was also enhanced in mouse lung, but one study found no effect in the rat. In studies with fetal rabbit and human lung in organ culture, PAPase activity increased with time and was not further stimulated (rabbit) by corticosteroids (Snyder et al. 1981a,b). Although this result argues against a direct inductive effect of glucocorticoid on PAPase in vivo, it should be noted that the lung explants in these experiments also demonstrated morphologic maturation and increasing PC synthetic rate in the absence of glucocorticoid (discussed further in Chap. 4).

In most of these studies, phosphatase activity was determined with aqueously-dispersed substrate. When PAPase was assayed using membrane-bound phosphatidic acid as substrate, activity was not significantly increased in the study by Possmayer et al. (1979). Recent studies indicate that there are two forms of PAPase in fetal lung distinguished by magnesium dependency, apparent molecular weight, and membrane association (Casola and Possmayer 1979, 1981c; Yeung et al. 1979). If the PAPase activity specific for membrane-bound substrate is the primary form involved in in vivo synthesis of diacylglycerol, as argued by Possmayer (1982), then the physiologic significance of glucocorticoid-induced PAPase activity with aqueous substrate is uncertain.

Nevertheless, there is considerable evidence that PAPase is an important enzyme in the differentiating fetal lung (reviewed by Bleasdale and Johnston 1982). Schultz et al. (1974) first described a developmental increase in PAPase activity of fetal rabbit lung. This finding has been confirmed for both rat and rabbit where microsomal PAPase activity (dependent on aqueously-dispersed phosphatidic acid) paralleled increasing PC content during gestation (Casola and Possmayer 1981a,b). Specific activity in cytosol preparations increased in the rat but not in the rabbit. Similar developmental changes also occurred with enzyme activity for membrane-dependent phosphatidic acid in both species. Furthermore, phosphatase activity has been identified in isolated lamellar bodies (Spitzer and Johnston 1978), surfactant (Benson 1980), and tracheal and amniotic fluid of the sheep and human (Rosenfeld et al. 1980; Herbert et al. 1978). In the latter studies, activity increased during late gestation in a manner similar to that seen for the L/S ratio. Finally, PAPase activity in adult liver is influenced by a variety of metabolic and surgical procedures, and activity is increased by administration of cortisol both in vivo and in isolated liver (Glenny and Brindley 1978; Lehtonen et al. 1979). Thus, PAPase may be an important enzyme in the control of glyceride and phospholipid biosynthesis in both liver and lung. The developmental profile in fetal lung and association of PAPase with lamellar bodies support the possibility that PAPase is a target enzyme for glucocorticoids during development. Further information on different forms and intracellular localization of the enzyme are needed to establish this point with certainty.

The third enzyme in this group is lyso PC:acylCoA acyltransferase. Since PC synthesized in the lung by the choline incorporation pathway is primarily unsaturated, it is apparent that the remodeling of PC to form saturated PC is important in surfactant biosynthesis. Also, since saturation of PC increases during gestation, it is tempting to consider that one or both of the remodeling enzymes has a regulatory role. Although both deacylation-reacylation and deacylation-transacylation may be occurring in fetal lung, most of the remodeling of PC in adult lung type II cells appears to result from reacylation (reviewed by Batenburg 1982). In microsomes from fetal rabbit lung, the specific activity of this enzyme increases during gestation (Rooney et al. 1976b; Tsao and Zachman 1977), supporting a possible physiologic role in increasing saturated PC synthesis.

Three groups have reported a modest increase in pulmonary lyso-PC:acyl-CoA acyltransferase activity in fetal rabbits 6 to 48 h after corticosteroid treatment. In two studies, there was no stimulation 72 h after treatment. Gross et al. (1984) found no stimulation of acyltransferase activity in rats, whereas both cholinephosphate cytidylyltransferase activity and choline incorporation were enhanced. Thus, the effect of glucocorticoids on lysoPC acyltransferase activity is confirmed in the rabbit, but further study is needed in other species.

c) Report of a positive effect. The remaining enzymes in Table 2.3 fall within this category and more data are required to establish inducibility. The results with cholinephosphotransferase are controversial. After injection of fetal rabbits with 9-fluoroprednisolone, Farrell (1973) observed a similar time-dependent increase in cholinephosphotransferase activity, choline incorporation into PC, and lung PC content. However, as previously pointed out (Possmayer 1982; Van Golde 1982), cholinephosphotransferase was assayed in this study using dipalmitoylglycerol as substrate; this disaturated diacylglycerol is not utilized by the enzyme (Rooney et al. 1976a). It is possible that the increased enzyme activity in treated animals may have reflected increased amounts of endogenous diacylglycerol rather than enzyme in the microsomal preparations. However, four other groups have not detected a corticosteroid-induced increase in cholinephosphotransferase of rabbit lung in assays using no added substrate, dipalmitoylglycerol, or dioleoylglycerol as substrate. The reported stimulation of activity in two other species (using unsaturated diacylglycerol as substrate) remains to be confirmed.

The enzyme lyso-PC:lyso-PCacyltransferase contributes to saturated PC synthesis via the remodeling pathway. Whereas Possmayer et al. (1979) found a 46 % increase in this acyltransferase activity, Rooney et al. (1979) detected no change using a similar treatment protocol. The specific activity of the enzyme in control tissue differs 4-fold between the two studies, suggesting the possibility that differences in assay systems may have influenced the response seen to hormone treatment.

Lipoprotein lipase, which catalyzes the hydrolysis of triglycerides from the circulation, may be involved in supplying long-chain fatty acids needed for synthesis of surfactant. One study in fetal rats found increased lipase activity after dexamethasone treatment (Mostello et al. 1981). In adult rats, administration of dexamethasone (200 μg/kg) for 8 days increased lipoprotein lipase activity in lung (70 %) but not in heart or adipose tissue (Hamosh et al. 1976). Neither study examined the effect of treatment on surfactant content or synthesis. The relative importance of de novo fatty acid synthesis vs. the circulating sources (including fatty acids released from triglycerides) for phospholipid synthesis in the developing lung is not yet established. However, fetal lung cultured in the absence of serum or fatty acids synthesizes PC at a rate comparable to that occurring in vivo and is responsive to corticosteroids (Chap. 4). This would appear to indicate that de novo synthesis is the major source of fatty acids and that hormonal induction of lipoprotein lipase is not physiologically important for surfactant production in the fetus.

The significance of the various data on enzyme activities after in vivo glucocorticoid treatment will eventually be established by additional studies both in vivo and in vitro. In the case of cholinephosphate cytidylyltransferase, for example, enzyme activity (in the absence of cofactor) is also increased by glucocorticoid treatment of explants from both rabbit and rat (Khosla et al. 1983; Gross et al. 1984). The activity of PAPase has also been assayed in explant cultures (Snyder et al. 1981a,b); although there was no stimulation by corticosteroids, future experiments will need to test both aqueous and membrane-associated substrate. Ultimately, definitive information on enzyme induction by glucocorticoids will require studies in isolated fetal type II cells involving determination of enzyme activity and the rate of synthesis of both enzyme protein and its mRNA.

2.6.2 Other Proteins

There is preliminary evidence that corticosteroids influence proteins other than enzymes involved in PC synthesis. As discussed in Chap. 8, both in vivo and in vitro studies indicate that glucocorticoids induce beta-adrenergic re-

Table 2.3. Studies of in vivo corticosteroid effects on enzymes of phospholipid biosynthesis in fetal lung. Reactions catalyzed by each enzyme are illustrated in Fig. 2.5

Enzyme	Species	Treatment	Response	Note	References
Choline kinase (EC 2.7.1.32)	Mouse	Dexamethasone (maternal)	None	Single, low dose	Oldenborg & Van Golde 1977
	Rabbit	Cortisol (fetal)	None		Rooney et al. 1976a
		Cortisol (Maternal)	None		Tsao et al. 1979
		9-Fluoroprednisolone (fetal)	None		Farrell 1973
	Rat	Betamethasone (maternal)	↓20 %		Rooney et al. 1979
			None		Gross et al. 1984
Cholinephosphate cytidylyltransferase (EC 2.7.7.15)	Rabbit	Cortisol (fetal)	↑22 % at 48 h	Cytosol without lipid cofactor	Rooney et al. 1976
		Betamethasone (maternal)	↑50 %	Cytosol without cofactor	Rooney et al. 1979
		Cortisol (maternal)	None		Freese & Hallman 1983 Hallman 1984
			↓36 % at 72 h	Homogenate without cofactor	Tsao et al. 1979
		9-Fluoroprednisolone (fetal)	None	?cofactor	Farrell 1973
	Rat	Betamethasone (maternal)	↑96 % at 48 h	Cytosol without cofactor	Gross et al. 1984
			None	With cofactor	
	Mouse	Dexamethasone (maternal)	↑17 % at 72 h	Cytosol with cofactor	Brehier & Rooney 1981
			↑37 %	Without cofactor	
		Dexamethasone (maternal)	None	Microsomal without cofactor	Oldenborg & Van Golde 1977
Cholinephosphotransferase (EC 2.7.8.2)	Rabbit	9-Fluoroprednisolone (fetal)	↑50 % at 6 and 72 h	No ↑ at 24 h	Farrell & Zachman 1973
				Saturated diacylglycerol as substrate	Farrell 1973
		Betamethasone (maternal)	None	At 12–48 h	Brehier et al. 1977 Possmayer et al. 1977, 1979
		Cortisol (fetal) or Betamethasone (maternal)	None	At 48 h	Rooney et al. 1975, 1976a, 1979
		Cortisol (maternal)	None	At 72 h	Tsao et al. 1979

	Mouse	Dexamethasone (maternal)	$\uparrow$27 % at 72 h	No $\uparrow$ at 48 h	Brehier & Rooney 1981
			$\uparrow$63 % at 72 h		Oldenborg & Van Golde 1977
	Rat	Dexamethasone (fetal)	$\uparrow$183 % at 6–12 h	Anencephalic fetuses	Farrell et al. 1977
Phosphatidate phosphatase (PA-Pase) (EC 3.1.3.4)	Rabbit	Betamethasone (maternal)	$\uparrow$100 %	Homogenate and microsomes with aqueous phosphatidic acid (PA) (see Fig.2.7)	Brehier et al. 1977
			$\uparrow$68 % at 24 h	Homogenate and aqueous PA	Possmayer et al. 1979
			None	Membrane-bound PA	
			$\uparrow$50 % at 48 h	Homogenate and aqueous PA	Rooney et al. 1979
			$\uparrow$50–58 %	Microsomes and aqueous PA	Freese & Hallman 1983 Hallman 1984
	Mouse	Dexamethasone (maternal)	$\uparrow$25 % at 48 h	Homogenate and aqueous PA	Brehier & Rooney 1981
	Rat	Betamethasone (maternal)	None at 48 h	Homogenate and aqueous PA	Gross et al. 1984
Phosphatidate cytidylyltransferase (EC 2.7.7.41)	Rabbit	Betamethasone (maternal)	$\uparrow$90–128 %	At 42 h	Freese and Hallman 1983; Hallman 1984
	Rat	Betamethasone (maternal)	None	At 48 h	Gross et al. 1984
Lyso PC:acyl–CoA acyltransferase (EC 2.3.1.23)	Rabbit	Dexamethasone (fetal)	$\uparrow$29 %	At 6 h	Das et al. 1981
		Betamethasone (maternal)	$\uparrow$33 %	At 24 h	Possmayer et al. 1979
		Cortisol (fetal)	None	At 72 h	Rooney et al. 1975
			$\uparrow$33 %	At 48 h	Rooney et al. 1976a
		Cortisol (maternal)	None	At 72 h	Tsao et al. 1979
	Mouse	Dexamethasone (maternal)	$\uparrow$100 %	At 72 h	Oldenborg & Van Golde 1977
	Rat	Betamethasone (maternal)	None	At 48 h	Gross et al. 1984

Continued

Table 2.3 (contd.)

Enzyme	Species	Treatment	Response	Note	References
Lyso PC:lyso PC acyltransferase (EC not listed)	Rabbit	Betamethasone (maternal)	↑46 %	At 24 h	Possmayer et al. 1979
			None	At 48 h	Rooney et al. 1979
		Cortisol (maternal)	None	At 72 h	Tsao et al. 1979
	Mouse	Dexamethasone (maternal)	None	At 72 h	Oldenborg & Van Golde 1977
Lysophosphatidic acid acyltransferase	Rabbit	Cortisol (fetal)	None	At 72 h	Rooney et al. 1975
Glycerophosphate phosphatidyltransferase (EC 2.7.8.5) + Phosphatidylglycerophosphatase (EC 3.1.3.27)	Rabbit	Betamethasone (maternal)	↑28 %	At 24 h	Possmayer et al. 1979
			None	At 42 h	Hallman 1984
		Cortisol (fetal)	↑53 %	At 72 h	Rooney et al. 1975
			None	At 48 h	Rooney et al. 1976a
		Betamethasone (maternal)	None	At 12–48 h	Brehier et al. 1977
	Rat	Betamethasone (maternal)	None	At 48 h	Gross et al. 1984
CDP-ethanolamine: diacylglycerol ethanolaminephosphotransferase (EC 2.7.8.1)	Rabbit	Betamethasone (maternal)	None	At 24 h	Possmayer et al. 1979
CDP-diacylglycerol: inositol phosphatidyltransferase (EC 2.7.8.11)	Rabbit	Betamethasone (maternal)	None	At 42 h	Freese and Hallman 1983; Hallman 1984
		Cortisol (fetal)	None	At 72 h	Rooney et al. 1975
	Rat	Betamethasone (maternal)	None	At 48 h	Gross et al. 1984
Lipoprotein lipase	Rat	Dexamethasone (maternal) (osmotic minipump infusion)	↑ 8–170 %	At 2½–4 days	Mostello et al. 1981
Phospholipase A_2 (EC 3.1.1.4)	Rabbit	Dexamethasone (fetal)	↑ 42 %	At 6 h	Das et al. 1981
PalmitoylCoA synthetase (EC 6.2.1.3)	Rabbit	Dexamethasone (fetal)	↑26 %	At 6 h; also rate of synthesis	Das et al. 1981

ceptor in fetal rabbit lung. This response occurs within 24 h and with physiologic concentrations of corticosteroids. In addition, there are preliminary indications that corticosteroids may enhance coupling of receptor to adenylate cyclase, suggesting a further level of glucocorticoid involvement in adrenergic responsiveness. The marked increase in beta-adrenergic receptor capacity during normal development, and the precocious rise with corticosteroid treatment, argue for the physiologic importance of glucocorticoid regulation of this protein. Increased receptor concentration on alveolar epithelial cells enhances the sensitivity to effects of both endogenous and exogenous catecholamines.

In a recent study, Frank et al. (1985) report that prenatal dexamethasone treatment increases the activity of lung antioxidant enzymes. During late gestation, there is a developmental increase in the activity of superoxide dismutase, catalase, and glutathione peroxidase in lungs of both rats (Frank et al. 1985; Tanswell and Freeman 1982) and rabbits (Frank and Groseclose 1984). Treatment of pregnant rats with 0.2 mg/kg of dexamethasone at 48 and 24 h prior to delivery on day 20 of gestation stimulated the specific activities of superoxide dismutase, catalase and glutathione peroxidase by 19, 43 and 45 %, respectively. These increases in enzyme activity are equivalent to 1–2 days of gestation; parallel effects are seen for saturated PC content. The authors speculate that prenatal glucocorticoid treatment may have a similar effect in the human and accordingly might provide some protection against hyperoxemia-induced lung injury in premature infants.

An alternative approach to examining glucocorticoid effects on lung proteins is two-dimensional gel electrophoresis after incubation of lung fragments with [^{35}S]methionine. Phelps and Gianoppoulos (1984) recently reported results from exposure of fetal lung to glucocorticoid both in vivo and in vitro. Exposure of 24 day rabbit lung explants to dexamethasone for 3 days did not affect the overall incorporation rate of [^{3}H]amino acids or [^{35}S]methionine into trichloroacetic acid-precipitable protein. On two-dimensional gel electrophoresis, nearly 400 different proteins were resolved. Exposure of lung to glucocorticoid either in vivo (0.2 mg/kg dexamethasone on days 25 and 26) or in culture (0.25 μM) reproducibly increased incorporation of [^{35}S]methionine into four proteins with approximate molecular weight of 20,000, 22,000, 24,000 and 42,000 daltons. Increased labeling of an additional protein (molecular weight 100,000 daltons) was seen in cultured tissue but not with in vivo treatment. In populations of cells enriched for type II cells, prior exposure to glucocorticoid in vivo increased labeling in three of the four proteins observed with whole lung tissue. In addition, labeling was enhanced in a doublet protein (35,000 daltons) which may represent surfactant apoprotein. These findings suggest that glucocorticoids induce synthesis of specific proteins in type II cells and other pulmonary cell types.

A similar electrophoretic study has also been carried out with fibroblasts cultured from fetal rat lung (Floros et al. 1985). Dexamethasone treatment did not alter the rate of methionine incorporation into total secreted proteins, but enhanced labeling of two proteins of apparent molecular weights of 30,000–35,000 daltons and a pI of 6.2–6.4. The effect was observed after as little as 4 h of treatment, and optimal response was seen with 10 nM dexa-

The growth inhibitory action of glucocorticoids is well documented in animals; representative studies are listed in Table 2.4. Administration of corticosteroid to newborn animals inhibits DNA synthesis and growth in many tissues, and also impairs later immune responsivity and locomotor activity. At least three different modes of glucocorticoid action probably operate with regard to growth. When corticoids are given to the fetus or pregnant animals, placental function is impaired due to precocious aging (degeneration), and this interferes with the supply of substrate and oxygen to fetal tissues. With betamethasone treatment of the pregnant rabbit, for example, growth stops in the placenta, lung and liver, and slows in the brain (Table 2.4). Second, in lymphoid cells, glucocorticoids inhibit glucose uptake and synthesis of DNA and protein causing cell death and tissue involution. This effect involves early stimulation of new protein synthesis and obviously is not reversible at later times of hormone exposure. A third action of glucocorticoids on tissue growth in the newborn animal is more specific for cell division. In the liver, for example, glucocorticoid inhibits cell proliferation but not RNA or protein synthesis, and the effect is completely reversible upon removal of excess corticosteroid (Henderson et al. 1971; Henderson and Loeb 1974). DNA synthesis in heart, skeletal muscle, kidney and lung is also relatively sensitive to inhibition by corticosteroids. By contrast, several other tissues are not affected at the same dose of corticosteroid (Table 2.4). It is likely that the decreased body weight after corticosteroid treatment is in part a direct result of the growth inhibition in the "sensitive" tissues.

Growth inhibition by glucocorticoid is dose related. This has been examined most carefully in the case of liver cell proliferation (Loeb 1976). In dose-response experiments with hydrocortisone treatment of weanling rats, accumulation of liver DNA was inhibited by as little as 3 mg hydrocortisone/kg/day and a maximal effect was observed with about 10-fold higher doses. Although circulating levels of cortisol were not determined in these studies, the lower doses of hydrocortisone probably produced plasma levels within the physiologic stress range. The well recognized action of glucocorticoids to inhibit growth of cultured fibroblasts is a receptor-mediated process which occurs with relatively low concentrations of hormone. Thus, it seems likely that endogenous corticoids may influence the rate of growth in various organs in addition to causing involution of lymphoid tissues.

The physiologic relevance of growth inhibition by corticosteroids is supported by observations on the time course (Loeb 1976). With repeated daily administration of hydrocortisone, there is little if any weight gain and no increase in liver DNA content. When hormone treatment is stopped, both body weight and liver DNA begin to increase within 2 days and there is a subsequent period of accelerated growth which results in "catch-up" to levels in untreated controls. There is also catch-up growth of the lung after birth for rabbits treated in utero with hydrocortisone (Kotas et al. 1974). The catch-up in body weight implies that accelerated hyperplasia occurs in all affected tissues. Thus, growth inhibition with corticosteroid treatment is a fully reversible event which probably also occurs to some extent during normal development.

In many of the other studies of growth inhibition shown in Table 2.4, extremely high doses of corticosteroids were used. Under these circumstances,

Table 2.4. Growth inhibitory and other adverse effects of glucocorticoids in developing animals

Investigator	Animal	Steroid (dose)	Cortisol equivalents (mg/kg/day)	Inhibitory effects
Loeb & Yeung 1973	Weanling rat	Cortisone (0.5 mg)	8	DNA synthesis in: heart, liver, muscle, kidney and lung
Loeb, personal communication		(5 mg)	80	DNA synthesis in brain, testis, spleen and intestine
Loeb 1976		0.2-10 mg daily for 6 days	3-150	Somatic growth and liver DNA
Carson et al. 1973	Fetal rabbit	Cortisol (2 mg)	100	Somatic growth, lung growth
Wellman and Volk 1972	Fetal rabbit	Cortisone × 2-7 days	4	Placental growth
Barrada et al. 1980	Fetal rabbit	Betamethasone × 2 days (0.8 mg)	7	Growth of placenta, lung, liver and brain
Weichsel 1974	Newborn rat	Cortisol (0.6 mg)	92	Somatic growth, thymic growth, brain thymidine kinase
Cotterell et al. 1972	Newborn rat	Cortisol × 4 days (0.2 mg)	30	Somatic growth, thymic growth, brain growth
Shapiro 1968	Newborn rat	Cortisol (1 mg)	150	Somatic growth, immune response, myelination and locomotor activity
DeSouza & Adlard 1973	5-day rat	Dexamethasone (0.01 and 0.2 mg) or Cortisol (0.5 mg) × 5 days	25-500	Somatic growth, brain growth
Gumbinas et al. 1973	6-day rat	Methylprednisolone (0.8 mg)	335	Somatic growth, brain growth, and myelinization
Johnson et al. 1981	Fetal monkey	Betamethasone (2 mg × 13 days)	7	Somatic growth, adrenal and thymus weight
Liggins & Howie 1972	Pregnant human	Betamethasone (12 mg)	5 (1.7 to fetus)	None for body weight

high circulating levels of corticoid would occur and persist for extended periods. In such situations catch-up of growth would be delayed and potentially less compensatory. It is also possible that extremely high doses of circulating corticosteroids would interfere with cell proliferation by mechanisms other than that which occurs with lower concentrations of steroids. It is clear from some studies such as that of Shapiro (1968) that exposure to a high dose of glucocorticoid during development has long-term effects on function. In terms of neurologic effects, pharmacological doses of glucocorticoids have immediate effects on brain cell division, differentiation, myelination and electrophysiological activity; later delayed effects include alterations in circadian rhythm, biogenic amine levels, stress responsiveness and behavior (reviewed by Weichsel 1977).

The relevance of these corticosteroid effects in small animals to the human situation is uncertain for two reasons. First, the human fetus receiving prenatal therapy is exposed to much less corticosteroid than in the animal studies (Table 2.4). The dose of betamethasone to the fetus, calculated as cortisol equivalents, is less than 2 mg/kg/day. The lowest concentration of hydrocortisone inhibiting DNA synthesis in rat liver was about 3 mg/kg/day. Doses of corticosteroid in the other postnatal studies have ranged between 25 and 500 mg/kg. Second, the human fetus has elevated glucocorticoid levels for a relatively short time during the period of fetal and postnatal development. By contrast, the short lifespan of the rat condenses the developmental period and corticosteroid exposure occurs over a relatively longer portion of development. This would magnify any effects of corticoid treatment on both growth and subsequent organ function.

Thus, the human fetus receiving prenatal glucocorticoid therapy is exposed to relatively low levels of circulating glucocorticoid for a very brief period in comparison with the treatment protocols utilized in young rats. Accordingly, it seems extremely unlikely that the severe growth inhibition and developmental sequelae seen in animals is relevant to the human situation. This conclusion is supported by the finding that peak plasma levels of glucocorticoid in the treated human infant are within the physiologic stress range (Chap. 6). These considerations argue strongly against the possibility of adverse effects of prenatal betamethasone (at the recommended dose) on tissue or body growth in the newborn infant.

The studies in rhesus monkeys (Macaca mulatta) most closely resemble the human situation. Johnson et al. (1981) administered betamethasone daily to pregnant animals for 13 days and examined the fetus either at that time (133 days gestation) or a month later at term. This treatment regimen involves somewhat higher doses of maternal glucocorticoid than in the human (Table 2.4), and the amount of betamethasone transferred from mother to fetus in the monkey is not known. After 13 days of this treatment, body and organ weights were significantly reduced in the treated fetus. When organ weights were expressed per body weight, there was a reduction only for the adrenal and thymus. When the pregnancies were allowed to proceed to term, treated fetuses were also smaller than control animals and had decreased weight per body weight for the adrenal and spleen. In contrast with these results, there was no reduction of body or organ (including brain) weight and no histologic changes in the brain associated with 3 days of treatment with 2 mg of dexamethasone (Kessler et al. 1982; Sumi et al. 1984) or betamethasone (Johnson et al. 1978, 1979). Thus, it is clear that prolonged exposure of the monkey fetus to corticosteroid inhibits growth; this finding cautions against excessive doses or treatment periods in pregnant women.

2.8 Effect of Gender

It has been recognized for some time that RDS occurs more frequently and has a higher mortality rate in male than female infants. Consistent with these clinical observations, Naeye et al. (1974) found that lungs of female fetuses were more mature histologically than lungs of male fetuses at 25–32 weeks gestation. These findings led to the concept that the male disadvantage for neonatal survival applied also to lung development. Moreover, recent evidence suggests that males may be less responsive to glucocorticoids for prevention of RDS than females (discussed in Chap. 5).

2.8.1 Differences Observed

The influence of gender on lung maturation has been examined in three animal models during the past five years. Table 2.5 summarizes differences observed between sexes in several indices of lung maturation in vivo. In the first study addressing this question, Kotas and Avery (1980) found greater deflation stability in female vs. male rabbit lungs. The gender difference persisted after corticosteroid treatment of the fetuses in utero. In these experiments, the untreated fetuses were injected with saline during surgery at 24 days gestation. Accordingly, the fetuses were stressed and exposed to elevated endogenous corticoids (see Chap. 4). It was unclear from these initial data, therefore, whether the difference between sexes represented a developmental lag and/or decreased glucocorticoid responsiveness in males vs. females.

Subsequent studies have established that there is less saturated PC in lavage fluid from males compared with females of undisturbed animals. At 28 days gestation, Nielson and Torday (1981) found approximately 50 % more saturated PC in female fetuses; a similar but less striking gender difference was observed by Freese and Hallman (1983) for both control and betamethasone-treated rabbits. In a study with rats, Adamson and Kind (1984a, c) found less saturated PC and fewer lamellar bodies in lung tissue of male vs. female lungs.

In striking contrast to the data for rabbits and rats, Truog et al. (1981) describe delayed lung development in female monkey fetuses. In groups of male and female fetuses of similar mean gestational age and birthweight, the females had less lavage phospholipid (per g dry lung and per tissue phospholipid) and less surface active material than the males. There was no difference between the two groups in lung weight, Vmax or tissue phospholipid (tissue saturated PC was not determined). However, males had a better respiratory score at birth than females, consistent with the presence of more surfactant in airways. Johnson et al. (1982) reported no differences between the sexes in the

Table 2.5. Gender differences in lung maturation: in vivo studies

Measurement	Species and age	Results: Untreated fetuses, Male	Results: Untreated fetuses, Female	Results: Corticosteroid-treated fetuses, Male	Results: Corticosteroid-treated fetuses, Female	References
Deflation stability at 10 cmH_2O (% of volume at 35 cmH_2O)	Rabbit 27 days	41 ± 2.5	49 ± 1.5[a]	69 ± 1.4	80 ± 3.6[a]	Kotas & Avery 1980
Air/tissue ratio	Rabbit 27 days	0.32 ± 0.016	0.35 ± 0.014	0.47 ± 0.024	0.61 ± 0.022[a]	Kotas & Avery 1980
Lavage saturated PC/sphingomyelin ratio	Rabbit 28 days	0.90 ± 0.13	1.38 ± 0.23[a]			Nielsen & Torday 1981
		1.80 ± 0.11	2.11 ± 0.10[a]	2.20 ± 0.20	2.76 ± 0.02[a]	Freese & Hallmann 1983
Lavage phospholipid (mg/g dry lung)	Monkey (135-150 days)	17 ± 14	7 ± 8[a]			Truog et al. 1981
Tissue saturated PC (µg P/mg dry weight)	Rat 20 days	0.38 ± 0.02	0.49 ± 0.03[a]			Adamson & King 1984a
Epithelial cells with lamellar bodies (%)	Rat 20 days	7.6 ± 3.0	19.9 ± 4.1[a]			Adamson & King 1984b

[a] $p < 0.05$ female vs. male

increase in Vmax for Rhesus monkeys exposed to daily treatment with betamethasone for 2 weeks. By contrast, Kessler et al. (1982) state that only male Rhesus fetuses responded to 3 days therapy with dexamethasone. These findings suggest that the primate is not an appropriate model for the sex differences in the human.

The gender difference is age-dependent. In fetal rabbits, a male-female difference in saturated PC/sphingomyelin ratio was found for lavage fluid at 26 and 28 days and for amniotic fluid at 28 days. No differences were detected earlier or later in gestation (Nielson and Torday 1981; Ward et al. 1983). Similarly in the fetal rat, differences in saturated PC content and the cellular composition of lung occurred on days 19 and 20, but not later in gestation (Adamson and King 1984c). Thus, sex-related differences in lung maturation exist during much of the third trimester but disappear before term. Differences in lung morphology between sexes have also been noted in fetal rabbits (Kotas and Avery 1980). The parallel developmental pattern for sex-related differences in lung structure and saturated PC content in the rat have led Adamson and King (1984a, b) to postulate that cellular differentiation and intercellular communication are the major determinants of the gender difference. This concept is supported by data of Torday (1984) which suggests that a sex difference in fibroblasts (production of cortisol and FPF) may contribute to delayed surfactant synthesis in the male fetus.

2.8.2 No Differences Found

The initial reports of gender differences in lung maturation stimulated a consideration of gender in subsequent investigations of lung physiology and biochemistry. As summarized in Table 2.6, gender differences have not been observed for a variety of measurements in lung of the rat, rabbit and monkey. These include lung tissue protein, DNA, glycogen, and phospholipid; phospholipid composition of lavage fluid; activity of several enzymes of phospholipid biosynthesis; the rate of both choline and glucose incorporation into PC; several hormone receptors; and tissue or plasma concentration of various hormones. In several instances measurements have been made in corticosteroid-treated animals as well as untreated fetuses. These findings would appear to rule out at least two possible explanations for the observed differences between genders: 1) The data for choline and glucose incorporation indicate that synthesis of PC is similar in male and female rabbits. The absence of a gender difference in both enzymes for phospholipid synthesis and tissue phospholipid content support this conclusion, although the latter measurement might not detect a small difference in surfactant content. In particular, the data for PAPase and cholinephosphate cytidylyltransferase are noteworthy, since both of these enzymes appear to have regulatory roles during normal development. Thus, the major sex difference in lung development of the rabbit may relate to surfactant secretion rather than synthesis. The data for tissue saturated PC in the rat, yet to be confirmed, suggest that decreased synthesis may indeed be a component of the gender difference in this species (Table 2.5). 2) Although endogenous glucocorticoids influence the rate of lung maturation (Chap. 4), there is no evidence to date that these hormones contribute directly to the gender difference. It is reported that plasma concen-

stimulate capillary growth in concert with alveolarization. Division of alveolar epithelial cells is slowed (withdrawal from the cell cycle into the G_0 phase) and differentiation accelerated. In those cells destined to be type I cells, glucocorticoids presumably stimulate specific proteins involved in the cytoskeletal structure, leading to extension and flattening of the cells along the alveolar surface. In pre-type II cells and already differentiated type II cells, glucocorticoids induce a limited number of proteins which directly or indirectly cause proliferation of the rough endoplasmic reticulum, depletion of lung glycogen, and increased synthesis of PC and other phospholipids. As a consequence of the latter effect, increased phospholipid cofactor is available and the activity of cholinephosphate cytidylyltransferase increases. This serves to amplify the effect to glucocorticoid on PC biosynthesis. Glucocorticoids also induce one or more of the acyltransferase enzymes which increases the production of saturated PC from the unsaturated species. The apoprotein for surfactant is also presumably induced by glucocorticoid so that its concentration increases in parallel with saturated PC. These events result in increased rate of synthesis and storage of surfactant, and, as a consequence, increased secretion of lamellar bodies from type II cells. The induction of beta-adrenergic receptor on alveolar epithelial cells increases the sensitivity of the cells to effects of endogenous catecholamines on both surfactant release and fluid reabsorption. Finally, the physiologic consequence of these glucocorticoid-induced biochemical and morphologic changes would be improved lung function and increased viability of prematurely delivered fetuses. Inherent in this proposal is the assumption that each of the actions of exogenous glucocorticoid represents accelerated occurrence of normal developmental events in the lung.

This global view of glucocorticoid effects is obviously highly speculative. The validity of various details will be tested in years to come as work in this area continues. There is an obvious need to identify specific proteins induced by glucocorticoids. Once this information is available, the mechanism of hormone regulation can be examined in greater detail. In particular, probes for both proteins (e.g., monoclonal antibodies) and their mRNAs (cDNA) will be invaluable tools in this process. At present, the best candidate for these types of studies is probably the apoprotein of surfactant. This protein has been partially characterized from several species, highly purified, and the amino acid sequence determined. Probes for this protein, combined with studies in isolated fetal type II cells, will generate additional detailed information regarding mechanisms of glucocorticoid regulation in the lung.

References

Adamson IYR, King GM (1984a) Sex differences in development of fetal rat lung. I. Autoradiographic and biochemical studies. Lab Invest 50:456

Adamson IYR, King GM (1984b) Sex differences in development of fetal rat lung. II. Quantitative morphology of epithelial-mesenchymal interactions. Lab Invest 50:461

Adamson IYR, King GM (1984c) Sex-related differences in cellular composition and surfactant synthesis of developing fetal rat lungs. Am Rev Respir Dis 129:130

Alescio T, Dani AM (1972) Hydrocortisone-increased glycogen deposition and its dependence on tissue interactions in mouse embryonic lung developing in vitro. J Embryol Exp Morph 27:155

Avery ME (1975) Pharmacological approaches to the acceleration of fetal lung maturation. Br Med Bull 31:13
Ballard PL (1979) Glucocorticoids and differentiation. In: Monographs on Endocrinology, Vol 12: Glucocorticoid Hormone Action, Baxter JD, Rousseau GG (eds), Springer, Berlin, Heidelberg, New York, pp 493–515
Ballard PL, Benson BJ, Brehier A, Carter JP, Kriz BM, Jorgensen EC (1980) Transplacental stimulation of lung development in the fetal rabbit by 3,5-dimethyl-3'-isopropyl-L-thyronine. J Clin Invest 65:1407
Ballard PL (1982) Hormonal aspects of fetal lung development. In: Lung Development: Biological and Clinical Perspectives, Vol II, Farrell PM (ed), Academic Press, New York, pp 205–253
Ballard PL (1983) Mode of action of glucocorticoids on lung maturation. Curr Prob in Clin Biochem 13:35
Ballard PL, Hovey ML, Gonzales LK (1984) Thyroid hormone stimulation of phosphatidylcholine synthesis in cultured fetal rabbit lung. J Clin Invest 74:898
Barrada MI, Blomquist CH, Kotts C (1980) The effects of betamethasone on fetal development in the rabbit. Am J Obstet Gynecol 136:234, 1980
Barrett CT, Sevanian A, Phelps DL, Gilden C, Kaplan SA (1978) Effects of cortisol and aminophylline upon survival, pulmonary mechanics, and secreted phosphatidyl choline of prematurely delivered rabbits. Pediatr Res 12:38
Batenburg JJ, Van Golde LMG (1979) Formation of pulmonary surfactant in whole lung and in isolated type II alveolar cells. In: Reviews in Perinatal Medicine, Vol 13, Scarpelli EM, Cosmi EV (eds), Raven Press, New York, pp 73–114
Batenburg JJ (1982) The phosphatidylcholine-lysophosphatidylcholine cycle. In: Lung Development: Biological and Clinical Perspectives, Vol 1, Biochemistry and Physiology, Farrell PM (ed), Academic Press, New York, pp 359–390
Baxter JD, Forsham PH (1972) Tissue effects of glucocorticoids. Am J Med 53:573
Beck JC, Mitzner W, Johnson JWC, Hutchins GM, Foidart J-M, London WT, Palmer AE, Scott R (1981) Betamethasone and the rhesus fetus: effect on lung morphometry and connective tissue. Pediatr Res 15:235
Benson BJ (1980) Properties of an acid phosphatase in pulmonary surfactant. Proc Natl Acad Sci USA 77:808
Blackburn WR, Kaplan HS, McKay DG (1965) Morphologic changes in the developing rat placenta following prednisolone administration. Am J Obstet Gynecol 92:234
Bleasdale JE, Johnston JM (1982) Phosphatidic acid production and utilization. In: Lung Development: Biological and Clinical Perspectives, Vol 1, Biochemistry and Physiology, Farrell PM (ed), Academic Press, New York, pp 259–294
Bourbon J, Jost A (1982) Control of glycogen metabolism in the developing fetal lung. Pediatr Res 16:50
Bourbon JR, Rieutort M, Engle MJ, Farrell PM (1982) Utilization of glycogen for phospholipid synthesis in fetal rat lung. Biochim Biophys Acta 712:382
Brandstrup N, Kretchmer N (1965) The metabolism of glycogen in the lungs of the fetal rabbit. Dev Biol 11:202
Brehier A, Benson BJ, Williams MC, Mason RJ, Ballard PL (1977) Corticosteroid induction of phosphatidic acid phosphatase in fetal rabbit lung. Biochem Biophys Res Commun 77:883
Brehier A, Rooney SA (1981) Phosphatidylcholine synthesis and glycogen depletion in fetal mouse lung: Developmental changes and the effects of dexamethasone. Exp Lung Res 2:273
Brown ER, Torday JS, Taeusch HW Jr (1978) Pharmacologic control of fetal lung development. Clin Perinatol 5:243
Brumley GW, Knelson JH, Schomberg DW, Crenshaw C Jr (1977) Whole and disaturated lung phosphatidylcholine in cortisol-treated, intrauterine growth-retarded and twin control lambs at different gestational ages. Biol Neonate 31:155
Buckingham S, McNary WF, Sommers SC, Rothschild J (1968) Is lung an analog of Moog's developing intestine? I. Phosphatases and pulmonary alveolar differentiation in fetal rabbits. Fed Proc 27:328 (abstract)
Bunton TE, Plopper CG (1984) Triamcinolone-induced structural alterations in the development of the lung of the rhesus macaque. Am J Obstet Gynecol 148:203
Carson S, Taeusch HW, Avery M (1973) Inhibition of lung cell division after hydrocortisone injection into fetal rabbits. J Appl Physiol 34:660

Casola PG, Possmayer F (1979) Pulmonary phosphatidic acid phosphatase. Properties of membrane-bound phosphatidate-dependent phosphatidic acid phosphatase in rat lung. Biochim Biophys Acta 574:212

Casola PG, Possmayer F (1981a) Pulmonary phosphatidic acid phosphohydrolase. Developmental patterns in rat lung. Biochim Biophys Acta 665:177

Casola PG, Possmayer F (1981b) Pulmonary phosphatidic acid phosphohydrolase. Developmental patterns in rabbit lung. Biochim Biophys Acta 665:186

Casola PG, Possmayer F (1981c) Separation and characterization of the membrane-bound and aqueously dispersed phosphatidate phosphatidic acid phosphohydrolase activities in rat lung. Biochim Biophys Acta 664:298

Comroe JH Jr (1977a) Premature science and immature lungs. Part I. Some premature discoveries. Am Rev Resp Dis 116:127

Comroe JH Jr (1977b) Premature science and immature lungs. Part II. Chemical warfare and the newly born. Am Rev Resp Dis 116:311

Comroe JH Jr (1977c) Premature science and immature lungs. Part III. The attack on immature lungs. Am Rev Resp Dis 116:497

Corbet AJ, Flax P, Alstan C, Rudolph AJ (1978) Effects of aminophyllin and dexamethasone on secretion of pulmonary surfactant in fetal rabbits. Pediatr Res 12:797

Cotterrell M, Balazs R, Johnson AL (1972) Effects of corticosteroids on the biochemical maturation of rat brain: Postnatal cell formation. J Neurochem 19:2151

Das DK, Ayromlooi J, Desiderio D, Tobias M, Steinberg H (1981) Effects of dexamethasone on the synthesis of dipalmitoyl phosphatidylcholine. Dev Pharmacol Ther 3:55

DeLemos RA, Shermeta DW, Knelson JH, Kotas R, Avery ME (1970) Acceleration of appearance of pulmonary surfactant in the fetal lamb by administration of corticosteroids. Am Rev Respir Dis 102:459

De Souza SW, Adlard BPF (1973) Growth of suckling rats after treatment with dexamethasone or cortisol. Arch Dis Child 48:519

Faridy EE, Thliveris JA, Morris GS (1981) Relationship between lung intra and extracellular DSPC in fetal and neonatal rats. Respir Physiol 45:55

Farrell PM (1973) Regulation of pulmonary lecithin synthesis. In: Respiratory Distress Syndrome, Academic Press, New York, pp 311–349

Farrell PM, Zachman RD (1973) Induction of choline phosphotransferase and lecithin synthesis in the fetal lung by corticosteroids. Science 179:297

Farrell PM, Blackburn WR, Adams AJ (1977) Lung phosphatidylcholine synthesis and cholinephosphotransferase activity in anencephalic rat fetuses with corticosteroid deficiency. Pediatr Res 11:770

Farrell PM, Hamosh M (1978) The biochemistry of fetal lung development. Clin Perinatol 5:197

Farrell PM (ed) (1982) Lung Development: Biological and Clinical Perspectives, Vol 1, Biochemistry and Physiology, Academic Press, New York

Floros J, Phelps DS, Smith BT (1985) Dexamethasone induces organ-specific developmental proteins (fsa, fsb) in rat lung fibroblasts. Electrophoresis 6:238

Forest MG (1979) Function of the ovary in the neonate and infant. Eur J Obstet Gynecol Reprod Biol 9:145

Frank L, Groseclose EE (1984) Preparation for birth into an o_2-rich environment: The antioxidant enzymes in the developing rabbit lung. Pediatr Res 18:240

Frank L, Lewis PL, Sosenko IRS (1985) Dexamethasone stimulation of fetal rat lung antioxidant enzyme activity in parallel with surfactant stimulation. Pediatrics 75:569

Freese WB, Hallman M (1983) The effect of betamethasone and fetal sex on the synthesis and maturation of lung surfactant phospholipids in rabbits. Biochim Biophys Acta 750:47

Gandelman R, vom Saal FS, Reinisch JM (1977) Contiguity to male foetuses affects morphology and behavior of female mice. Nature 226:722

Gardey-Levassort C, de Lauture M-O RD, Thiroux G, Olive G (1981) Current concepts: I. Catecholamines in developing rat lung. Life Sci 28:331

Giannopoulos G, Sommers-Smith SK (1982) Androgen receptors in fetal rabbit lung and the effect of fetal sex on the levels of circulating hormones and pulmonary hormone receptors. J Steroid Biochem 17:461

Gilden C, Sevanian A, Tierney DF, Kaplan SA, Barrett CT (1977) Regulation of fetal lung phosphatidyl choline synthesis by cortisol: Role of glycogen and glucose. Pediatr Res 511:845

Gilfillan AM, Chu AJ, Rooney SA (1984) Stimulation of phosphatidylcholine synthesis by exogenous phosphatidylglycerol in primary cultures of type II pneumonocytes. Biochim Biophys Acta 79:269

Glenny YHP, Brindley DN (1978) The effects of cortisol, corticotropin and thyroxine on the synthesis of glycerolipids and on the phosphatidate phosphohydrolase activity in rat liver. Biochem J 176:777

Gluck L (1976) Administration of corticosteroids to induce maturation of fetal lung. Am J Dis Child 130:976

Gonzales LW, Ballard PL, Ertsey R, Williams MC (1985) Hormonal stimulation of surfactant synthesis in explant cultures of human fetal lung. Clin Res 33:137A (abstract)

Gross I (1977) Nutritional and hormonal influences on lung phospholipid metabolism. Fed Proc 36:2665

Gross I, Ballard PL, Ballard RA, Jones CT, Wilson CM (1983) Corticosteroid stimulation of phosphotidylcholine synthesis in cultured fetal rabbit lung: evidence for de novo protein synthesis mediated by glucocorticoid receptors. Endocrinology 112:829

Gross I, Dynia DW, Wilson CM, Ingleson LD, Gewolb IH, Rooney SA (1984) Glucocorticoid-thyroid hormone interactions in fetal rat lung. Pediatr Res 18:191

Gumbinas M, Oda M, Huttenlocher P (1973) The effects of corticosteroids on myelination of the developing rat brain. Biol Neonate 22:355

Hallman M, Gluck L (1977) Development of the fetal lung. J Perinat Med 5:3

Hallman M, Epstein BL (1980) Role of myo-inositol in the synthesis of phosphatidylglycerol and phosphatidylinositol in the lung. Biochem Biophys Res Commun 92:1151

Hallman M (1984) Effect of extracellular myo-inositol on surfactant phospholipid in the fetal rabbit lung. Biochim Biophys Acta 795:67

Hamosh M, Yeager H, Shechter Y, Hamosh P (1976) Lipoprotein lipase in rat lung. Effect of dexamethasone. Biochim Biophys Acta 431:519

Heifetz A, Snyder JM (1981) The effects of hydrocortisone on the biosynthesis of sulfated glycoconjugates by human fetal lung. J Biol Chem 256:4957

Henderson IC, Fischel RE, Loeb JN (1971) Suppression of liver DNA synthesis by cortisone. Endocrinology 88:1471

Henderson IC, Loeb JN (1974) Hormone-induced changes in liver DNA synthesis: Effects of glucocorticoids and growth hormone on liver growth and DNA polymerase activity. Endocrinology 94:1637

Herbert WNP, Johnston JM, MacDonald PC, Jimenez JM (1978) Fetal lung maturation. Human amniotic fluid phosphatidate phosphohydrolase activity through normal gestation and its relation to the lecithin/sphingomyelin ratio. Am J Obstet Gynecol 132:373

Hitchcock KR (1980) Lung development and the pulmonary surfactant system: hormonal influences. Anat Rec 198:13

Johnson JW, Mitzner W, London WT, Palmer AE, Scott R, Kearney K (1978) Glucocorticoids and the rhesus fetal lung. Am J Obstet Gynecol 130:905

Johnson JW, Mitzner W, London WT, Palmer AE, Scott R (1979) Betamethasone and the rhesus fetus: Multisystemic effects. Am J Obstet Gynecol 133:677

Johnson JWC (1980) Betamethasone: Do side effects outweigh benefits? Contemporary Ob/Gyn 15:195

Johnson JW, Mitzner W, Beck JC, London WT, Sly DL, Lee PA, Khouzami VA, Cavalieri RL (1981) Long-term effects of betamethasone on fetal development. Am J Obstet Gynecol 141:1053

Johnson JWC, Beck JC, Mitzner W, London WT (1982) Male and female responses to betamethasone. Society for Gynecologic Investigation meeting, p 108 (abstract)

Jost A (1961) The role of fetal hormones in prenatal development. The Harvey Lectures, Academic Press, New York. Series 55:201.

Kauffman SL (1977a) Acceleration of canalicular development in lungs of fetal mice exposed transplacentally to dexamethasone. Lab Invest 36:395

Kauffman SL (1977b) Proliferation, growth and differentiation of pulmonary epithelium in fetal mouse lung exposed transplacentally to dexamethasone. Lab Invest 37:497

Kessler DL, Truog WE, Murphy JH, Palmer S, Standaert TA, Woodrum DE, Hodson WA (1982)

Experimental hyaline membrane disease in the premature monkey. Effects of antenatal dexamethasone. Am Rev Respir Dis 126:62
Khosla SS, Gobran LI, Rooney SA (1980) Stimulation of phosphatidylcholine synthesis by 17β-estradiol in fetal rabbit lung. Biochim Biophys Acta 617:282
Khosla SS, Brehier A, Eisenfeld AJ, Ingleson LD, Parks PA, Rooney SA (1983) Influence of sex hormones on lung maturation in the fetal rabbit. Biochim Biophys Acta 750:112
Kikkawa Y, Kaibara M, Motoyama EK, Orzalesi MM, Cook CD (1971) Morphologic development of fetal rabbit lung and its acceleration with cortisol. Am J Pathol 2:423
Kitterman JA, Liggins GC, Clements JA, Campos G, Lee CH, Ballard PL (1981) Inhibitors of prostaglandin synthesis, tracheal fluid, and surfactant in fetal lambs. J Appl Physiol: Respirat Environ Exercise Physiol 51:1562
Knelson JH (1971) Environmental influence on intrauterine lung development. Arch Intern Med 127:421
Kotas RV, Avery ME (1971) Accelerated appearance of pulmonary surfactant in the fetal rabbit. J Appl Physiol 30:358
Kotas RV, Mims LC, Hart LK (1974) Reversible inhibition of lung cell number after glucocorticoid injection into fetal rabbits to enhance surfactant appearance. Pediatrics 53:358
Kotas RV, Avery ME (1980) The influence of sex on fetal rabbit lung maturation and on the response to glucocorticoid. Am Rev Respir Dis 121:377
Kotas RV (1982) Physiologic assessment of lung surfactant. In: Lung Development: Biological and Clinical Perspectives, Vol 1, Biochemistry and Physiology, Farrell PM (ed), Academic Press, New York, pp 57–86
Lehtonen MA, Savolainen MJ, Hassinen IE (1979) Hormonal regulation of hepatic soluble phosphatidate phosphohydrolase. Induction by cortisol in vivo and in isolated perfused rat liver. Fed Europ Biochem Soc 99:162
Liggins GC (1969) Premature delivery of foetal lambs infused with glucocorticoids. J Endocrinol 45:515
Liggins GC, Howie RN (1972) A controlled trial of antepartum glucocorticoid treatment for prevention of the respiratory distress syndrome in premature infants. Pediatrics 50:515
Liggins GC, Kitterman JA, Campos GA, Clements JA, Forster CS, Lee CH, Creasy RK (1981) Pulmonary maturation in the hypophysectomized ovine fetus. Differential responses to adrenocorticotrophin and cortisol. J Dev Physiol 3:1
Loeb JN, Yeung LL (1973) Effects of cortisone on thymidine incorporation by various nonlymphoid tissues of the weanling rat. Proc Soc Exp Biol Med 143:502
Loeb JN (1976) Corticosteroids and growth. N Engl J Med 295:547
Maniscalco WM, Wilson CM, Gross I, Gobran L, Rooney SA, Warshaw JB (1978) Development of glycogen and phospholipid metabolism in fetal and newborn rat lung. Biochim Biophys Acta 530:333
Meisel RL, Ward IL (1981) Fetal female rats are masculinized by male littermates located caudally in the uterus. Science 213:239
Mendelson CR, Johnston JM, MacDonald PC, Snyder JM (1981) Multihormonal regulation of surfactant synthesis by human fetal lungs in vitro. J Clin Endocrinol Metab 53:307
Mitzner W, Johnson JWC, Scott R, London WT, Palmer AE (1979) Effect of betamethasone on pressure-volume relationship of fetal rhesus monkey lung. J Appl Physiol 47:377
Mitzner W, Johnson JW, Beck J, London W, Sly D (1982) Influence of betamethasone on the development of mechanical properties in the fetal rhesus monkey lung. Am Rev Respir Dis 125:233
Morishige WK, Joun NS (1982) Influence of glucocorticoids on postnatal lung development in the rat: possible modulation by thyroid hormone. Endocrinology 111:1587
Mostello DJ, Hamosh M, Hamosh P (1981) Effect of dexamethasone on lipoprotein lipase activity of fetal rat lung. Biol Neonate 40:121
Motoyama EK, Orzalesi MM, Kikkawa Y, Kaibara M, Wu B, Zigas CJ, Cook CD (1971) Effect of cortisol on the maturation of fetal rabbit lungs. Pediatrics 48:547
Naeye RL, Freeman RK, Blanc WA (1974) Nutrition, sex, and fetal lung maturation. Pediatr Res 8:200
Nelson GH, Eguchi K, McPherson JC (1976) Effects of gestational age, dexamethasone and metopirone on lecithin concentration in fetal lung tissue and amniotic fluid in rats and guinea pigs. Gynecol Invest 7:337

Nielsen HC, Torday JS (1981) Sex differences in fetal rabbit pulmonary surfactant production. Pediatr Res 15:1245

Nielsen HC, Zinman HM, Torday JS (1982) Dihydrotestosterone inhibits fetal rabbit pulmonary surfactant production. J Clin Invest 69:611

Oldenborg V, Van Golde LMG (1977) The enzymes of phosphatidylcholine biosynthesis in the fetal mouse lung. Effects of dexamethasone. Biochim Biophys Acta 489:454

Olson EB Jr (1979) Role of glucocorticoids in lung maturation. J Animal Sci 49:225

Padbury JF, Hobel CJ, Lam RW, Fisher DA (1981) Sex differences in lung and adrenal neurosympathetic development in rabbits. Am J Obstet Gynecol 141:199

Padbury JF, Hobel CJ, Gonzales FA, Fisher DA (1983) Ontogenesis and sex differences in rabbit fetal adrenal phenylethanolamine N-methyltransferase. Biol Neonate 43:205

Perelman RH, Engle MJ, Kemnitz JW, Kotas RV, Farrell PM (1982) Biochemical and physiological development of fetal Rhesus lung. J Appl Physiol: Respirat Environ Exercise Physiol 53:230

Phelps DS, Giannopoulos G (1984) Effect on dexamethasone on the synthesis of specific proteins in fetal rabbit lung in vivo and in organ culture. Exper Lung Res 7:195

Platzker ACG, Kitterman JA, Clements JA, Tooley WH (1972) Surfactant appearance and secretion in fetal lamb in response to dexamethasone. Pediatr Res 6:406 (abstract)

Platzker ACG, Kitterman JA, Mescher EJ, Clements JA, Tooley WH (1975) Surfactant in the lung and tracheal fluid of the fetal lamb and acceleration of its appearance by dexamethasone. Pediatrics 56:554

Possmayer F, Duwe G, Metcalfe R, Stewart-DeHaan J, Wong C, Heras JL, Harding PGR (1977) Cortisol induction of pulmonary maturation in the rabbit fetus. Its effects on enzymes related to phospholipid biosynthesis and on marker enzymes for subcellular organelles. Biochem J 166:485

Possmayer F, Casola P, Chan F, Hill S, Metcalfe IL, Stewart-DeHaan PJ, Wong T, Heras JL, Gammal EB, Harding PGR (1979) Glucocorticoid induction of pulmonary maturation in the rabbit fetus. The effect of maternal injection of betamethasone on the activity of enzymes in fetal lung. Biochim Biophys Acta 574:197

Possmayer F (1982) The perinatal lung. In: Biochemical Development of the Fetus and Neonate, Jones CT (ed), Elsevier Biomedical Press, Amsterdam, pp 337–391

Post M, Batenburg JJ, Smith BT, Van Golde LMG (1984a) Pool sizes of precursors for phosphatidylcholine formation in adult rat lung type II cells. Biochim Biophys Acta 795:552

Post M, Batenburg JJ, Van Golde LMG, Smith BT (1984b) The rate-limiting reaction in phosphatidylcholine synthesis by alveolar type II cells isolated from fetal rat lung. Biochim Biophys Acta 795:558

Post M, Smith BT (1984) Fibroblast-pneumonocyte factor purified with the aid of monoclonal antibodies stimulates cholinephosphate cytidylyltransferase activity in fetal type II cells. Pediatr Res 18:401A (abstract)

Quirk JG, Bleasdale JE, MacDonald PC, Johnston JM (1980) A role for cytidinemonophosphate in the regulation of glycerophospholipid composition of surfactant in developing lung. Biochem Biophys Res Commun 95:985

Robert MF, Bator AT, Taeusch HW Jr (1975) Pulmonary pressure-volume relationships after corticotropin (ACTH) and saline injections in fetal rabbits. Pediatr Res 9:760

Rooney SA, Gross I, Gassenheimer LN, Motoyama EK (1975) Stimulation of glycerolphosphate phosphatidyltransferase activity in fetal rabbit lung by cortisol administration. Biochim Biophys Acta 398:433

Rooney SA, Gobran I, Gross I, Wai-Lee TS, Nardone LL, Motoyama EK (1976a) Studies on pulmonary surfactant. Effects of cortisol administration to fetal rabbits on lung phospholipid content, composition and biosynthesis. Biochim Biophys Acta 450:121

Rooney SA, Wai-Lee TS, Gobran L, Motoyama EK (1976b) Phospholipid content, composition and biosynthesis during fetal lung development in the rabbit. Biochim Biophys Acta 431:447

Rooney SA, Gobran LI (1977) Alveolar lavage and lavaged lung tissue phosphatidylcholine composition during fetal rabbit development. Lipids 12:1050

Rooney SA (1979) Development of the pulmonary surfactant system during late fetal and early postnatal life. In: Mead Johnson Symposium on Perinatal and Developmental Medicine, No. 14: The Surfactant System and the Neonatal Lung. Mead Johnson and Co., Evansville, Indiana, pp 17–24

Rooney SA, Gobran LI, Marino PA, Maniscalco WM, Gross I (1979) Effects of betamethasone on phospholipid content, composition and biosynthesis in fetal rabbit lung. Biochim Biophys Acta 572:64
Rooney SA, Brehier A (1982) The CDPcholine pathway: cholinephosphate cytidylyltransferase. In: Lung Development: Biological and Clinical Perspectives, Vol 1, Biochemistry and Physiology, Farrell PM (ed), Academic Press, New York, pp 317–335
Rooney SA (1983) Biochemical development of the lung. In: The Biological Basis of Reproductive and Developmental Medicine, Warshaw JB (ed), Elsevier Biomedical Press, New York, pp 239–287
Rosenfeld CR, Andujo O, Johnston JM, Jimenez JM (1980) Phosphatidic acid phosphohydrolase and phospholipids in tracheal and amniotic fluids during normal ovine pregnancy. Pediatr Res 14:891
Russell BJ, Nugent L, Chernick V (1974) Effects of steroids on the enzymatic pathways of lecithin production in fetal rabbits. Biol Neonate 24:306
Sadiq HF, Devaskar UP (1984) Glucocorticoids increase pulmonary epidermal growth factor receptors in female and male fetal rabbit. Biochem Biophys Res Commun 119:408
Sanfacon R, Possmayer F, Harding PGR (1977) Dexamethasone treatment of the guinea pig fetus: Its effects on the incorporation of ^{3}H-thymidine into deoxyribonucleic acid. Am J Obstet Gynecol 127:745
Shapiro S (1968) Some physiological, biochemical, and behavioral consequences of neonatal hormone administration: Cortisol and thyroxine. Gen Compar Endocrinol 10:214
Schultz FM, Jimenez JM, MacDonald PC, Johnston JM (1974) Fetal lung maturation. I. Phosphatidic acid phosphohydrolase in rabbit lung. Gynecol Invest 5:222
Shelley HJ (1961) Glycogen reserves and their changes at birth and in anoxia. Br Med Bull 17:137
Smith BT, Torday JS, Giroud CJP (1974) Evidence for different gestation-dependent effects of cortisol on cultured fetal lung cells. J Clin Invest 53:1518
Smith BT, Bogues WG (1979) Effects of drugs and hormones on lung maturation in experimental animal and man. Pharmacol Ther 9:51
Smith BT (1984) Pulmonary surfactant during fetal development and neonatal adaptation: hormonal control. In: Pulmonary Surfactant, Robertson B, Van Golde LMG, Batenburg JJ (eds), Elsevier, Amsterdam, pp 357–381
Snyder JM, Johnston JM, Mendelson CR (1981a) The effect of cortisol on rabbit fetal lung maturation in vitro. Dev Biol 85:129
Snyder JM, Johnston JM, Mendelson CR (1981b) Differentiation of type II cells of human fetal lung in vitro. Cell Tissue Res 220:17
Sorokin S, Padykula HA, Herman E (1959) Comparative histochemical patterns in developing mammalian lungs. Devel Biol 1:125
Spitzer HL, Johnston JM (1978) Characterization of phosphatidate phosphohydrolase activity associated with isolated lamellar bodies. Biochim Biophys Acta 531:275
Sumi SM, Truog WE, Kessler DM (1984) Maternal corticosteroid therapy and the fetal brain in experimental hyaline membrane disease. Pediatr Res 18:440
Sundell HW, Tsiantos H, Relier JP, Dolanski E, Victorine L, Otten A, Strott C, Orth D, Chytil F, Stahlman MT (1973) Prevention of HMD with ACTH infusion in fetal lambs. Pediatr Res 7:407
Taeusch HW Jr, Heitner M, Avery M (1972) Accelerated lung maturation and increased survival in premature rabbits treated with hydrocortisone. Am Rev Respir Dis 105:971
Taeusch HW Jr, Avery ME (1977) Regulation of pulmonary alveolar development in late gestation and the perinatal period. In: Development of the Lung, Hodson WA (ed), Marcel Dekker, New York and Basel, pp 399–418
Tanswell AK, Freeman BA (1982) Antioxidant enzyme maturation in fetal rat lung. In vivo and in vitro observations. Am Rev Resp Dis 125:200
Thibeault DW, Emmanouilides GC, Dodge ME (1978) Pulmonary and circulatory function in preterm lambs treated with hydrocortisone in utero. Biol Neonate 34:238
Torday JS (1984) The sex difference in type II cell surfactant synthesis originates in the fibroblast in vitro. Exper Lung Res 7:187

Truog WE, Kessler DL, Palmer S, Murphy J, Woodrum DE, Hodson WA (1981) Differential effect of sex in experimental hyaline membrane disease in newborn monkeys. Am Rev Respir Dis 124:435

Tsai MY, Handschin B, Syverson BJ, Josephson MW, Brown DM (1984) Effect of prenatal dexamethasone on immunoreactive 6-ketoprostaglandin $F_{1\alpha}$ levels in fetal rat lungs. Pediatr Res 18:908

Tsao FHC, Zachman RD (1977) Phosphatidylcholine-lysophosphatidylcholine cycle pathway enzymes in rabbit lung. II. Marked differences in the effect of gestational age on activity compared to the CDP-choline pathway. Pediatr Res 11:858

Tsao FHC, Gutcher GR, Zachman RD (1979) Effects of hydrocortisone on the metabolism of phosphatidylcholine in maternal and fetal rabbit lungs and livers. Pediatr Res 13:997

Tye LM, Burton AF (1980) Effects of dexamethasone on fetal mouse development. Biol Neonate 38:260

Van Golde LMG (1976) Metabolism of phospholipids in the lung. Am Rev Respir Dis 114:977

Van Golde LMG (1982) The CDPcholine pathway: cholinephosphotransferase. In: Lung Development: Biological and Clinical Perspectives, Vol 1, Biochemistry and Physiology, Farrell PM (ed), Academic Press, New York, pp 337–358

Veyssiere G, Berger M, Jean-Faucher C, De Turckheim M, Jean C (1976) Levels of testosterone in the plasma, gonads, and adrenals during fetal development of the rabbit. Endocrinology 99:1263

Vilos GA, Challis JRG, Lye SJ, Possmayer F, Harding PG (1983) Accelerated prepartum maturation of the fetal sheep lung with physiological doses of adrenocorticotrophin. J Dev Physiol 5:341

vom Saal FS, Bronson FH (1980) Sexual characteristics of adult female mice are correlated with their blood testosterone levels during prenatal development. Science 208:597

Wang NS, Kotas RV, Avery ME, Thurlbeck WM (1971) Accelerated appearance of osmiophilic bodies in fetal lungs following steroid injection. J Appl Physiol 30:362

Ward IL, Weisz J (1980) Maternal stress alters plasma testosterone in fetal males. Science 207:328

Ward JA, Erenberg A, Roberts RJ (1983) Postnatal increase in airway surfactant in the premature rabbit exposed in utero to betamethasone. Dev Pharmacol Ther 6:388

Weichsel ME Jr (1974) Glucocorticoid effect upon thymidine kinase in the developing cerebellum. Pediatr Res 8:843

Weichsel ME Jr (1977) The therapeutic use of glucocorticoid hormones in the perinatal period: Potential neurological hazards. Ann Neurol 2:364

Weisz J, Ward IL (1980) Plasma testosterone and progesterone titers of pregnant rats, their male and female fetuses and neonatal offspring. Endocrinology 106:306

Wellman KF, Volk BW (1972) Fine structural changes in the rabbit placenta induced by cortisone. Arch Path 94:147

Yeung A, Casola PG, Wong C, Fellows JF, Possmayer F (1979) Pulmonary phosphatidic acid phosphatase. A comparative study of the aqueously dispersed phosphatidate-dependent and membrane-bound phosphatidate-dependent phosphatidic acid phosphatase activities of rat lung. Biochim Biophys Acta 574:226

3 Glucocorticoid Receptor

Shortly after the initial description of glucocorticoid effects on lung maturation it was proposed that these responses were mediated through glucocorticoid receptors. Subsequent studies in several laboratories have identified receptor in fetal and adult lung tissue and characterized the binding reaction. In this chapter I review briefly several general properties of glucocorticoid receptor in lung tissue, and then discuss in more detail various aspects of glucocorticoid binding which relate specifically to the lung.

The generally accepted model for glucocorticoid action in target cells is shown in Fig. 3.1. On entering the cell cytoplasm corticosteroid binds reversibly to receptor, a protein with high affinity binding sites for glucocorticoids. At physiologic temperatures this interaction alters receptor conformation (activation step), exposing binding sites with high affinity for specific regions of the chromatin. More than one form of unactivated receptor probably exists in vivo, and not all receptor-steroid complexes become activated. The extent of activation is a determinant of the amount of nuclear binding which occurs. Translocation of activated receptor-steroid complex to the nucleus, and interaction with chromatin, modulates gene expression. In most systems this involves increased synthesis of specific mRNAs, although negative regulation also occurs. Translation of these messages in the cytoplasm increases the amount of specific inducible proteins ("glucocorticoid domain") which in turn mediates the biologic response.

Since glucocorticoid receptors in different tissues appear to be functionally

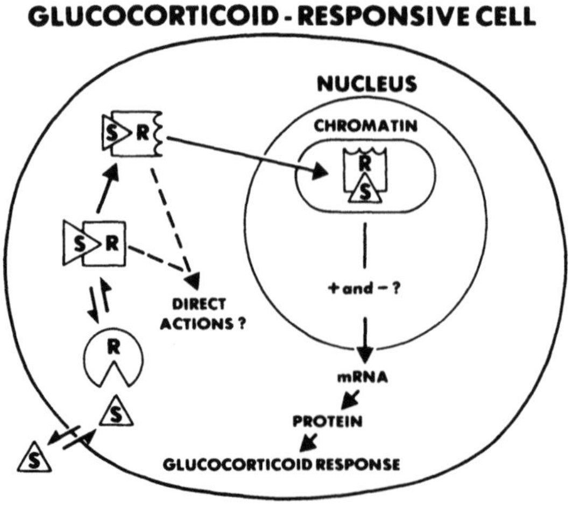

Fig. 3.1. Model of early events in glucocorticoid action within target cells. Abbreviations: *R*, receptor; *S*, steroid.
Cytoplasmic binding results in an activated receptor-steroid complex which binds to chromatin and stimulates synthesis of specific mRNAs. Steroid-receptor complex conceivably could also act at sites other than the chromatin. From Baxter and Rousseau (1979), by permission

identical, the reader is referred to an earlier monograph in this series entitled "Glucocorticoid Hormone Action" (Baxter and Rousseau 1979) for a detailed discussion of glucocorticoid receptors and the evidence supporting the scheme outlined in Fig. 3.1. In addition, previous reviews have described binding methodology, and both physiochemical and other properties of lung receptor (Ballard 1977a,b, 1979; Giannopoulos 1975c; Ballard 1982).

3.1 General Properties

3.1.1 Distribution

Glucocorticoid receptor has been detected in both fetal and adult lung of every species which has been examined. Most binding studies have used cytosol preparations; in some cases receptor has also been assayed in intact lung cells. Receptor capacity is similar in lung cytosol of most species, with somewhat higher levels in adult rat and rabbit (Table 3.1). In most of these species, glucocorticoids are known to influence lung maturation (see Table 2.1).

The concentration of receptor sites in lung and other tissues of three species is shown in Table 3.2. In each case lung contains a relatively high concentration of binding sites per mg cytosol protein. Similar results are obtained when binding data are expressed per DNA. Although the average concentration of binding sites per pulmonary cell is high compared with cells of other tissues, the relative distribution of receptor among the approximately 40 different cell types in lung is largely unexplored. As discussed in section B-III, receptor is known to be present in fibroblasts, alveolar epithelial cells and endothelial cells.

Table 3.1. Glucocorticoid receptor in lung of various species. Binding studies were performed in lung cytosol with [^{3}H] dexamethasone in the presence of sulfhydryl compound, if required

Source	Cytosol binding capacity (pmol/mg protein)	References
Fetal rat	0.35	Granberg & Ballard 1977
Adult rat	0.82	Granberg & Ballard 1977
Fetal rabbit (27 days)	0.43	Granberg & Ballard 1977 Giannopoulos, 1974
Adult rabbit (Adx)	0.53	Granberg & Ballard 1977 Giannopoulos, 1974
Fetal sheep (130-140 days)	0.36	Ballard & Ballard 1972
	0.48	Flint & Burton 1984
Fetal monkey (140-144 days)	0.37	Granberg & Ballard 1977
Fetal human (15-17 weeks)	0.27	Granberg & Ballard 1977
Adult hamster	0.26	Granberg & Ballard 1977
Adult mouse (Adx)	0.24	Granberg & Ballard 1977

Adx, adrenalectomized

Table 3.2. Receptor concentration in various tissues of three species. Data represent mean values for dexamethasone binding capacity (pmol/mg cytosol protein) from 2 to 6 experiments except for the human fetus (single specimen at 16 weeks gestation). From Granberg and Ballard (1977) (rat), Ballard et al. (1974) (rabbit), and Ballard and Ballard (1974) (human)

Tissue	Adult rat	Rabbit		Fetal human
		Fetal	Adult	
Lung	0.69	0.43	0.53	0.21
Thymus	0.89	0.08	0.65	
Liver	0.34	0.12	0.12	0.13
Spleen	0.28		0.27	
Brain	0.26	0.08	0.12	
Kidney	0.23	0.24	0.16	0.13
Uterus	0.19			
Heart	0.18	0.17	0.13	0.07
Prostate	0.11			
Adipose	0.10		0.14	
Stomach	0.09		0.19	
Bladder	0.09		0.11	
Testis	0.08		0.22	
Muscle	0.06	0.14	0.03	0.06
Seminal vesicle	0.01			
Small intestine	-	0.12	0.20	0.16
Placenta (fetal)	-	0.26		
Skin	-	0.22		0.22

3.1.2 Physiochemical and Binding Properties

Studies with lung tissue, though less extensive than for other systems, indicate that various physiochemical properties of lung receptor resemble those described for other sources of receptor. Receptor in lung tissue is a protein and migrates as a single peak on both sucrose gradients and gel filtration columns. The receptor-steroid complex in cytosol (rat, rabbit, and human) sediments with values of 7S and 4S in low and high salt solutions, respectively; complexes extracted from nuclei with concentrated salt solutions after intact cell binding sediment at 4S (Toft and Chytil 1973; Giannopoulos 1973, 1975a; Iacobelli et al. 1978). Nuclear uptake of lung receptor-steroid complex in vitro is dependent on an activation step (heating, precipitation with ammonium sulphate, or exposure to 0.4 M KCl). On incubation of intact cells with corticosteroid at 37 °C, receptor is lost from the cytoplasmic fraction and increases in the nucleus where approximately 70 % of receptor is located at equilibrium (Giannopoulos et al. 1973; Giannopoulos 1975a, b; Ballard and Ballard 1972, 1974; Ballard et al. 1978; Ballard et al. 1984). The binding activity in lung cytosol fulfills criteria for glucocorticoid receptors in terms of appropriate binding kinetics and a limited number of sites which have a high affinity and specificity for steroids with glucocorticoid activity (Giannopoulos et al. 1974; Ballard 1977a, b, 1979; Giannopoulos 1975c). The relative affinity of various steroids for lung receptor is presented in Tables 3.5 and 6.5.

3.2 Specific Properties

3.2.1 Sulfhydryl Groups

Receptor of lung as well as other tissues contains sulfhydryl groups. Oxidation of these groups, or exposure to sulfhydryl blocking agents, reduces glucocorticoid binding in cytosol preparations. This loss is prevented and reversed by the presence of a sulfhydryl compound in the reaction mixture (Granberg and Ballard 1977).

In certain species, receptor in lung cytosol is particularly sensitive to oxidation of sulfhydryl groups compared with other tissues. Figure 3.2 shows the binding activity in cytosol of adult rat lung prepared in the presence and absence of dithiothreitol. At 2 °C, dexamethasone binding capacity decreased with a $t_{1/2}$ of 40 min in the absence of steroid or sulfhydryl compound. This rapid inactivation of unbound receptor is prevented by the presence of dithiothreitol and is reversed by later addition. Once the receptor-glucocorticoid complex is formed, sulfhydryl compounds do not affect the stability of receptor. This observation indicates that binding of steroid prevents the oxidation of receptor sulfhydryl groups. It is not known whether the sulfhydryl groups are located adjacent to the steroid binding site or at a distant location on the protein.

The sulfhydryl sensitivity of lung receptor compared with binding in other tissues of the adult rat is shown in Table 3.3. Whereas receptor in some tissues is not affected by the absence of a sulfhydryl compound during cytosol binding experiments, lung receptor is rapidly inactivated in the absence of dithiothreitol. The variability between tissues may be explained in part by differences in the concentration of endogenous sulfhydryl compounds available to stabilize receptor. The data of Table 3.3 indicate in general an inverse correla-

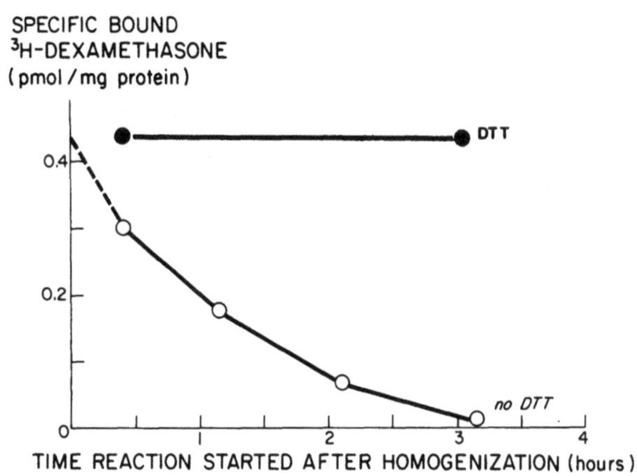

Fig. 3.2. The effect of dithiothreitol (DTT) on binding activity in cytosol of adult rat. Cytosol was prepared in the presence and absence of 3 mM DTT with addition of [^{3}H]dexamethasone at the intervals shown. The binding reaction proceeded for 4 h at 2 °C. Data from Granberg and Ballard (1977), by permission

Table 3.3. Endogenous sulfhydryl groups and the effect of dithiothreitol on dexamethasone binding in cytosol of rat tissues. Incubations were carried out with 30 nM [^{3}H] dexamethasone in the presence and absence of 3 mM dithiothreitol for 4 h at 2 °C. Data from Granberg and Ballard (1977)

Tissue	Activity in absence of dithiothreitol (%)[a]	Non-protein sulfhydryl groups (nmol/ml cytosol)
Liver	100	1,507
Kidney	100	247
Heart	100	393
Testis	100	818
Muscle (upper leg)	89	123
Seminal vesicle	76	53
Brain	61	247
Thymus	55	325
Bladder	21	25
Spleen	16	-
Stomach	15	290
Prostate	13	55
Adipose (periuterine)	9	46
Lung	7	158
Uterus	5	96

[a] Percent of binding in the presence of dithiothreitol

tion between endogenous sulfhydryl concentration and the effect of dithiothreitol. Liver in particular contains a high concentration of glutathione and other sulfhydryl-containing compounds. When liver cytosol was boiled, and the supernatant added to lung cytosol, binding activity was stable in the absence of added dithiothreitol (Granberg and Ballard 1977).

The requirement for sulfhydryl compound to stabilize lung receptor is also variable among species. As shown in Table 3.4, receptor in lung cytosol of adult rat, fetal monkey, adult hamster, and adult mouse was unstable in the absence of dithiothreitol. By contrast, sulfhydryl compound had little influence on binding in cytosol of fetal rat, rabbit and human, and adult rabbit. In part, the species variability may also relate to the concentration of endogenous non-protein sulfhydryl compounds. The rapid inactivation of receptor in rat lung cytosol in the absence of sulfhydryl compounds accounts for the low levels or absence of binding reported in some studies (Ballard et al. 1974b; Giannopoulos 1974, 1975c; Mulay et al. 1982).

The presence of dithiothreitol in lung cytosol also affects the K_D. With cytosol of adult rat lung, the K_D for dexamethasone binding was 2.5 nM with dithiothreitol compared with 12.6 nM without dithiothreitol (Granberg and Ballard 1977). This effect probably results from greater inactivation of receptor in reaction systems with low concentrations of dexamethasone than in those with higher concentrations where the binding reaction is faster and more receptor is stabilized in the bound form.

The possible importance of receptor sulfhydryl groups in vivo is uncertain. It is conceivable that the degree of oxidation/reduction of sulfhydryl groups

Table 3.4. Cytosol sulfhydryl content and effect of dithiothreitol on dexamethasone binding in lung of various species. The concentration of binding sites was determined with 30 nM [^{3}H]dexamethasone in cytosol with and without 3 mM dithiothreitol. Data from Granberg and Ballard (1977)

Source of tissue	Activity in absence of dithiothreitol (%)[a]	Non-Protein sulfhydryl groups (nmol/ml cytosol)
Fetal rat (20 days)	94	340
Adult rat (Adx)	7	168
Fetal rabbit (27 days)	95	290
Adult rabbit (Adx)	96	666
Fetal monkey (140–144 days)	20	-
Fetal human (15–17 weeks)	90	-
Newborn premature human	92	-
Adult hamster	18	134
Adult mouse (Adx)	9	146

Adx, adrenalectomized
[a] Percent of binding in presence of dithiothreitol

could serve as a mechanism to regulate the concentration of active receptor. It has been proposed that endogenous sulfhydryl groups may serve as a messenger in hormonal regulation of certain enzymes (Gilbert 1982).

3.2.2 Corticosteroid Affinity and Specificity: Species Differences

Among various tissues of a given species, the absolute and relative binding affinities of various corticosteroids are quite similar. This has led to the assumption that glucocorticoid receptor in different tissues is functionally identical (Feldman et al. 1978). Recent studies have addressed this question between species (Giannopoulos and Keichline 1981; Ballard et al. 1984). Table 3.5

Table 3.5. Binding affinity of various corticosteroids in lung of different species according to Giannopoulos and Keichline (1981). The binding affinities relative to corticosterone were determined by competition for ^{3}H-triamcinolone acetonide binding in lung cytosol

Steroid	Fetal rat	Adult rat	Fetal rabbit	Adult rabbit	Fetal mouse	Fetal human	Fetal guinea pig
K_D							
Triamcinolone acetonide (nM)	3.9	–	1.6	–	3.7	2.8	12.7
Relative binding affinity (%)							
Triamcinolone acetonide	566	600	2 080	1 664	425	921	3 455
Corticosterone	100	100	100	100	100	100	100
Deoxycorticosterone	34	36	18	5	39	28	36
Cortisol	24	40	318	379	36	142	298
ll-Deoxycortisol	8	14	56	50	8	23	152
Progesterone	38	26	16	5	41	31	38

presents data for corticosteroid binding in cytosol preparations from lung of rabbit, man, mouse, rat, and guinea pig. The K_D for triamcinolone acetonide binding varies by a factor of 8 between these species. In general, the K_D correlates directly with the relative concentration of circulating corticosteroid in these species; total plasma corticoids are high in the guinea pig (Jones 1974), relatively low in the rabbit (Mulay et al. 1973; Hümmelink and Ballard 1984), and intermediate in rat, mouse and human (D'Agostino et al. 1982; Barlow et al. 1974; Murphy 1983).

There are also major differences in the relative affinities of corticosterone and cortisol (Table 3.5). Cortisol has a greater affinity than corticosterone in the rabbit, human and guinea pig, while the reverse is true for the rat and mouse. A species difference also occurs in epithelial cell lines derived from rat lung (L-2) and human lung (A-549). Corticosterone has a higher affinity than cortisol in the cells of rat origin, whereas as the two corticosteroids have a similar affinity in the cells of human origin (Ballard et al. 1978). For both the rat and rabbit, at least, there are apparently no developmental changes in binding affinities. Corticosterone is the major endogenous glucocorticoid of the rat and mouse, whereas cortisol is predominant in the human and guinea pig. In the rabbit, cortisol is the major circulating corticoid in the fetus, but corticosterone is more abundant in the adult.

In experiments with cultured fetal lung, the K_D for nuclear binding of dexamethasone was 0.7 nM in the rabbit and 6.8 nM in the rat (see Table 3.7). This species difference for binding in intact cells at 37 °C is of greater magnitude but in the same direction as for cytosol binding. As discussed further below, there is a similar species difference in the concentration of dexamethasone required for half-maximal stimulation of choline incorporation into PC.

These observations are consistent with evolutionary changes in pulmonary glucocorticoid receptors in response to the composition and concentration of endogenous corticosteroids. Since glucocorticoid receptors of various tissues in a given species are similar in steroid specificity and affinity, these findings with lung receptor presumably are representative of species differences for receptor of all target tissues. The unique situation in the rabbit, where the ratio of circulating cortisol:corticosterone changes during development, may indicate the importance of the glucocorticoid milieu in the fetus in relationship to evolutionary changes in receptor properties.

3.2.3 Distribution Among Cell Types

The distribution of glucocorticoid receptor among the many different cell types in the lung has been examined by autoradiography. Beer et al. (1983) exposed explants of adult mouse lung to [^{3}H]dexamethasone for 90 min at 37 °C. In preliminary dose-response experiments, specific binding in the nuclear fraction was half-maximal at about 4 nM and the capacity was ~3 fmol/µg DNA; these values are comparable to results in cultured rat lung (Ballard et al. 1984). In autoradiographs, nuclear localization of silver grains was observed in alveolar cells (including type II cells), endothelial cells of vessels of all sizes, smooth muscle cells surrounding bronchioles and bronchi, and fibroblasts of the lamina propria underlying bronchiolar epithelium. In contrast, epithelial cells of bronchioles and bronchi contained only randomly dispersed labeling. These findings are consistent with the indirect evidence for the presence of receptor among most pulmonary cell types: 1) the relatively high concentration of receptor in lung tissue compared with other tissues, and 2) the generalized distribution of both glucocorticoid receptor and responsiveness among mammalian tissues and cell types (Table 3.2). At present there are no comparable autoradiographic studies of receptor distribution among cells of the fetal lung.

The type II alveolar cell and mesenchymal fibroblast are of major interest with regard to glucocorticoid effects on surfactant production in the fetus. As discussed in Chap. 9 and 10, glucocorticoids may act directly in type II cells and/or in fibroblasts (via fibroblast pneumonocyte factor) to stimulate surfactant synthesis in the type II cell. Dexamethasone binding sites have been demonstrated in isolated type II cells, cell lines which apparently originated from type II cells, and lung fibroblasts. These data are shown in Table 3.6, along with results for whole lung tissue and mixed populations of pulmonary cells. The organotypic cultures derived from fetal rat lung contain approximately 90 % type II cells after culturing for 2–3 weeks in gelatin sponges (Douglas and Teel 1976). Populations of lung cells containing 81–96 % type II epithelial cells were prepared from adult rats using elastase, density gradient centrifugation, and adherence in primary culture (Dobbs and Mason 1979). The F-42 and L-2 epithelial cell lines were derived from lungs of adult rat by gradient and cloning techniques, respectively, and early passages of these cell

Table 3.6. Dexamethasone binding in lung tissue and in various populations of lung cells. Mean ± SE values for 4 to 12 experiments are shown. Data from Ballard et al. (1978), Granberg and Ballard (1977), and Ballard et al. (1984)

	Specific binding in cytosol		Specific nuclear binding in intact cells	
	Sites/cell	K_D (nM)	Sites/cell	K_D (nM)
Fetal rat lung				
Fresh tissue (21 days)	8,000	4.7±1.1	8,400±440	6.8±0.6
Organotypic cultures			13,500±1,780	10.2±0.8
Adult rat lung				
Fresh tissue	20,600±800	2.5±0.4		
Heterogenous cells, freshly isolated			7,500±840	6.9±1.1
Heterogenous cells, cultured 1-2 weeks			26,500±750	7.9±0.2
Isolated type II cells			5,700±650	8.2±1.9
L-2 and F-42 cells[a]	15,100±300	1.8±0.4	57,100±8,900	8.0±0.6
Human lung				
Fetal fibroblastic cells			15,100±300	5.0±0.4
A-549 cell line[b]	32,900±2,300	2.5±0.3	48,100±1,700	10.8±1.3

[a] Equivalent results were obtained for both L-2 and F-42 cells of passage 20-29 (cytosol binding) and passage 36-51 (intact cell nuclear binding)

[b] Cells of passage 16-120

lines resemble type II cells morphologically (Douglas and Kaighn 1974; Hitchcock-O'Hare et al. 1976). The A-549 cell line was established from a human alveolar cell carcinoma, and may have originated from a transformed type II cell.

As shown in Table 3.6, specific binding of [^{3}H]dexamethasone was detected in all populations and lines of lung cells which were examined. Binding by adult type II cells has been confirmed by Keller et al. (1981). The K_D values for both cytosol and intact cell binding were similar among the different cell types. Binding has been further characterized in the L-2 and A-549 cell lines. In both cell lines, binding capacity was similar for synthetic (dexamethasone and triamcinolone acetonide) and natural (cortisol and corticosterone) glucocorticoids in cytosol preparations. Competition by various unlabelled steroids in these cell lines was characteristic of glucocorticoid binding to receptor in lung tissue of the rat and human, respectively (Ballard et al. 1978).

The concentration of binding sites in cultured heterogeneous rat cells, L-2 and F-42 cells, and A-549 cells is considerably greater than detected in freshly isolated cells. These differences reflect an increase in cell size and protein content during culture. When binding capacity is expressed per mg protein, values for freshly isolated and cultured cells are similar (Ballard et al. 1978).

In both fetal and adult lung, values for binding capacity and K_D in whole tissue and isolated populations of type II cells are similar. This indicates that type II cells contain approximately the same number of receptors per cell as the average for all lung cell types. Also, as expected, the K_D for dexamethasone binding is similar in type II cells, fibroblasts, and whole tissue. It therefore appears that receptor in different pulmonary cell types is functionally identical and probably present at similar concentrations. Thus, studies of glucocorticoid binding in whole lung tissue reflect binding which occurs in fibroblasts and type II cells.

3.2.4 Ontogeny

The developmental pattern for glucocorticoid receptor has been examined in the rat, rabbit, sheep and human. In the rat, the number of dexamethasone binding sites in lung cytosol increases from approximately 4,000 to 8,000 per cell during the last few days of fetal life (Fig. 3.3). There is a further increase after birth, reaching a value of about 19,000 binding sites per cell in lungs of adult adrenalectomized rats. In lungs of intact animals, a lower concentration is found (13,650 sites/cell), reflecting the influence of endogenous corticosteroids on both nuclear translocation of cytoplasmic receptor, and possibly total receptor content (down regulation). The presence of endogenous corticosteroids, however, does not interfere with determination of total receptor capacity in the cytosol. Because of the higher affinity of dexamethasone than corticosterone, equilibrium binding under these conditions represents an exchange assay which measures total binding sites.

The postnatal increase in cytosol receptor concentration of rat lung is influenced by thyroid hormones (Morishige 1982). In the newborn, receptor concentration in lung cytosol is similar for euthyroid and hypothyroid pups. Whereas binding capacity increased 50 % during the next 10 days in euthyroid

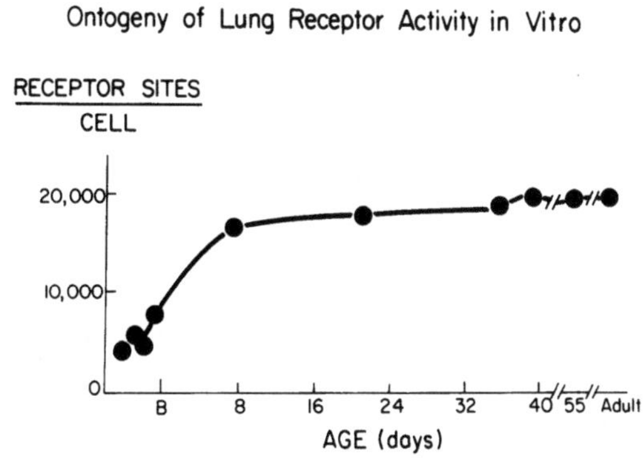

Fig. 3.3. Developmental pattern for glucocorticoid receptor in cytosol of rat lung. Dose response binding with [^{3}H]dexamethasone was carried out in the presence of DTT at the ages shown. Values after birth are from adrenalectomized animals. Data from Granberg and Ballard (1977), by permission

animals, no increase occurred in hypothyroid rats. Administration of T_3 to the hypothyroid rats increased receptor concentration to control levels within 2 days; this effect was dose-dependent and stimulation was observed with as little as 0.01 μg T_3. The normal postnatal increase in cytosol receptor occurs at the same time that endogenous T_3 and T_4 levels increase. These findings indicate a possible role of endogenous thyroid hormones in the postnatal, but not prenatal, rise in cytosol receptor concentration.

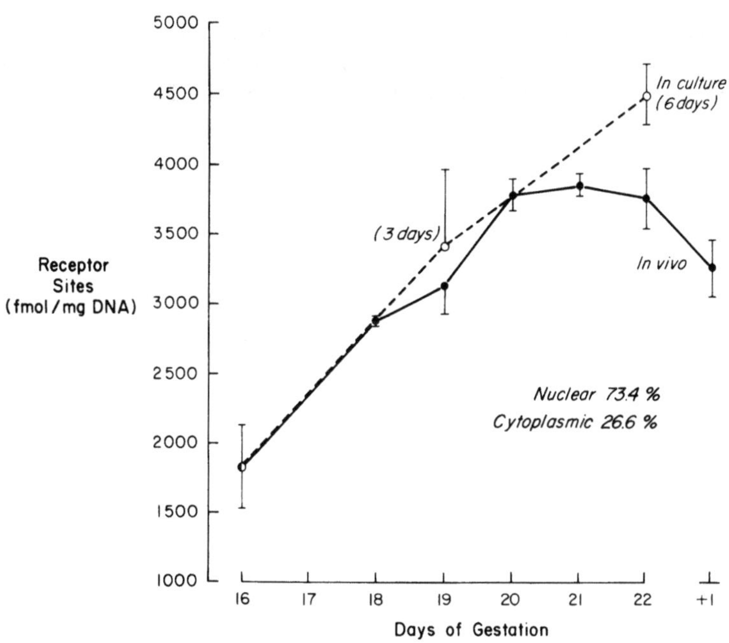

Fig. 3.4. Dexamethasone binding in fetal rat lung during late gestation. Binding capaicty was determined in nuclear plus cytoplasmic fractions of freshly explanted fetal lung *(solid line)* and in 16-day lung cultured for 3 or 6 days in medium containing 1 % fetal calf serum *(dashed line)*. From Ballard et al. (1984), by permission

The ontogeny of glucocorticoid receptor has also been studied in intact lung cells (Ballard et al. 1984). As shown in Fig. 3.4, there is a developmental increase in dexamethasone binding sites when assayed in explants of fetal rat lung at 37 °C. In this experimental approach, cytoplasmic and nuclear fractions are prepared in the cold after equilibrium binding has occurred. This allows an estimate of total cell receptor sites and cytoplasmic: nuclear distribution under physiologic conditions. In this study there was a 103 % increase in receptor concentration between days 16 and 22 of gestation, similar to the results using cytosol. At term there are on the average 12,200 binding sites per cell. Binding capacity also increased during culture of 16-day fetal lung (Fig. 3.4).

In the rabbit, dexamethasone binding capacity of lung tissue increases 47 % between days 23 and 30 of gestation (term = 31 days) (Fig. 3.5). There was no developmental change in non-specific binding, nuclear:cytoplasmic distribution, or the K_D. The average concentration of binding sites in fetal rabbit lung at 30 days gestation with this assay is about 6,500/cell. A similar developmental increase has been observed for uptake of [^{3}H]cortisol into nuclei of lung slices at 37 °C (Giannopoulos et al. 1972). In studies with cytosol from fetal rabbit lung, little or no increase in receptor concentration was found when data were expressed per mg of protein or g tissue (Ballard and Ballard 1972; Giannopoulos 1974; Ballard et al. 1984). When cytosol binding data are expressed per mg DNA, however, there is a 49 % increase during the last week of gestation (Ballard et al. 1984). These results apparently reflect an increase in extracellular mass (e.g., blood volume) during development.

An analogous situation for the ontogeny of receptor apparently occurs in fetal liver (Cake et al. 1981). Glucocorticoid receptor concentration in rat hepatocytes is low until day 19 of gestation when the level increases several fold. A

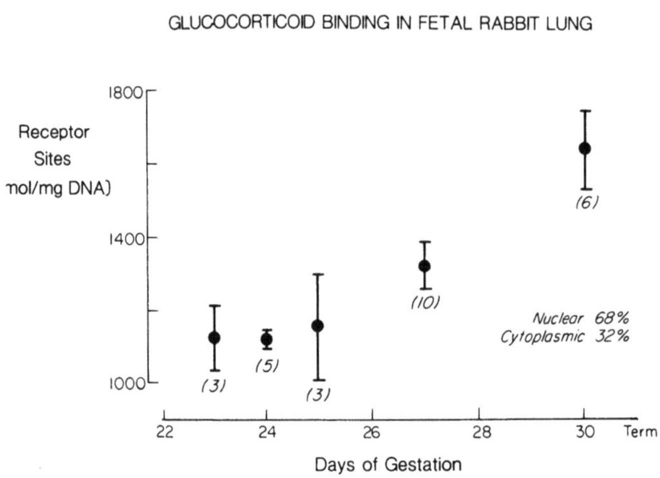

Fig. 3.5. Dexamethasone binding in explants of fetal rabbit lung in late gestation. Binding capacity in nuclear plus cytoplasmic fractions was assayed in explants of fetal rabbit lung cultured at 37 °C. Reprinted from Ballard et al. (1984), by permission

similar rise in receptor is observed after 3 days culture of isolated cells (15-day gestation) in medium supplemented with charcoal-treated calf serum. Moreover, induction of both tyrosine aminotransferase and glycogen accumulation by dexamethasone correlates closely with receptor concentration.

The influence of gender on glucocorticoid binding in lung has been investigated because of reports that maturation of the surfactant system is slower in male than female fetuses, and that male fetuses may be less responsive to glucocorticoid treatment (Nielsen and Torday 1981; Kotas and Avery 1980). Studies with fetal rabbit lung, both in culture (Gross et al. 1983; Ballard et al. 1984) and in cytosol (Giannopoulos and Sommers-Smith 1982), failed to find any differences in the binding capacity or K_D for males vs. females. Thus, the reported influence of sex is apparently not related to differences in glucocorticoid receptor.

Flint and Burton (1984) examined dexamethasone binding capacity in lung cytosol of the fetal lamb. They found a progressive increase in binding sites (per mg protein) between day 54 (0.14 pmol) and day 100 of gestation (~0.95 pmol), and then a decline to a value of about 0.42 pmol at term. Hypophysectomy at 119–128 days did not affect receptor concentration at term. The decrease in receptor during the third trimester may reflect increasing serum protein within the lung as well as increasing circulating corticosteroids which would promote nuclear localization and cytoplasmic depletion. The results in hypophysectomized animals, however, argue against the latter possibility as a major influence.

In the human, as in other species, glucocorticoid receptor was detected at the earliest points of gestation examined (Fig. 3.6). In lung of human fetuses at 15–17 weeks gestation, cytosol binding capacity was 0.27–0.33 pmol/mg protein (Ballard and Ballard 1974; Iacobelli et al. 1978). Receptor concentration in specimens obtained during the second trimester were similar. In a brief communication, Szabo et al. (1980) report lower levels of specific cortisol binding in human lung cytosol and a decline during the second trimester; these levels may result from both a suboptimal cortisol concentration (10 nM) and metabolism during the assay (see Chap. 4). With lungs of older fetuses and infants, less binding was detected (Fig. 3.6); however, this finding may represent an artifact associated with delivery and demise. Lungs from aborted fetuses and from premature infants dying in the newborn period have rela-

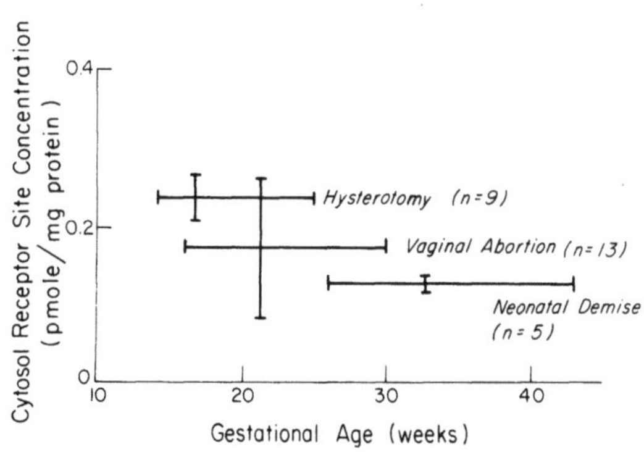

Fig. 3.6. Glucocorticoid receptor in cytosol of human fetal and neonatal lung. Binding capacity was determined with [^{3}H]dexamethasone in cytosol at 2 °C. The range of gestational ages is indicated by the *horizontal lines* at the mean concentration. *Vertical lines* represent the SE at the mean gestational age for specimens in each group. Data from Ballard and Ballard (1974), by permission

tively high concentrations of endogenous corticoids (Ballard and Ballard 1974) which presumably results from the stress associated with abortion, prematurity, neonatal illnesses, and death. The high levels of endogenous corticoids would deplete the cytoplasm of receptors and result in less binding on assay in vitro. Thus, the actual developmental pattern for receptor during the third trimester in the human fetal lung is uncertain, but it is unlikely that there is a decrease in average receptor concentration per cell.

The developmental increase in glucocorticoid binding capacity for fetal rat, rabbit and lamb lung could reflect appearance of receptor in specific pulmonary cell types during development, greater receptor concentration in certain cell types, or a similar increase in all pulmonary cells. In fetal liver, for example, hepatocytes appear to acquire receptor later in development than hematopoetic cells (Cake et al. 1981). The factors controlling receptor concentration in fetal lung (and liver) are not known, but it is noteworthy that binding capacity increases during culture in medium with no added hormones and only a low level of serum. The topic of autoregulation during development is discussed further in Chap. 4. Although the physiologic significance of increasing pulmonary receptor concentration is uncertain, this event could amplify the effect of endogenous corticosteroids in fetal lung during late gestation. Data comparing receptor concentration and the rate of choline incorporation into PC support this possibility (Ballard et al. 1984). In rabbit fetuses of 27-days gestation, the rate of choline incorporation was higher in those lungs with a greater concentration of receptor. A positive slope between the two parameters was found both for inter- and intra-litter comparisons. These studies indicate that receptor concentration may be linked with the rate of surfactant synthesis in preterm pups.

3.3 Evidence for Receptor Mediation of Corticosteroid Effects

The identification of glucocorticoid receptor in fetal lung indicated that this organ was a potential target tissue for corticosteroids. Studies with cultured lung tissue have established that most, if not all, effects of glucocorticoids result from a direct action of glucocorticoids in fetal lung (in contrast to indirect effects secondary to hormonal action in other tissues). Furthermore, recent data support the earlier proposals that these effects are mediated by glucocorticoid receptors.

3.3.1 Studies in Cultured Lung

Stimulation of choline incorporation and PC content by corticosteroid has been examined in organ cultures of fetal rat (Gross and Wilson 1982; Ballard et al. 1984), fetal rabbit (Snyder et al. 1981; Gross et al 1983), and in the human fetus (Ekelund et al. 1975a, b; Mendelson et al. 1981; Gonzales and Ballard 1984; Zsolnai and Gyevai 1984). Figure 3.7 shows dose-response curves for stimulation of choline incorporation by cortisol and dexamethasone in explants of 24-day gestation fetal rabbit lung cultured for 2 days. A response occurs with corticosteroid concentrations in the nM range, and the effect pla-

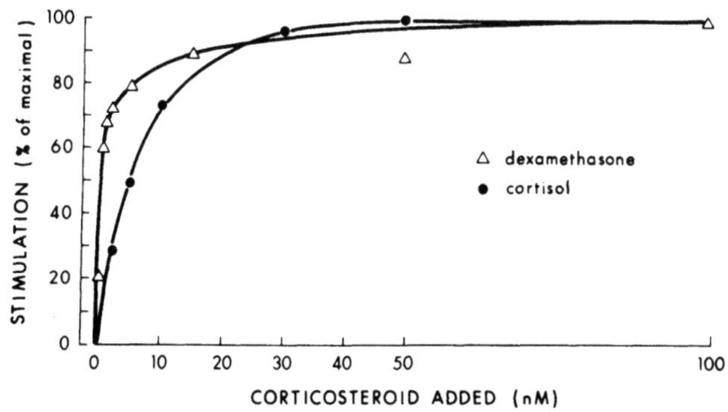

Fig. 3.7. Dose-response curves for stimulation of choline incorporation into PC by dexamethasone and cortisol. Explants of 24-day gestation fetal rabbit lung were cultured for 48 h in the presence of steroid at the concentrations shown. Data from Gross et al. (1983), by permission

teaus at higher concentrations. Half-maximal stimulation by dexamethasone occurs at a concentration of 0.7 nM, whereas half-maximal stimulation by cortisol is achieved at 6.8 nM (Table 3.7). A similar dose-response relationship for cortisol was found with cultures of 19-day rabbit lung maintained for 6 days in the presence of 10 % fetal calf serum (Snyder et al. 1981). Rat lung is nearly 10-fold less sensitive to dexamethasone than rabbit tissue, consistent with the higher K_D for binding in the rat.

Precise quantitative interpretation of the response data are complicated by the difficulty of assessing free corticosteroid concentration. The data for stimulation of choline incorporation in Fig. 3.7 and Table 3.7 reflect the concentration of hormone added to the culture medium. Calculations based on [^{3}H]corticosteroid binding indicate that corrections for tissue-bound hormone would not substantially affect the values for half-maximal stimulation of choline incorporation. Thus, the data of Table 3.7 indicate a linear relationship between occupancy of receptor by glucocorticoid and stimulation of choline incorporation. These results resemble those found for other corticosteroid responsive systems (Baxter and Rousseau 1979).

The close correlation between binding and response data are consistent with a direct action of steroid on PC synthesis in type II cells without secon-

Table 3.7. Corticosteroid binding and response in fetal lung tissue. Dose-response studies were carried out with fetal rabbit (25–27 days) and rat (18 days) lung in culture. Mean ± SE values for n = 3 – 7 are shown. Data from Gross et al. (1983), and Ballard et al. (1984)

Species	Steroid	K_D for nuclear binding (nM)	Half-maximal stimulation of choline incorporation (nM)
Rabbit	Dexamethasone	0.7 ± 0.6	0.7 ± 0.1
	Cortisol	7.3 ± 0.1	6.8 ± 0.5
Rat	Dexamethasone	6.8 ± 0.6	6.6 ± 1.9

dary mediation through cyclic AMP (Chap. 8) or other factors, such as fibroblast pneumonocyte factor (Chap. 9). In biological systems which respond to hormones acting through cAMP, there is generally a substantial difference in response curves for binding and effect (which is more sensitive to hormone). By mathematical analysis, Strickland and Loeb (1981) concluded that separation of dose curves for hormone binding and response is obligatory in systems involving secondary mediators.

Dose-response studies performed with fetal lung cells in monolayer culture have generated conflicting results. In an initial study with cells cultured from 28-day fetal rabbit lung, stimulation of choline incorporation was observed at a cortisol concentration of 10 nM (but not at 1 nM), and the response was half-maximal at ~200 nM (Torday et al. 1975). In a subsequent study, similar preparations of lung cells were cultured for 10 days in medium containing 10 % fetal calf serum which had been charcoal treated to remove endogenous corticosteroids. DNA accumulation was half-maximally stimulated at a cortisol concentration of ~0.2 nM, while choline incorporation into saturated PC showed a bi-phasic response with stimulation at 1 and 10 nM, but not at higher concentrations (Torday 1980). The discrepancy between these studies is unresolved, but probably relates to the different culture conditions. In cultured rabbit fibroblasts (Smith and Giroud 1975), the rate of thymidine incorporation was stimulated by cortisol in cells from 20-day fetal lung, and was suppressed in cultures prepared from 28-day lung. The half-maximal response for both of these processes appears to occur between 10 and 100 nM cortisol, with the effect plateauing by 10 μM. In cultures of human fibroblasts, half-

Table 3.8. Effect of various steroids on choline incorporation and dexamethasone binding in cultured fetal rabbit lung according to Gross et al. (1983)

Steroid	Choline incorporation (% of dexamethasone effect)[a]	[^{3}H]dexamethasone nuclear binding (% inhibition)[b]
Dexamthasone	100	88 ± 1
Cortisol	96 ± 3	62 ± 2
Cortisone	92 (91,92)	41 ± 5
Corticosterone	43 (32,53)	19 ± 5
Dehydrocorticosterone	27 (26,27)	11 ± 4
Progesterone	0	2 ± 7
17α-Hydroxyprogesterone	0	0 ± 3
17β-Estradiol	0	− 6 ± 6
Testosterone	0	− 12 ± 2

[a] Data are expressed as the stimulation of choline incorporation into PC by the various steroids as a percentage of that produced by dexamethasone and are the mean of 2 to 4 experiments. Explants of 24-day lung were exposed to the steroids at a concentration of 100 nM for 48 h

[b] Explants of 24-day fetal lung were exposed to [^{3}H]dexamethasone (10.3 nM) with or without unlabeled competing steroid (100 nM) for 2 h at 37 °C, and specific nuclear binding was assessed. Data are the mean ± SE of 4 to 7 experiments

maximal stimulation of fibroblast penumonocyte factor occurred at a cortisol concentration of about 30 nM (Smith 1978), consistent with data for glucocorticoid binding in this species.

In contrast to the results with cultured lung of rat and rabbit, Mendelson et al. (1981) reported that relatively high concentrations of cortisol were required for stimulation of choline incorporation in human lung. Tissue from a 22-week abortus was incubated for 4 days in medium containing insulin, prolactin and increasing concentrations of cortisol. Stimulation was first observed at a cortisol concentration of 5 μM and the response did not plateau at 50 μM, the highest concentration tested. The high dose of cortisol required in this study probably reflects rapid metabolism of cortisol to inactive cortisone by human lung tissue, whereas this reaction is primarily in the reverse direction for pulmonary fibroblasts (discussed in Sect. 4.3.4). This interpretation is supported by the observation that dexamethasone, which is not substantially metabolized by lung, demonstrates optimal activity at a concentration of about 10 nM in human lung (Gonzales and Ballard 1984).

A second line of evidence for receptor mediation is the specificity of the response for steroids with corticosteroid activity (Torday et al. 1975; Gross et al. 1983). Data for stimulation of choline incorporation and for nuclear binding in explants of fetal rabbit lung are shown in Table 3.8. Choline incorporation was stimulated by dexamethasone, cortisol, cortisone (through conversion to cortisol), corticosterone and dehydrocorticosterone (by conversion to corticosterone). These steroids all competed for binding of [^{3}H]dexamethasone with a relative potency similar to that for stimulation choline incorporation. At the doses used, there was no effect of progesterone, 17α-hydroxyprogesterone, estradiol, or testosterone on choline incorporation, and these steroids did not compete with [^{3}H]dexamethasone for binding.

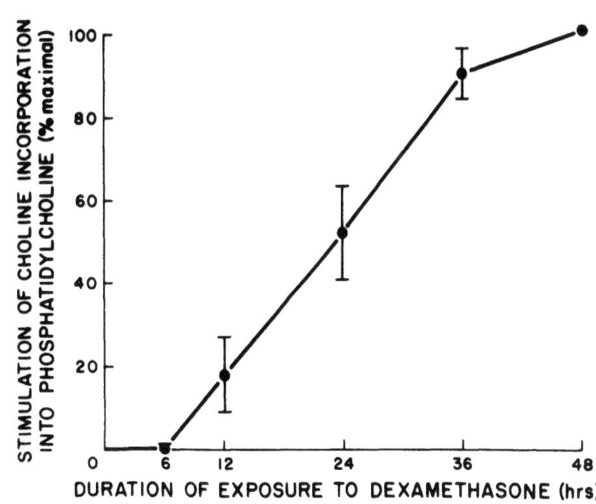

Fig. 3.8. Choline incorporation after various times of exposure to dexamethasone. Explants of 24-day fetal rabbit lung were cultured for 48 h in the presence of 100 nM dexamethasone for the times indicated. Data from Gross et al. (1983), by permission

phosphatidylcholine in cortisol-treated, intrauterine growth retarded and twin control lambs at different gestational ages. Biol Neonate 31:155
D'Agostino JB, Vaeth GF, Henning SJ (1982) Diurnal rhythm of total and free concentrations of serum corticosterone in the rat. Acta Endocrinol 100:85
Dobbs LG, Mason RJ (1979) Pulmonary alveolar type II cells isolated from rats. Release of phosphatidylcholine in response to β-adrenergic stimulation. J Clin Invest 63:378
Douglas WH, Kaighn ME (1974) Clonal isolation of differentiated rat lung cells. In Vitro 10:230
Douglas WH, Teel RW (1976) An organotypic in vitro model system for studying pulmonary surfactant production by type II alveolar pneumonocytes. Am Rev Resp Dis 113:17
Ekelund L, Arvidson G, Astedt B (1975) Cortisol-induced accumulation of phospholipids in organ culture of human fetal lung. Scand J Clin Lab Invest 35:419
Ekelund L, Arvidson G, Emanuelsson H, Myhrberg H, Åstedt B (1975b) Effect of cortisol on human fetal lung in organ culture. Cell Tissue Res 163:263
Farrell PM, Zachman RD (1973) Induction of choline phosphotransferase and lecithin synthesis in the fetal lung by corticosteroids. Science 179:297
Feldman D, Funder J, Loose D (1978) Is the glucocorticoid receptor identical in various target organs? J Steroid Biochem 9:141
Flint APF, Burton RD (1984) Properties and ontogeny of the glucocorticoid receptor in the placenta and fetal lung of the sheep. J Endocr 103:31
Giannopoulos G, Mulay S, Solomon S (1972) Cortisol receptors in rabbit fetal lung. Biochem Biophys Res Commun 47:411
Giannopoulos G (1973) Glucocorticoid receptors in lung. I. Specific binding of glucocorticoids to cytoplasmic components of rabbit fetal lung. J Biol Chem 248:3876
Giannopoulos G, Mulay S, Solomon S (1973) Glucocorticoid receptors in lung. II. Specific binding of glucocorticoids to nuclear components of rabbit fetal lung. J Biol Chem 248:5016
Giannopoulos G (1974) Variations in the levels of cytoplasmic glucocorticoid receptors in lungs of various species at different developmental stages. Endocrinology 94:450
Giannopoulos G, Hassan Z, Solomon S (1974) Glucocorticoid receptors in fetal and adult rabbit tissues. J Biol Chem 249:2424
Giannopoulos G (1975a) Glucocorticoid receptors in lung. Mechanism of specific glucocorticoid uptake by fetal rabbit lung nuclei. J Biol Chem 250:2896
Giannopoulos G (1975b) Glucocorticoid receptors in lung. Comparison between nonactivated and activated forms of the cytoplasmic glucocorticoid binding protein and their relationship to the nuclear binding protein of fetal rabbit lung. J Biol Chem 250:2904
Giannopoulos G (1975c) Early events in the action of glucocorticoid in developing tissues. J Steroid Biochem 6:623
Giannopoulos G, Keichline D (1981) Species-related differences in steroid-binding specificity of glucocorticoid receptors in lung. Endocrinology 108:1414
Giannopoulos G, Sommers-Smith SK (1982) Androgen receptors in fetal rabbit lung and the effect of fetal sex on the levels of circulating hormones and hormone receptors. J Steroid Biochem 17:461
Gilbert HF (1982) Biological disulfides: The third messenger? J Biol Chem 257:1286
Gonzales LK, Ballard PL (1984) Glucocorticoid and thyroid hormone stimulation of phosphatidylcholine (PC) synthesis in cultured human fetal lung. Pediatr Res 18:310A (abstract)
Granberg JP, Ballard PL (1977) The role of sulfhydryl groups in the binding of glucocorticoids by cytoplasmic receptors of lung and other mammalian tissues. Endocrinology 100:1160
Gross I, Wilson CM (1982) Fetal lung in organ culture. IV. Supraadditive hormone interactions. J Appl Physiol: Respirat Environ Exercise Physiol 52:1420
Gross I, Ballard PL, Ballard RA, Jones CT, Wilson CM (1983) Corticosteroid stimulation of phosphatidylcholine synthesis in cultured fetal rabbit lung: Evidence for de novo protein synthesis mediated by glucocorticoid receptors. Endocrinology 112:829
Hitchcock-O'Hare KE, Meymaris E, Bonaccorso J, Vanburen SB (1976) Separation and partial characterization of surface-active fractions from mouse and rat lung homogenates. Identification of a possible marker system for pulmonary surfactant. J Histochem Cytochem 24:487
Hümmelink R, Ballard PL (1984) Endogenous corticosteroids and lung maturation in the fetal rabbit. Pediatr Res 18:139A (abstract)
Iacobelli S, Ranelletti F, Sica G, Barile G (1978) Glucocorticoid receptors in human fetal lung. J Endocrinol Invest 1:209

Jones CT (1974) Corticosteroid concentrations in the plasma of fetal and maternal guinea pigs during gestation. Endocrinology 95:1129
Kauffman SL (1977) Acceleration of canalicular development in lungs of fetal mice exposed transplacentally to dexamethasone. Lab Invest 36:395
Keller GH, Ladda RL (1981) Correlation between phosphatidylcholine labelling and hormone receptor levels in alveolar type II epithelial cells: effects of dexamethasone and epidermal growth factor. Arch Biochem Biophys 211:321
Kotas RV, Avery ME (1980) The influence of sex on fetal rabbit lung maturation and on the response to glucocorticoids. Am Rev Resp Dis 121:377
Liggins GC, Kitterman JA, Campos GA, Clements JA, Forster CS, Lee CH, Creasy RK (1981) Pulmonary maturation in the hypophysectomised ovine fetus. Differential responses to adrenocorticotrophin and cortisol. J Devel Physiol 3:1
Mendelson CR, Johnston JM, MacDonald PC, Snyder JM (1981) Multihormonal regulation of surfactant synthesis by human fetal lung in vitro. J Clin Endocrinol Metab 53:307
Morishige WK (1982) Thyroid hormone influences glucocorticoid receptor levels in the neonatal rat lung. Endocrinology 111:1017
Mulay S, Giannopoulos G, Solomon S (1973) Corticosteroid levels in the mother and fetus of the rabbit during gestation. Endocrinology 93:1342
Mulay S, Varma DR, Solomon S (1982) Influence of protein deficiency in rats on hormonal status and cytoplasmic glucocorticoid receptors in maternal and fetal tissues. J Endocrinol 95:49
Murphy BEP (1983) Human fetal serum cortisol levels at delivery. A review. Endocrine Rev 4:150
Nielsen HC, Torday JS (1981) Sex differences in fetal rabbit pulmonary surfactant production. Pediatr Res 15:1245
Platzker ACG, Kitterman JA, Mescher EJ, Clements JA, Tooley WH (1975) Surfactant in the lung and tracheal fluid of the fetal lamb and acceleration of its appearance by dexamethasone. Pediatrics 56:554
Smith BT (1978) Fibroblast-pneumonocyte factor: intercellular mediator of glucocorticoid effect on fetal lung. In: Stern L (ed), Intensive Care in the Newborn, Vol II, Masson, Boston, pp 25–32
Smith BT, Giroud CJP (1975) Effects of cortisol on serially propagated fibroblast cell cultures derived from the rabbit fetal lung and skin. Pharmacology 53:1037
Snyder JM, Mendelson CR, Johnston JM (1981) The effect of cortisol on rabbit fetal lung maturation in vitro. Dev Biol 85:129
Strickland S, Loeb NJ (1981) Obligatory separation of hormone binding and biological curves in systems dependent on secondary mediators of hormone action. Proc Natl Acad Sci USA 78:1366
Szabo I, Vertes M, Bodis J, Lanyi E, Sauerhering E (1980) Steroid receptors in human fetal lung. Lancet, October 4, p 751.
Toft D, Chytil F (1973) Receptors for glucocorticoids in lung tissue. Arch Biochem Biophys 157:464
Torday JS (1980) Glucocorticoid dependence of fetal lung maturation in vitro. Endocrinology 107:839
Torday JS, Smith BT, Giroud CJP (1975) The rabbit fetal lung as a glucocorticoid target tissue. Endocrinology 96:1462
Vilos GA, Challis JRG, Lye SJ, Possmayer F, Harding PG (1983) Accelerated prepartum maturation of the fetal sheep lung with physiological doses of adrenocorticotrophin. J Dev Physiol 5:341
Warburton D (1983) Chronic hyperglycemia with secondary hyperinsulinemia inhibits the maturational response of fetal lamb lungs to cortisol. J Clin Invest 72:433
Zsolnai B, Gyevai A (1984) Induction of lamellar body synthesis by corticosteroids in first-trimester human fetal lung. Gynecol Obstet Invest 17:258

4 Role of Endogenous Corticosteroids

The effects of corticosteroid treatment appear to represent precocious development of normal biochemical, physiologic and morphologic events in pulmonary differentiation (Chap. 1 and 2). Most, if not all, of these effects are mediated through receptor, indicating that physiologic concentrations of glucocorticoid are sufficient to produce a response (Chap. 3). Glucocorticoids also regulate developmental processes in a variety of other tissues of fetal and newborn animals (Ballard 1979a). These considerations support the concept that endogenous corticoids influence the timing of normal lung development and that administration of glucocorticoid mimics the action of endogenous hormone. In this chapter I review the evidence that endogenous glucocorticoids have a physiologic role in lung maturation. Previous discussions of this topic include reviews by Taeusch and Avery (1977), Smith (1979), and Ballard (1982a).

4.1 Temporal Associations

4.1.1 Plasma and Amniotic Fluid Corticosteroids

With only one apparent exception, concentrations of corticosteroids in fetal plasma increase during late gestation in association with the final events in lung development. In some species both total and free corticoids rise, whereas in others only the free concentration increases. The temporal patterns for circulating corticoids in several species are presented for comparison.

4.1.1.1 Sheep

The development of surgical techniques for chronic in utero preparations of fetal sheep has provided a popular and useful experimental model for investigating the ontogenesis of endogenous hormones. Accordingly, there is abundant information on the pattern of corticosteroid concentrations in the fetal sheep (Alexander et al. 1968; Bassett and Thorburn 1969; Comline et al. 1970; Paisey and Nathanielsz 1971; Nathanielsz et al. 1972; Thorburn et al. 1972; Alexander et al. 1973; Fairclough and Liggins 1975; Wintour et al. 1975; Magyar 1980a; Magyar et al. 1981; Challis et al. 1981; Ballard et al. 1982b; Rose et al. 1982; Hennessy et al. 1983). The major circulating corticosteroid is cortisol. Plasma concentrations of corticosterone, 11-deoxycortisol and 11-deoxycorticosterone are in the order of 2, 2, and <1 % of that for cortisol at term.

An example of the prepartum surge in fetal corticoids is shown in Fig. 4.1. In this study there was a slow increase in plasma corticoids (approximately 0.014 μg/dl/day) between 110 and about 130 days gestation. After 130 days, in

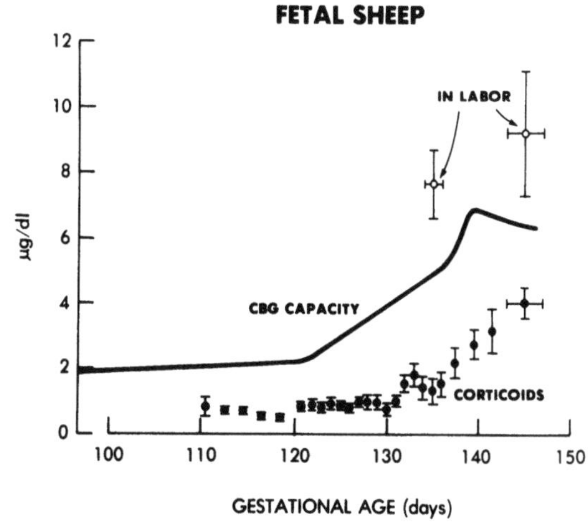

Fig. 4.1. Plasma corticoids in fetal sheep during the third trimester. Mean ± SE values for 4–12 samples are shown. The concentrations for animals in labor are higher ($p < 0.05$) than for sheep not in labor at the same gestational age. The profile for CBG capacity is shown for comparison. Data from Ballard et al. (1982b), by permission

the absence of labor, the daily increment was 0.21 μg/dl. Corticoid concentrations are similarly high for both preterm and term fetuses on the day prior to spontaneous delivery. After birth (not shown), total corticoid concentrations decrease rapidly and eventually reach the adult level by about one month of age (Ballard et al. 1982b). There is a similar temporal pattern for corticosterone in the fetus. In part, the rapid increase in corticoids just before birth may reflect hemoconcentration, since the total serum protein concentration increases about 25 % in the five days before delivery (Ballard et al. 1982b). By contrast, maternal plasma levels of corticoids are constant during gestation (cortisol <1 μg/dl) except for a rise beginning approximately 3 days before delivery. The concentration of maternal corticoids have no apparent relationship over time with fetal levels. According to Hennessy et al. (1983), placental transfer from mother to fetus is sufficient to account for all of the fetal cortisol from 100–121 days, but represents <12 % of the fetal pool after 136 days gestation.

The plasma concentration of *free* cortisol also increases in the fetus (Fairclough and Liggins 1975; Ballard et al. 1982b). Unbound corticoids represent about 12 % of the total concentration during the first half of the third trimester (Table 4.1). The increase in unbound corticoids occurs later than for total cortisol, beginning around 135 days of gestation. This delay apparently results from an earlier increase in corticosteroid binding globulin (CBG) (beginning approximately 120 days) than for total corticoids (Fig. 4.1). The increase in CBG is caused by yet unidentified pituitary hormone(s) (Ballard et al. 1982b; Ballard et al. 1983). Thus, the rise in unbound cortisol occurs only during the last 2 weeks of gestation, with most of the increase occurring in the last few days before delivery. There is a similar rise with preterm labor. Compared with the level at 115 days, there is a 16- and 21-fold increase in unbound cortisol at preterm and term delivery, respectively. This change is sufficient to increase occupancy of lung glucocorticoid receptors several-fold.

The temporal pattern for fetal unbound cortisol resembles that for terminal lung development. For example, surfactant is first detected in tracheal fluid at

Table 4.1. Unbound plasma corticoids in fetal sheep. Data calculated from assays of albumin, CBG capacity, and corticoids (primarily cortisol) in plasma from chronically catheterized fetuses (Ballard et al. 1982b)

Gestational age (days)	n	Unbound corticoids	
		% of total corticoids	Concentration (μg/dl)
114–115	7	12.7	0.09 ± 0.01
119–120	6	12.1	0.10 ± 0.02
125	8	11.8	0.10 ± 0.01
129–130	10	11.8	0.09 ± 0.01
134–135 (no labor)	6	7.6	0.11 ± 0.02
139–140 (no labor)	4	6.3	0.19 ± 0.04
136–138 (day before spontaneous birth)	5	17.5	1.41 ± 0.38
142–149 (day before spontaneous birth)	5	14.5	1.87 ± 0.22

about 130 days, and increases exponentially until term (Mescher et al. 1975). There is no detectable change in free corticoid concentrations when surfactant first becomes evident in tracheal fluid. This finding suggests that, in the sheep at least, endogenous cortisol does not induce the initial appearance of surfactant, but rather exerts its influence during the last week of gestation when there are major increases in lung volume and saturated PC content (Kitterman et al. 1981). As discussed below (Sect. 4.1.2), values for these two parameters correlate closely with cortisol levels.

4.1.1.2 Rat and Mouse

In contrast to the pattern of fetal sheep, plasma corticosterone decreases during the last few days of gestation in both the rat (Martin et al. 1977; Holt and Oliver 1968; Dupouy et al. 1975) and mouse (Dalle et al. 1978). In the fetal rat, for example, total corticosteroids increase from 13 μg/dl at 5 days before delivery to a peak level of 45 μg/dl 2 days later, and then decrease to <5 μg/dl at birth. There is a similar temporal pattern for fetal adrenal weight (mg/g body weight) and adrenal content of corticosteroid, indicating that changes in plasma corticoids reflect primarily adrenal production rather than clearance rate (Martin et al. 1977; Dalle et al. 1978). In both species, plasma corticoid binding capacity also decreases dramatically during the last few days of fetal life, resulting in a several-fold increase in free (and albumin-bound) corticosteroids (Van Baelen et al. 1977; Savu et al. 1977; Martin et al. 1977). Corticosteroid levels in the rat are shown in Table 4.2, along with developmental data related to lung maturation. In these two species, therefore, a precipitous decrease in plasma CBG produces a rise in free circulating corticosteroid concentrations in late gestation.

Pulmonary development in the mouse has not been well characterized. An early study by Buckingham and Avery (1962) found that low surface tension

Table 4.2. Plasma corticosteroids and indices of lung maturity in the fetal rat. The corticosteroid data are from Martin et al. (1977). PC synthesis was measured by the rate of [^{14}C]choline incorporation (Farrell et al. 1977). Data for tissue content of saturated PC are from Gross et al. (1978). Amniotic fluid PC (acetone-precipitable) results are from Nelson et al. (1976)

Gestational age (days)	Plasma corticosteroids		PC synthesis in lung (cpm/mg lung/h)	Lung saturated PC (μg P/mg protein)	Amniotic fluid PC (μg/dl)
	Total	Free + albumin-bound			
17	13.3	–	1690	–	158
18	34.3	1.6	1670	–	179
19	45.1	3.1	1790	0.84	257
20	34.8	3.1	2310	0.99	584
21	23.5	5.9	3730	1.29	1254
22	6.9	2.2	4240	1.62	–

in extracts of lung did not develop until the last day of gestation. Kauffman (1977) reported an increase in the proportion of type II cells containing lamellar bodies between days 17 and 18 of gestation (18 vs. 48 %).

4.1.1.3 Rabbit

The relationship of endogenous corticosteroids to lung development appears to be more complex in this species. In the adult, corticosterone is the major circulating corticoid, although cortisol appears to be preferentially secreted by the adrenal in response to chronic ACTH treatment (Kass et al. 1954). In the fetus, the concentration of cortisol exceeds that for corticosterone, but the relative amounts vary during late gestation. Mulay et al. (1973) reported variable levels of corticosterone and a 50 % increase in cortisol of fetal plasma during the last week of gestation. These results may have been influenced by stress associated with performing a laparotomy under local anesthesia. By equilibrium dialysis, a greater proportion of cortisol was unbound with increasing

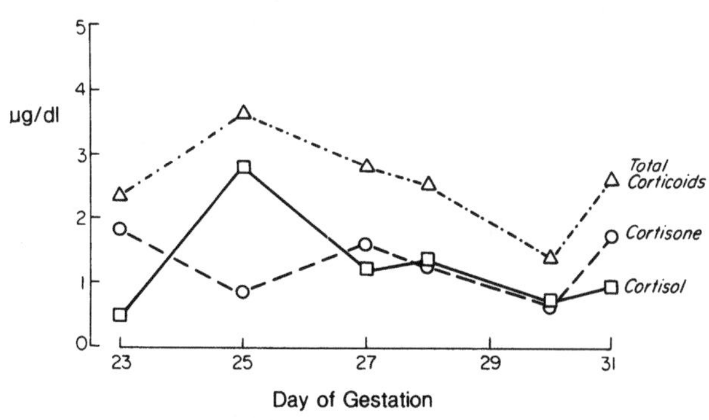

Fig. 4.2. Concentration of cortisol and cortisone in fetal rabbit plasma during the last 9 days of gestation. Each point represents mean values for 5–10 samples. Total corticoids are the calculated sum of cortisol and cortisone. Data adapted from Barr et al. (1980)

gestation and the calculated concentration of free cortisol increased 3-fold in the last week.

Subsequent investigations have re-examined corticoid levels and binding proteins in the fetal rabbit. In these studies there was a decrease in cortisol during the last week of gestation (to 25-33 % of the maximal levels) beginning on day 25 (Fig. 4.2) or day 23 (Hümmelink and Ballard 1984). The concentrations of cortisone (Fig. 4.2) and corticosterone (Hümmelink and Ballard 1984) also decrease during this interval, whereas maternal cortisol concentration increases several-fold (Mulay et al. 1973; Barr et al. 1980). The ratio of cortisol to corticosterone in fetal plasma was 3.7:1 between 21 and 28 days, and 1.5:1 thereafter. As shown in Fig. 4.3, the cortisol binding capacity of fetal plasma decreases markedly between 23 days (36 μg/dl) and term (2.1 μg/dl). During the same period, the plasma concentration of albumin increases from 1.13 g/dl to 2.29 g/dl. Despite the decrease in CBG, the concentration of unbound cortisol actually decreases during the last week from (approximately 0.04 μg/dl to 0.02 μg/dl) (Hümmelink and Ballard 1984). A similar decline occurs for unbound cortisone which is a physiologically active corticosteroid in rabbit lung through conversion to cortisol (discussed in Sect. 4.3.2). Thus, these findings suggest that both total and free plasma corticoids in the fetal rabbit decrease during late gestation when alveolarization and pulmonary surfactant synthesis are occurring.

However, it is likely that other factors are operating in the case of the rabbit to increase both the supply of cortisol and the responsiveness of lung cells. The ability of lung tissue to convert cortisone to cortisol increases with gestational age (discussed in Sect. 4.3.4) and cortisone is present in plasma at a concentration similar to that for cortisol (Fig. 4.2). The concentration of glucocorticoid receptors in lung cells increases in late gestation (Chap. 3) and this

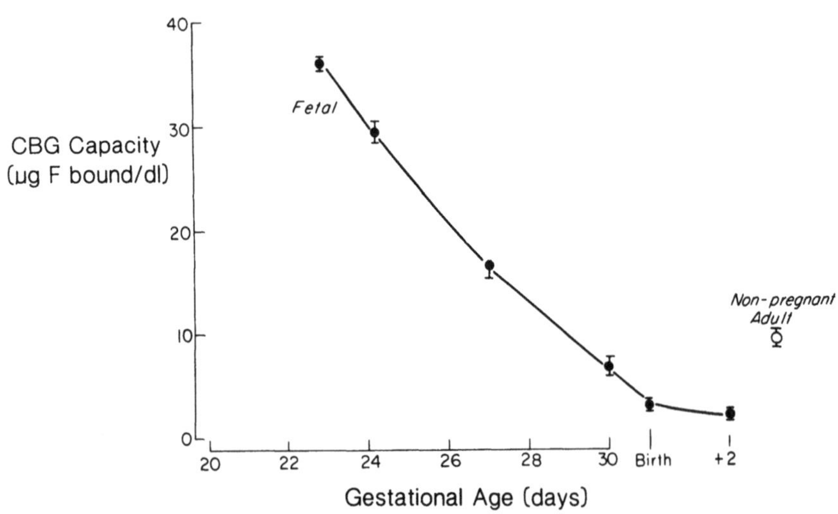

Fig. 4.3. Plasma CBG capacity in the fetal and newborn rabbit. Data from Hümmelink and Ballard (1984)

event would increase the concentration of receptor-cortisol complexes in nuclei of lung cells independent of an increase in circulating cortisol. It is also possible that *free* cortisol is not the physiologically important form of steroid for fetal rabbit lung. Thus, the role of endogenous corticoids in maturation of the fetal rabbit lung remains uncertain at present. Information about the concentration of receptor-cortisol complex within nuclei of type II cells and fibroblasts would help resolve this question.

4.1.1.4 Non-human Primates

The developmental profile for serum cortisol in Rhesus monkeys *(Macaca mulatta)* is shown in Fig. 4.4. Similar results are found for samples obtained at cesarean section of undisturbed fetuses and for repeated in utero sampling of instrumented fetuses. Between 110 and 150 days gestation, fetal cortisol is constant at a mean level of 8–10 μg/dl. There is a progressive rise in cortisol after 150 days and a further increase associated with spontaneous labor. Cortisol also increases in amniotic fluid of Rhesus monkeys during the third trimester (Patrick et al. 1976), but there are no significant changes in maternal cortisol which is 2- to 3-fold greater than the fetal concentration (Beamer et al. 1972; Seron-Ferre et al. 1978a; Ballard, unpublished data). In a study of three baboon fetuses, Oakey (1974) found a cortisol concentration of 4 μg/dl or less at 116 and 132 days gestation and a level of 15 μg/dl at 168 days. An abrupt rise in the L/S ratio occurs at about 170 days gestation in the baboon (Gluck et al. 1974).

The cortisol binding capacity in serum of the fetal Rhesus monkey decreases during the third trimester when total cortisol is increasing (Fig. 4.5). This combination of changes would produce even greater developmental increases in free cortisol than for the total concentration. Thus, there is a sub-

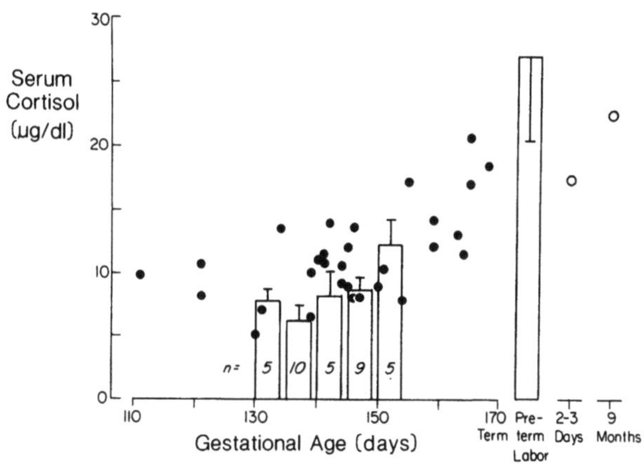

Fig. 4.4. Plasma cortisol in the fetal Rhesus monkey during the third trimester. The *solid circles* are results for umbilical blood of individual fetuses delivered by cesarean section, and the *open circles* are mean values of 4 samples each (Ballard, unpublished data). The *bars* show mean and SE values for fetal blood from chronically catheterized fetuses at the gestational age ranges shown (Jaffe et al. 1978)

ong and Murphy 1976). Results for both total corticoids and cortisol suggest that the major increase in plasma concentration occurs during the last 5 weeks of pregnancy (Smith and Shearman 1974a, b; Murphy 1982b). The temporal pattern appears similar in infants delivered with and without labor (Murphy 1982b).

An alternative approach to assessing fetal corticoid production is determination of corticosterone sulfate levels in maternal plasma and urine (Fencl et al. 1980b). This corticosteroid is produced by the fetal adrenal and not substantially metabolized nor produced by the placenta. Maternal levels increase during the last two trimesters, with a further rise during labor, and are relatively low in women with anencephalic fetuses. In one woman with no adrenals, concentrations of corticosterone sulfate were in the normal range, and there was a pronounced rise in the week before spontaneous delivery. It is suggested that cortisol production by the fetus follows a similar pattern.

There is no detailed information on the concentration of *free* cortisol during human development. However, levels may be approximated based on information about the ontogeny of serum albumin and CBG. Total serum protein and albumin levels increase throughout the third trimester (Bland 1972), and CBG binding capacity increases late in gestation (Ballard 1979b). Thus, it is likely that the temporal pattern for total serum cortisol also applies to free cortisol, although the magnitude of the increase may be somewhat less because of increased binding.

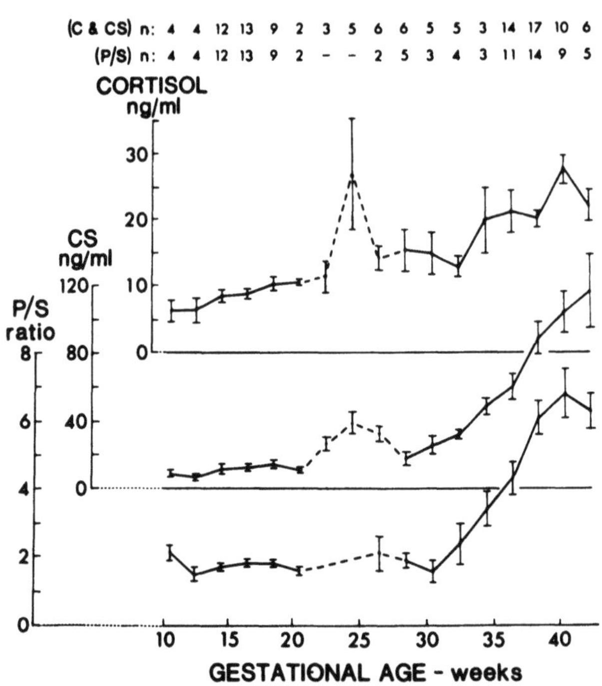

Fig. 4.6. Developmental patterns for cortisol (C), corticoid conjugates (CS), and the palmitic/stearic ratio (P/S) in human amniotic fluid. The correlation coefficient (Pearson's) is 0.76 for CS vs. P/S and 0.58 for C vs. P/S. From Murphy (1978), by permission

An increase in amniotic fluid cortisol between early and late gestation has been confirmed by several investigators (Fencl and Tulchinsky 1975; Murphy et al. 1975; Sivakumaran et al. 1975; Tan et al. 1976; Gewolb et al. 1977; Murphy 1978) and recently reviewed (Schindler 1982). A relationship between amniotic fluid L/S ratio and cortisol (conjugated plus unconjugated) was noted by Fencl and Tulchinsky (1975). Murphy (1978) extended this line of investigation by determining separately unconjugated cortisol and conjugated corticosteroids (cortisol plus corticosterone) in samples of amniotic fluid. As shown in Fig. 4.6, unconjugated cortisol increases in a linear fashion through gestation, while conjugated corticosteroids increase more rapidly beginning around 30 weeks. The palmitic/stearic ratio (P/S), another index of surfactant production, also increased after 30 weeks and had a positive correlation with conjugated corticosteroid values ($r = 0.79$). This relationship is particularly noteworthy since the fetal adrenal is felt to be the major source (via fetal urine) of corticosteroid sulphate in amniotic fluid (Giroud 1971; Fencl et al. 1980a).

A close correlation has been reported between amniotic fluid and lung fluid concentrations for both cortisol and cortisol sulphate (Fencl et al. 1980a). If the secretion of cortisol by fetal lung reflects levels of the steroid within the tissue, then these data are consistent with a developmental increase in cortisol levels within fetal lung. Although lung is apparently not a major source of amniotic fluid corticoids, the gestational rise in amniotic fluid corticosteroids may reflect a similar increase in both fetal plasma and pulmonary tissue. This conclusion is supported by the finding of low cortisol concentrations in amniotic fluid and umbilical arterial plasma of anencephalic fetuses (Fencl et al. 1976).

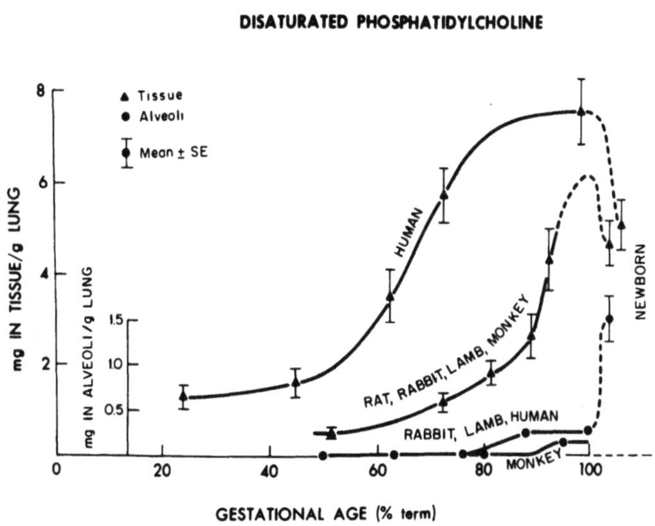

Fig. 4.7. Concentrations of saturated PC in lung tissue and alveolar spaces plotted against gestational age for human and other species. Values are calculated from various literature sources. From Clements and Tooley (1977), by permission

The developmental pattern for lung content of saturated PC in humans and other species is illustrated in Fig. 4.7. Differentiated type II cells (Stahlman and Gray 1978) and surface active material are first detected in lung tissue at 20–24 weeks gestation. Secretion of surfactant into alveolar spaces, as reflected by amniotic fluid assays, begins to increase around 32 weeks gestation. Thus, in the human, the initial appearance of differentiated Type II cells and surfactant occurs relatively early in gestation. Later in pregnancy the accumulation of alveolar surfactant is temporally associated with an increase in both plasma and amniotic fluid cortisol. It has not been feasible to carry out the more definitive study of comparing the amniotic fluid L/S ratio with serum cortisol in individual unstressed fetuses. There are also no data available regarding the rate of saturated PC synthesis in human lung during the third trimester.

4.1.1.6 Other Species

There is a prepartum increase in the concentration of corticosteroids in fetal plasma of goats (Thorburn et al. 1972), cattle (Fairclough et al. 1975), pigs (Dvorak 1972; Randall 1983) and guinea pigs (Jones 1974). In the case of the guinea pig, at least, the concentration of free cortisol has also been shown to increase (Jones, 1974; Dalle and Delost 1980). The developmental pattern of circulating corticosteroids in these species, presumably reflecting fetal adrenal secretion, is generally similar to that in the sheep; however, there is little information on the timing of lung development.

4.1.2 Biochemical Correlations

The relationship between endogenous cortisol concentrations and indices of lung maturation have been examined in studies with both rabbits and sheep.

4.1.2.1 Rabbit Studies

It is now well documented that surgical procedures in the pregnant rabbit accelerate both biochemical and morphologic development of the fetal lung (Ballard et al. 1978; Hitchcock 1979; Robert et al. 1975; Rooney et al. 1979; Rooney et al. 1976; Russell et al. 1974). Surgery with fetal injection affects the rate of choline incorporation into PC, lung PAPase activity, lung deflation stability, lung weight:body weight ratio, and morphologic appearance. It appears that surgery with saline injection is a greater stimulus than surgery alone. Figure 4.8 illustrates the increase in both choline incorporation and plasma corticoids in fetal rabbits subjected to surgery with or without injection of saline. The assays were carried out 48 h after surgery, indicating that there is a prolonged stress response to the surgical procedure. The involvement of corticoids in the response to stress is supported by the observation that metopirone, and to a lesser extent maternal adrenalectomy, reduced the morphologic maturation resulting from surgery (Hitchcock 1979).

A correlation is also observed between the concentration of plasma corticoids and the activity of lung PAPase, an enzyme which is induced by corticosteroid treatment (Fig. 4.9). Endogenous corticoids were measured in con-

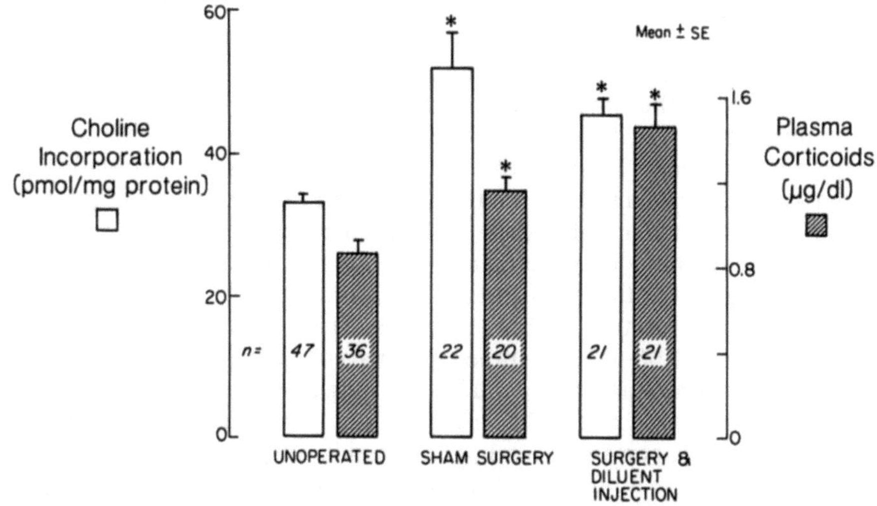

Fig. 4.8. Effect of surgical procedures in the pregnant rabbit on fetal corticoids and choline incorporation by lung tissue. The measurements were performed in fetuses at 26 days gestation 48 h after surgery. *Asterisks*, $p < 0.05$ vs. unoperated animals. From Ballard (1982a), by permission

trol fetuses, those subjected to surgery, and fetuses exposed to maternal treatment with DIMIT which increases plasma corticoids in both mother and fetus (Ballard et al. 1980). These and other findings are consistent with the proposal that fetal stress accelerates lung development, at least in part, through stimulation of endogenous corticosteroids.

4.1.2.2 Sheep Studies

Investigations in the sheep have compared endogenous corticoid levels with lung maturity in unstressed fetuses. These data are particularly convincing because of the strong correlations which have been observed. The large and rela-

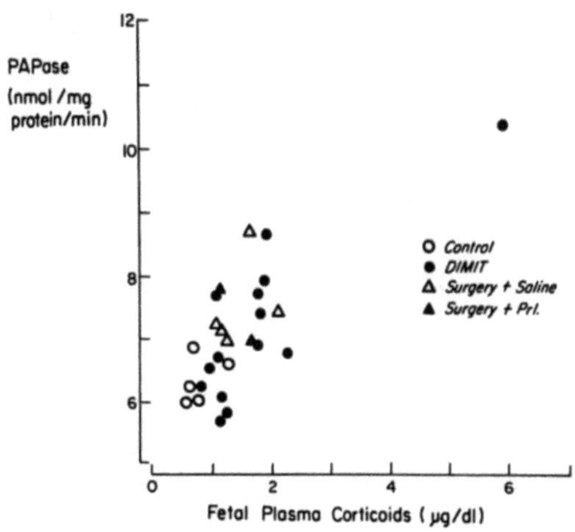

Fig. 4.9. Relationship of fetal corticoids to phosphatidic acid phosphatase (PAPase) activity in lung of 26-day fetal rabbits. The data are mean values for litters of 4–8 fetuses from unoperated rabbits receiving injections of diluent (control), or DIMIT, and operated animals whose fetuses received injections of saline or prolactin. The correlation coefficent is 0.76 ($p < 0.01$). From Ballard et al. (1980)

tively rapid increase in plasma cortisol during the last 7–10 days of gestation produces considerable variability in cortisol levels between fetuses of the same gestational age. This is in part due to the fact that fetal cortisol is more closely related to the time before delivery than to gestational age.

Erenberg et al. (1979) studied five fetuses which were delivered at gestational ages between 138 and 142 days. There was a positive correlation between serum cortisol and both the tracheal fluid L/S ratio ($r = 0.96$, $p < 0.01$) and the specific activity of PAPase in lung homogenate ($r = 0.99$, $p < 0.001$).

A subsequent study by Kitterman et al. (1981) compared a number of indicators of lung maturation with cortisol concentrations in 12 fetal lambs delivered by cesarean section at 123–149 days. There were significant positive correlations ($r = 0.66–0.93$) between plasma cortisol and measurements in 1) pressure-volume studies (V_{40} and V_{10}), 2) lung tissue saturated PC (as a percent of total phospholipids and as mg/g wet lung), 3) lavage fluid saturated PC (as mg/g wet lung, percent of total phospholipids, and percent of saturated PC in tissue plus lavage fluid), and 4) the total (tissue plus lavage fluid) saturated PC. In 8 of 9 measurements with a significant correlation, the r value was greater with fetal cortisol than with gestational age. Fig. 4.10 presents the data for total saturated PC plotted vs. both gestational age and plasma cortisol. There is a wide variation in total saturated PC during late gestation and a close correlation with cortisol, but not gestational age. In addition, morphologic maturation of the lung, as judged by the size of potential air spaces and thickness of alveolar septae, related closer to fetal cortisol concentration than gestational age. Maternal estrogen, maternal progesterone, and fetal prolactin values did not correlate with either age or the various indicators of lung development. These findings illustrate the wide range of pulmonary maturity, as judged by both lung volume and saturated PC content, among fetal sheep during the last few days of normal gestation. Since presumably all fetuses are similarly mature at term, the terminal maturational events must occur over a period as short as a few days. The apparent rapidity of lung maturation in vivo

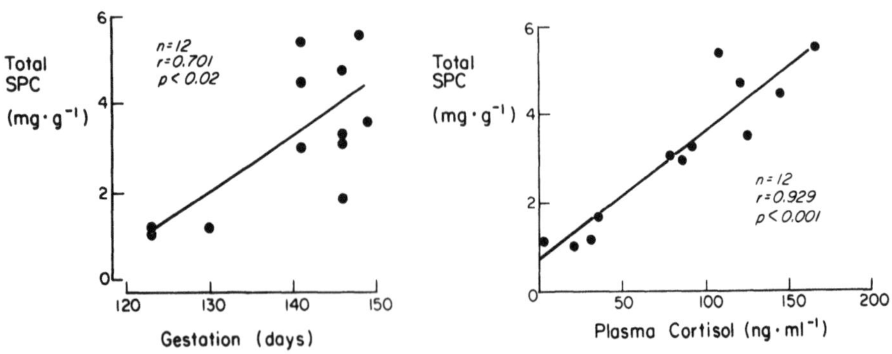

Fig. 4.10. Relationship between lung content of saturated PC (SPC) and both gestational age and plasma cortisol in the fetal sheep. Saturated PC was determined in lung tissue and lavage fluid at cesarean section of undisturbed fetuses. There is considerable variation in the values at late gestation and a close correlation with plasma cortisol. Data from Kitterman et al. (1981), by permission

is consistent with the time course of response to administered glucocorticoids prior to term (Platzker et al. 1975). The strong correlations with plasma cortisol are persuasive evidence for the involvement of endogenous cortisol in this process.

4.2 Experimental Manipulations

4.2.1 Increased Corticosteroid Levels

Experimental maneuvers which increase the concentration of endogenous corticosteroids have been shown to accelerate pulmonary maturation. As discussed in the preceding section, maternal laparotomy and fetal manipulation, with or without injection of saline into the fetus, increases both corticoid levels and lung maturity. Kotas (1973) demonstrated that inoculation of fetal rabbits in utero with *Staphylococcus aureus* enhanced lung pressure-volume properties. Although corticoids were not measured, the injection itself would increase circulating levels.

Infusion of ACTH to premature fetal lambs and rabbits enhances lung maturity and neonatal survival (Liggins 1969; Sundell et al. 1973; Robert et al. 1975; Sundell et al. 1979; Vilos et al. 1983). The doses in the sheep studies ranged from 0.5 μg/h (given in both a pulsatile and continuous form) to supraphysiologic doses of 5 μg/h. The experimental conditions and plasma cortisol levels achieved in these studies are presented in Table 3.9. The highest cortisol values after ACTH are similar to the concentrations found normally at term in the fetal lamb. The results using pulsed ACTH are of particular relevance to the question of the role of endogenous corticosteroids in normal lung development. Compared with nontreated twins, fetuses receiving pulsed ACTH for 72 h prior to delivery at 130 days gestation displayed greater detensibility and deflation stability in pressure-volume studies, and more PC in pulmonary lavage fluid (Vilos et al. 1983). Although it is likely that these effects are mediated through cortisol, it is also possible that ACTH has a direct effect in the lung or stimulates other hormones.

4.2.2 Ablation Procedures

Several experimental approaches to abolishing adrenocortical function have been utilized. In fetal sheep, hydranencephaly produced by ligation of both carotid arteries resulted in low plasma cortisol and delayed appearance of surfactant in tracheal fluid (Platzker et al. 1976). Decapitation of fetal rats (Blackburn et al. 1972; Blackburn et al. 1973) and rabbits (Chiswick et al. 1973; Meyrick et al. 1975) resulted in thicker and more cellular alveolar septae, fewer lamellar bodies and more glycogen in type II cells, and evidence of less surface active material than in control fetuses. When decapitated fetuses were treated with ACTH (Chiswick et al. 1973) or dexamethasone (Farrell et al. 1977), there was an increase in lamellar bodies and rate of choline incorporation, respectively. In pigs, fetal decapitation was associated with non-inflatable lungs at term delivery of live animals (Stryker and Dziuk 1975).

The breakdown of lung glycogen in both fetal rats and rabbits is delayed by in utero decapitation and fully restored by administration of cortisol to the fetuses (Bourbon and Jost 1982). By contrast, suppression of thyroid function by thyroidectomy or methimazole did not affect glycogen metabolism. The timing of the decapitation is of particular interest. Glycogen breakdown, expressed as glycogen content per gram of protein, normally begins by days 20.5 and 27 in the rat and rabbit, respectively. Decapitation had to be performed before day 18.5 and 24 in the rat and rabbit, respectively, to significantly influence glycogen breakdown. This finding might reflect a slow decrease in circulating corticosteroids after decapitation (cortisol values were not reported) or delayed expression (e. g., 3 days in the rabbit) of glucocorticoid action in the lung.

Interpretation of these ablation experiments, with relationship to endogenous corticosteroids, is difficult because of the decrease in many hormones secondary to ablation of the hypothalamus and pituitary. Also, the neck ligature used for decapitation obstructs the trachea and severs the spinal cord. Both the central nervous system and retention of lung fluid, with its associated effects on fetal breathing patterns, alter the rate of lung growth and maturation (Kitterman 1984; Liggins et al. 1981b; Wigglesworth and Desai 1979).

Metopirone, an inhibitor of adrenal 11 β-hydroxylase activity, has been employed as a means to more selectively reduce fetal corticosteroid concentration (Nelson et al. 1976; Vidyasagur and Chernick 1975). In rabbits, this treatment was associated with some reduction in the amount of tissue surfactant, but other indices of pulmonary maturation were unaffected. These experiments are difficult to interpret because of the rapid clearance of metopirone in rabbits and the lack of data on plasma corticoids after treatment. In two pregnant baboons treated with continuous infusion of metopirone for 5 days in late gestation, there was a delay in the expected increase in amniotic fluid L/S ratio. Similar treatment in five other animals did not affect deflation stability in pressure-volume studies or the minimal surface tension of lung extract (Kling and Kotas 1975).

Vilos et al. (1985) have recently reported that accelerated lung maturation (distensibility and lavage PC) after ACTH infusion is blocked by simultaneous administration of metopirone, consistent with mediation through endogenous cortisol. They also find that treatment of one twin in utero produces a mature pressure-volume curve at preterm birth in the infused fetus but not in the untreated twin. These results suggest that the mechanics of labor per se are not involved in the maturation of lung occurring with normal labor and birth.

The effect of hypophysectomy and replacement hormone therapy was studied in sheep by Liggins et al. (1981a). A group of 22 fetuses was hypophysectomized by a cryosurgical approach at 99–122 days pregnancy. Successful ablation of pituitary function was indicated by brain histology, low plasma levels of prolactin and cortisol, and nonresponsiveness to TRH. The animals remained undisturbed until term when the fetuses were infused with either $ACTH_{1-24}$ or cortisol sodium succinate for 72–84 h. An untreated group of hypophysectomized fetuses were delivered at the same gestational age without surgery or infusion. Pressure-volume studies and lipid analyses of the fetal lung were compared with a group of intact fetuses.

Lung weight as a percent of body weight was decreased in the hypophysectomized groups receiving cortisol or ACTH compared with intact controls. Adrenal weight was less than 50 % of control in hypophysectomized animals without treatment or receiving cortisol, but was normal in animals infused with ACTH. Cortisol infusion produced fetal plasma cortisol concentrations of about 18 μg/dl, whereas maximal concentrations with ACTH infusion were approximately 9 μg/dl.

The results of this study are presented in Table 4.4. Compared with intact fetuses, hypophysectomy alone decreased lung volume at both 40 and 5 cmH_2O pressure, decreased the content of total phospholipids and saturated PC in lung tissue, and markedly reduced the amount of saturated PC in lavage fluid. These findings indicate that hypophysectomy impairs the synthesis and release of surfactant, as well as structural development. Treatment with cortisol did not affect any of the parameters studied. With infusion of ACTH, however, there was an increase in lung volumes, tissue total phospholipid, and lavage fluid saturated PC compared to untreated hypophysectomized fetuses. The increase in distensibility and alveolar saturated PC with ACTH treatment suggest increased release of surfactant.

These data clearly demonstrate retarded lung maturation in hypophysectomized fetuses, supporting the proposed role of endogenous hormones in this process. By term, the degree of lung maturation in the hypophysectomized fetuses was comparable to that of intact fetuses at approximately 130 days gestation (Kitterman et al. 1981). This indicates a very slow rate of lung maturation in the absence of all pituitary hormones. The failure of cortisol infusions to stimulate lung development is perhaps not unexpected in view of the accumulating evidence that the lung is under multi-hormonal regulation. The surpris-

Table 4.4. Effects of hypophysectomy (HPX) and treatment with cortisol or $ACTH_{1-24}$ on lung development in fetal sheep (Liggins et al. 1981a). Data are means ± SD

	Controls (n = 7)	HPX (n = 6)	HPX + cortisol (n = 6)	HPX + ACTH (n = 6)
Gestational age at delivery (days)	144.5 ± 3.5	152.2 ± 2.9	155.0 ± 2.1	154.2 ± 3.9
Lung volume (ml/kg)				
40 cm H_2O	15.1 ± 6.1	4.5 ± 2.6[a]	6.4 ± 5.1[a]	12.3 ± 2.6[b,c]
5 cm H_2O	10.7 ± 4.0	3.3 ± 2.4[a]	3.1 ± 2.9[a]	8.5 ± 2.5[b]
Lung tissue				
Phospholipids (mg/g)	15.2 ± 2.8	10.1 ± 1.2[a]	12.4 ± 3.2	14.8 ± 3.8[b]
Saturated PC (mg/g)	3.62 ± 0.76	1.44 ± 0.37[a]	1.73 ± 0.68[a]	2.42 ± 0.79[a]
(mg/mg DNA)	0.51 ± 0.13	0.15 ± 0.06[a]	0.21 ± 0.10[a]	0.30 ± 0.23[a]
Lung lavage				
Saturated PC (mg/g)	0.63 ± 0.48	0.04 ± 0.06[a]	< 0.01[a]	0.13 ± 0.10[a,b,c]
(% phospholipid)	47.3 ± 11.1	32.2 ± 11.5	32.0 ± 16.6	46.4 ± 9.3

[a] $P < 0.05$ control vs. HPX groups
[b] $P < 0.05$ HPX vs. cortisol and ACTH groups
[c] $P < 0.05$ cortisol vs. ACTH groups

ing finding in this study was the effectiveness of ACTH vs. cortisol on lung maturity. The authors suggest that the response to ACTH could be mediated by adrenal products other than cortisol (e. g., catecholamines) or by direct ACTH effects in the lung. Other differences between the two treated groups may have affected the outcome. Cortisol concentrations prior to infusion were higher in the ACTH group (approximately 2.8 μg/dl) than in the cortisol-induced group (approximately 1.4 μg/dl). Also, ACTH was infused for 84 h compared with 72 h for cortisol, and different cortisol concentrations were achieved.

The lungs of the hypophysectomized lambs were also examined with regard to structural maturity (Crone et al. 1983). By morphometric analysis of alveolar wall thickness and relative numbers of Type I and Type II cells, lungs of hypophysectomized fetuses at term resembled those of 123-day fetuses. Thus hypophysectomy markedly retarded both structural and biochemical aspects of lung development. Treatment with either ACTH or cortisol resulted in lungs morphologically similar to intact animals at term. This finding contrasts sharply with the failure of cortisol to enhance lung distensibility and phopholipid content, and suggests that cortisol stimulated structural but not functional development whereas ACTH enhanced both parameters. These results may indicate a time effect for different actions of cortisol in the lung, or may reflect the involvement of other hormones in some but not all effects of cortisol.

4.2.3 Studies with Cultured Lung Tissue

The experience with fetal lung in culture is relevant to the question of the role of endogenous corticosteroids in the maturational process. Early studies with organ culture of lung and other fetal tissues demonstrated that differentiation continues under these in vitro conditions (Chen 1954; Sorokin 1961; Alescio and Dani 1972; Funkhouser et al. 1976; Minor 1979). However, these experiments utilized culture medium containing relatively high concentrations of serum which exposed the tissue to corticosteroids and other endogenous hormones. More recently, attention has turned to the contribution of serum and hormones in the differentiation which is observed in vitro. Contrasting results have been obtained in different culture systems, leaving the question of autoregulation vs. hormonal requirement unresolved.

Torday (1980) examined the synthesis of DNA and saturated PC in monolayer cultures obtained by trypsin treatment of fetal rabbit lung. The cells were cultured in Ham's F-10 medium supplemented with 10% calf serum, charcoal-treated calf serum, or adrenalectomized calf serum. Cells cultured in the presence of calf serum continued to grow and demonstrated increasing rates of saturated PC synthesis during 12 days of culture. These increases did not occur when cells were cultured in medium supplemented with serum which was either charcoal-treated (removing corticosteroids and other low molecular weight compounds) or from adrenalectomized calves. Addition of cortisol to cultures containing charcoal-treated serum restored both saturated PC and DNA synthesis, whereas steroids without glucocorticoid activity were inactive. It was concluded that maturation of rabbit lung cells in culture is de-

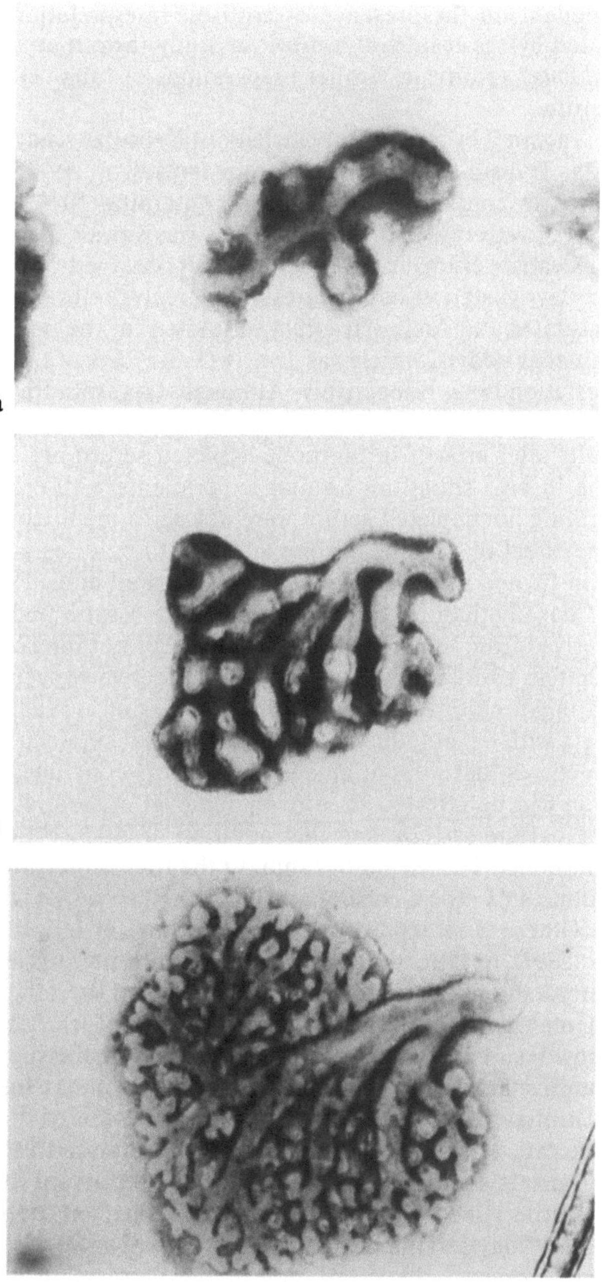

a

b

c

Fig. 4.11 a–c. Morphologic development of fetal rat lung in organ culture. Intact, individual lungs of 14-day fetuses were cultured in Waymouth's medium containing 1 % bovine serum. Photomicrographs (× 25) of lung before culture (**a**), after 1 day in culture (**b**), and 4 days in culture (**c**). From Gross and Wilson (1983), by permission

pendent on the presence of cortisol. Interpretation of these data is complicated by the results of a previous study (Smith et al. 1974), in which cortisol *inhibited* growth in similar preparations of lung cells cultured with untreated serum.

Tanswell et al. (1983a) carried out a similar study with lung cells from fetal rats. Trypsin-dispersed cells from fetuses of 18–22 days gestation were cultured to confluence in medium containing 10% carbon-treated calf serum. Cell growth under these conditions was slower than with medium containing untreated serum. At confluence, cells obtained from fetuses of 18, 19, 20 and 22 days gestation had progressively greater rates of choline incorporation into saturated PC. A similar effect was noted for the percentage of cells containing lamellar bodies, which was 2 %, 18 % and 26 % of the cells in 18, 19 and 22-day gestation lung, respectively. Although data from freshly isolated lung tissue or cells at the various gestational ages were not presented for comparison, the results after growth in hormone-depleted serum are in general agreement with the in vivo situation. Similar experiments with cells grown in medium containing nondepleted serum were not performed. However, in a separate paper, the effect of dexamethasone addition to cultures grown in medium with carbon-treated serum was examined (Tanswell et al. 1983b). Low concentrations of dexamethasone (0.055 nM) stimulated saturated PC synthesis in cultures derived from lungs of 18 and 20 days, but not for 22 days. This dose is approximately 10-fold less than the lowest effective concentration of dexamethasone in organ culture of fetal rat lung (Gross et al. 1983). Interpretation of these data with dexamethasone is difficult because of variable and biphasic response curves that were attained. The authors conclude that fetal lung differentiation can be arrested in vitro by removal of steroid and other hormones from the culture system, and that addition of glucocorticoids can partially reverse this effect. These findings support the results of Torday (1980) with monolayer cultures of rabbit cells.

Other recent studies with organ culture of lung suggest that differentiation proceeds in vitro under conditions where there is little or no serum present. Gross and Wilson (1983) maintained fetal rat lung in organ culture supplemented with 1% fetal calf serum. Under these conditions, there was both growth and morphologic differentiation of the tissue as illustrated in Fig. 4.11. During the six days in culture the DNA content increased nearly 3-fold and considerable airway branching with formation of terminal air sacs is evident. The rate of choline incorporation into saturated PC as a function of time in culture is shown in Fig. 4.12. Independent of the initial age of the tissue at culturing, incorporation increases at the same equivalent gestational age (18–20 days). This developmental pattern is very similar to that observed in vivo; however, the magnitude of the increase in both rate of synthesis and content of saturated PC during culture is less than observed in vivo. Nuclear binding capacity for dexamethasone also increased during culture by an amount equivalent to that in vivo. Because of the low concentrations of hormones in this culture system (concentrations of cortisol, T_3 and T_4 were 0.4, 0.015 and 1.7 nM, respectively), the authors suggest that circulating hormones in vivo modulate the process of lung maturation but are not necessary for continued differentiation. This interpretation implies that the temporal pattern of

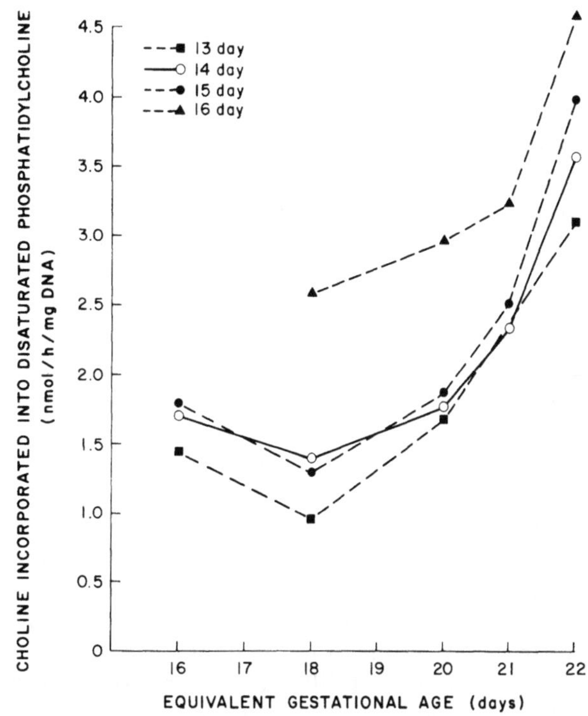

Fig. 4.12. Choline incorporation into saturated PC by explant of 13– through 16-day fetal rat lung in culture. Lung was cultured as described for Fig. 4.11 and data are mean values for 1–4 experiments. From Gross and Wilson (1983), by permission

lung development is determined by intrapulmonary (genetic) factors which are influenced but not dependent upon circulating hormones.

Organotypic cultures (in gelatin sponges) prepared with 20-day fetal rat lung cells were examined by Simpson et al. (1985). Differentiation of epithelial cells was equivalent in cultures fed with medium containing 10 % charcoal-treated fetal calf serum versus untreated serum. Aronson (1984) cultured explants of 13-day fetal rat lung in serum-free medium. After 5 days of culture, birefringent granules were observed by polarized light microscopy. The birefringence pattern resembled that seen with a population of adult lung cells enriched for type II cells, suggesting the appearance of intracellular lamellar bodies during culture without added hormones.

Two groups have examined PC synthesis in organ cultures of fetal rabbit lung. In the study by Gross et al. (1983), lung from 24-day gestation fetuses was cultured in serum-free Waymouth's medium in an atmosphere of 95 % oxygen. Under these conditions, the rate of PC synthesis began to increase after 2 days of culturing in the absence of any hormone. Repeated washings of the tissue at the time of culture initiation decreased but did not eliminate this rise in PC synthesis. Since endogenous cortisol would be removed from the tissue under these conditions, these results indicate that the change during culture occurs in the absence of glucocorticoid.

Snyder et al. (1981b) and Longmuir et al. (1981) cultured rabbit using Waymouth's medium and an atmosphere of 95 % air. With 19-day tissue grown in the absence of serum, there was no increase in the rate of choline incorporation (per mg protein) by day 11 compared with day 1; however, the rate did double in the last 4 days after an initial decline. Explants exposed to culture medium containing 10 % fetal calf serum had an overall (day 11 vs. day 1) increase in choline incorporation and PC content, beginning after 7 days of culture, which closely mimicked the in vivo pattern. It is worth noting that 10 % fetal calf serum in the culture medium (Tanswell et al., 1983; Gross and Wilson, 1983) would provide considerably less cortisol to the tissue than occurs in vivo (see Sect. 4.1.1.3). By light and electron microscopy, cultures maintained without serum showed intact and viable cells, no apparent capillaries or other blood vessels, enlargement of ductal lumina, and the appearance of cuboidal epithelial cells with lamellated inclusions. Type I cells were only rarely observed. The overall tissue structure after 6 days of culture was considered to be very similar to that of 25-day fetuses, implying that morphologic maturation occurred in the absence of serum or added hormones. Similar structural development was observed after culture of 23-day lung for 6 days with 10 % serum.

The findings of Snyder et al. (1981b) for PC synthesis are somewhat different from the results of Gross et al. (1983). However, it can be noted that the oxygen environment differed, and that the cultures were initiated with different gestational age material. It is possible that fetal lung at 19 days gestation has not been exposed to endogenous corticoids and other hormones to a significant extent, and therefore is dependent on the presence of serum in the culture medium. By contrast, lung at 24 days gestation may have already been partially stimulated by the endogenous hormonal milieu.

In studies with human tissue, Snyder and co-workers (Snyder et al. 1981a; Mendelson et al. 1981; Heifetz and Snyder 1981; Okazaki et al. 1982) maintained lung explants from abortuses at 16–22 weeks in culture for up to 10 days. In the absence of serum or any hormones, there was a several-fold increase in PC synthesis and content during the incubation period (Table 4.5). The addition of cortisol, in the presence of prolactin or insulin plus prolactin, caused an earlier increase in the rate of PC synthesis during culture. Surpri-

Table 4.5. Development of the surfactant system in cultured human fetal lung (Mendelson et al. 1981). Lung explants from a 20-week human fetus were cultured on lens paper-covered steel grids floating on Waymouth's MB 752/1 medium without serum or added hormones

Incubation days	Choline incorporated into PC (nmol/24 h/mg protein)	PC content (nmol/P/mg protein)
2	7.0	133
4	9.0	163
6	16.4	290
8	37.8	316

singly, none of the hormonal combinations increased the percent of PC which was saturated. By light and electron microscopy, both the pre-alveolar epithelium and mesenchymal tissues were well maintained during culture. At the beginning of the incubation, epithelial cells contained few small microvilli, abundant glycogen, little rough endoplasmic reticulum or golgi apparatus, and no apparent lamellar bodies. By 6 days in culture, in the absence of hormones and both with and without serum, most of the ductal epithelial cells resembled mature type II cells, as evidenced by increased endoplasmic reticulum and golgi apparatus, decreased glycogen, prominent microvilli, and lamellated inclusions. Results were similar during culture in serum-free Waymouth's medium and in medium containing heat-inactivated fetal calf serum. Addition of cortisol, in either the presence or absence of calf serum, resulted in more and larger lamellar bodies within the epithelial cells, consistent with the biochemical data. Since mature type II cells are normally found in human fetal lung only after 24 weeks (Stahlman and Gray, 1978), the authors conclude that accelerated differentiation occurs during culture and is further stimulated by glucocorticoid. This conclusion is supported by a recent study of second trimester human lung by Gonzales et al. (1985). In similar experiments with lung tissue from 7–12 week abortuses, however, Zsolani and Gyevai (1984) found no spontaneous appearance of lamellar bodies in epithelial cells after culture for 3 weeks in the presence of 20 % serum; addition of dexamethasone during the last 5 days produced fully developed lamellar bodies. Considered together, these various results indicate that the amount and degree of differentiation during explant culture without hormones may depend on the gestational age of the tissue. Moreover, responsiveness to corticosteroid, during organ culture at least, is apparently acquired as early as the end of the first trimester.

The stimulus for accelerated development during organ culture is not known. It is possible that the change in oxygen tension from in vivo to in vitro acts as a stimulus for hypertrophy of type II cells such as occurs with injury. Alternatively, lung maturation may be under an inhibitory influence in vivo. It is noteworthy that undifferentiated lungs from fetal rats (Funkhouser et al. 1976) and rabbits (Snyder et al. 1981b) which are maintained in organ culture develop ductal epithelium composed primarily of type II cells. While it is clear that morphologic changes occur in culture in the absence of added hormones, it is not established that these changes are identical to those occurring normally in vivo (see Chap. 1).

One possibility for the altered morphologic pattern in culture is that both culture per se and exposure to glucocorticoid, to an even greater extent, synchronize differentiation of epithelial cells. This would result in virtually all cells accumulating lamellar bodies and other features characteristic of type II cells at the same time. In vivo differentiation, by contrast, proceeds more slowly and with considerable variability between cells, resulting in a mixed pattern of epithelial cells at any given time. The failure to observe type I cells in cultured lung tissue has not been explained. It is possible that with longer times in culture differentiation of type I from type II cells might occur. Alternatively, the conditions in vitro may not be suitable for appearance of type I cells. For example, the close proximity of endothelial cells may be important in vivo for type II cell division and differentiation into type I cells. In cultured tissue, however, endothelial cells are relatively sparse initially, do not proliferate, and, in fact, tend not to survive with continued culture. Another possibility is that additional circulating factors or hormones, other than cortisol or prolactin, are necessary for development of the type I cell.

4.3 Sources of Increased Corticosteroids

Endogenous corticosteroids could influence the timing of lung development through increased availability to lung cells and/or through increased sensitivity of cells to hormonal influence. In most species, it is clear that the lung is exposed to rising concentrations of circulating corticoids with advancing gestation. This section reviews several possible mechanisms for increasing both circulating and tissue concentrations of corticosteroids. In addition, the possible role of increasing glucocorticoid receptor concentration within lung cells is discussed as a mechanism for amplifying glucocorticoid effects.

4.3.1 Steroidogenesis

As noted in Sec. 4.1.1, plasma concentrations of total corticosteroids increase during gestation in fetuses of most species. Where the question has been studied (e.g., in the sheep), it is clear that this rise reflects increased adrenal production of corticoids rather than a decreasing metabolic clearance rate (Liggins 1976; Bassett and Thorburn 1973). However, the events responsible for increased fetal adrenocortical activity are uncertain. Although plasma concentrations of immunoreactive ACTH increase during late gestation in the fetal sheep, the rise occurs after the start of the cortisol surge. Except near term, the fetal adrenal shows little response to administered ACTH. Several possible mechanisms for the developmental change in adrenal function have been considered experimentally. These include a developmental increase in secretory capacity of the fetal adrenal (via an increase in 17α-hydroxylase activity, a shift in the ratio of cortisol to corticosterone production, and/or increased responsiveness to ACTH), decreasing inhibition of ACTH function by higher molecular weight precursors from the pituitary, development of pulsatile ACTH secretion, and possible adrenocorticotrophic effects of other hormones such as prolactin, α-MSH, enkephalins, prostaglandins and growth hormone (Nathanielsz et al. 1972; Jones et al. 1977a; Jones et al. 1977b, Liggins et al. 1977; Glickman et al. 1979; Llanos et al. 1979; Glickman and Challis, 1980; Magyar et al. 1980b; Roebuck et al. 1980; Challis et al. 1982). Although the details of the process remain controversial (see Challis et al. (1984) for review), it is clear that the fetal rather than the maternal adrenal is responsible for the rise in fetal corticoids in the sheep. In other species, most notably in the human, the maternal adrenal may make a substantial contribution to the fetal supply of cortisol. Maternal concentrations of both total and free cortisol increase during gestation and rise abruptly during labor (Ballard 1979b; Lefebvre et al. 1970; Carr et al. 1981), and passage of cortisol from mother to fetus readily occurs (discussed in Chap. 6).

4.3.2 Plasma Binding

In the rat and mouse, adrenal size and plasma concentrations of total corticosterone decrease in late gestation. In these species, however, there is an increasing concentration of free cortisol due to a decline in plasma CBG. It appears that the change in plasma binding of corticosteroid is the major mechanism for increasing the hormone supply to the lung and other responsive tissues. The factors responsible for the decrease in CBG are not known.

Developmental changes in levels of CBG also contribute to the timing of the cortisol rise in the fetal sheep. In this species, cortisol binding capacity in plasma increases several-fold during the last trimester (Fairclough and Liggins 1975; Ballard et al. 1982b). Because the rise in CBG precedes the increase in total plasma cortisol concentrations, levels of free cortisol do not begin to increase until several days after total corticoids increase. The developmental rise in CBG requires an intact fetal pituitary, but the responsible hormone(s) has not been identified (Ballard et al. 1982b; Ballard et al. 1983).

The concentration of free corticoids may also be influenced by changes in serum albumin concentrations. In many species there is an increase in albumin concentration in the fetus during late gestation (e.g., rabbit, sheep and human). This change would tend to decrease the concentration of free corticosteroids, but the relative impact is probably slight.

4.3.3 Tissue Uptake and Responsiveness

As discussed in Chap. 3, there is an increase in glucocorticoid receptor concentration in lung cells of the rat and rabbit during late fetal life. Since the interaction between glucocorticoid and receptor is a second order reaction, formation of steroid-receptor complex would be enhanced by greater receptor concentration per se. Accordingly, glucocorticoid stimulation of lung maturation in these species could conceivably occur without any elevation of circulating free cortisol concentrations. The relative importance of this mechanism for the effects of endogenous corticosteroids remains to be defined.

A second theoretical possibility for increasing the uptake of glucocorticoids would be developmental changes in the permeability of lung cells to protein-bound steroids. Although there is considerable evidence that only unbound corticoids are physiologically active in most tissues, there are also data suggesting that protein-bound hormone is taken up by liver cells (reviewed in Ballard 1979b). Furthermore, recent studies with other steroid hormones argue for physiologic activity of protein-bound steroid (Siiteri et al. 1982). Thus, it is conceivable that increasing uptake of corticosteroid bound to either albumin or CBG could occur in the developing fetal lung and contribute to the supply of available glucocorticoid.

Glucocorticoid responsiveness in the lung may also result in part from developmental changes in intracellular processes other than receptor. Such events could be under either genetic or hormonal regulation. This possibility is supported by the observed effect of gestational age on the responsiveness of PC synthesis in fetal lung to glucocorticoid (Smith et al. 1974b; Gross et al. 1983).

4.3.4 Cortisone:Cortisol Interconversion

Interconversion of (inactive) cortisone and (active) cortisol is catalyzed by the enzyme 11-β-hydroxysteroid dehydrogenase (E.C. 1.1.1.146). This enzyme is known to occur in various tissues of animals and man. The conversion of cortisone to cortisol in both peripheral tissues and in the lung influences the availability of cortisol to lung cells.

4.3.4.1 Metabolism in Placenta and Membranes

It has been recognized for many years that cortisone is the predominant corticosteroid in human placenta and in fetal plasma (De Courcy et al. 1952; Bro-Rasmussen et al. 1962), whereas relatively low levels occur in adult serum. Cortisone is also present in relatively high concentrations in fetal plasma of other species, such as the Rhesus monkey (Kittinger 1974) and the rabbit (Barr et al. 1980). The difference in the cortisone:cortisol ratio on the two sides of the placenta results in large part from metabolism of maternal cortisol in the placenta. Oxidative activity (i.e., cortisol to cortisone conversion) is observed in human placental tissue from as early as 8 weeks gestation until term, whereas little, if any, reductive activity is present; labor and parturition do not influence the rate of cortisone production by placenta (Osinski 1960; Levitz et al. 1978; Bernal et al. 1980; Murphy 1981; Giannopoulos et al. 1982; Bernal et al. 1982). Most of the circulating pool of cortisone in the fetal monkey is also felt to arise from placental metabolism of maternal cortisol (Kittinger 1974; Mitchell et al. 1981; Mitchell et al. 1982). As in other tissues, placental 11-β-hydroxysteroid dehydrogenase is localized in the microsomal fraction and the direction of the reaction is influenced by the relative concentrations of NADP and NADPH and in some cases NAD and NADH. Most studies of placental enzymes have utilized incubation of minced tissues without additional cofactors; these results presumably reflect the direction and magnitude of the reaction in vivo.

Studies of dehydrogenase activity in human fetal membranes (amnion and chorion) have revealed primarily reductive activity (cortisone to cortisol) (Tanswell et al. 1977; Tanswell and Smith 1978; Bernal et al. 1980; Murphy 1981; Giannopoulos et al. 1982). The more recent studies with this tissue indicate that the activity detected in membrane preparations is primarily due to contaminating decidua (Bernal et al. 1980; Murphy 1981; Giannopoulos et al. 1982). Net production of cortisol from cortisone is found as early as 13 weeks gestation in the human; some, but not all, studies find an increase in activity during gestation. It has been proposed that reduction of cortisone in the membranes (decidua) might account for the developmental pattern of the cortisol:cortisone ratio in amniotic fluid. According to Murphy (1977) the ratio of (unconjugated) cortisol:cortisone increases from 0.33 at 11–16 weeks to 3.8 by 36–40 weeks gestation. Similar values are reported by Smith et al. (1977a). The concentration of cortisol in amniotic fluid also increases during gestation, as previously discussed.

In the sheep, cortisol concentration in amniotic fluid rises during the third trimester while that of cortisone falls. A positive correlation between the cortisol:cortisone ratio and concentration of saturated PC in amniotic fluid is reported by Smith et al. (1977b). Since there is little passage of maternal steroids across the sheep placenta during the third trimester, amniotic fluid cortisone in this species may arise primarily from peripheral metabolism of cortisol derived from the fetal adrenal rather than from the maternal adrenal as occurs in primates.

The factors regulating both oxidative and reductive steroid metabolism in decidua are unknown. Increased production of cortisol might result from either increased metabolism of cortisone to cortisol or decreased conversion in the reverse direction. Relative concentrations of NADP and NADPH might change during gestation and, in part, influence production rates.

The possible relationship of amniotic fluid cortisol to lung maturation in the human has been examined. Among infants born at less than 32 weeks gestation, the cortisol:cortisone ratio was lower in eight infants who developed RDS compared with four who did not (Smith et al. 1977a). In a subsequent study, lower values for steroid reductive activity in amniotic membranes were generally found for infants who developed RDS compared with control infants (Tanswell and Smith 1978). These observations support the concept that cortisol production by the decidua is a major source of free cortisol in amniotic fluid. Cortisol in amniotic fluid could be available to the fetus by swallowing, absorption through fetal skin, or transfer via membrane vasculature (Migeon et al. 1961; Carson et al. 1979; Murphy 1982a).

Both cortisone and cortisol are present in relatively low concentrations in amniotic fluid (0.1–0.5 μg/dl) of third trimester rabbits; between 28 and 30 days, however, cortisol increases coincident with the increase in maternal cortisol level (Barr et al. 1980). The transfer of corticosteroid from amniotic fluid to the fetal circulation has been studied in anesthetized rabbits by Lugg and Nicholas (1983). After injection, radiolabeled cortisone disappeared from amniotic fluid with a halftime of about 30 min. By 60 min, the concentration of labeled cortisol in the fetal circulation was 18 % of the initial concentration of cortisone in the amniotic fluid. Of the labeled steroid remaining in amniotic fluid at 60 min, the majority represented cortisol. When radiolabeled cortisol was injected into amniotic fluid, there was a relatively slow decrease in total radioactivity and little conversion to cortisone; at 60 min the plasma concentration of cortisol was about 48 % of the initial amniotic fluid level. These findings are similar to the kinetics for radiolabeled cortisol in the fetal sheep (Carson et al. 1979). The slower clearance of cortisol might result from binding by CBG in amniotic fluid whereas cortisone has a low affinity for binding. Thus, under these experimental conditions, both amniotic fluid cortisone, and to a lesser extent cortisol, are sources of cortisol for the fetal rabbit. Based on the kinetic data, it would appear that most of the fetal cortisol of amniotic origin arises from conversion of cortisone by fetal tissues.

4.3.4.2 Metabolism in Fetal Lung

The presence of 11-β-hydroxysteroid dehydrogenase activity in lung tissue has been known for a number of years (Koerner 1966). Studies over the past decade have examined the properties, regulation, ontogeny, and relationship to fetal lung maturation. It has been proposed that conversion of cortisone to cortisol within lung tissue is a major source of glucocorticoid for pulmonary cells. The evidence for this mechanism is substantial in some species but remains controversial in the case of the human.

Assay of 11-β-hydroxysteroid dehydrogenase activity has involved lung perfusion or incubation of either intact tissue or subcellular fractions with tritiated corticosteroid. After the incubation, steroids are extracted and separated by thin layer or column chromatography. In many studies there have been either parallel incubations with labeled cortisone and labeled cortisol, or simultaneous incubation with both steroids labeled with different isotopes (^{3}H vs. ^{14}C). This approach has allowed simultaneous determination of the dehydrogenase activity in both directions and calculation of net reductive or oxidative activity. The data have alternately been expressed as percent conversion for a specified time interval of incubation, or more rigorously as rate of conversion (moles of steroid formed per min per unit protein or DNA). Since the total amount of steroid formed can be substantial, appropriate concentrations of substrate are required; the Km for both cortisone and cortisol in vitro is in the range of 2–4 μM (Nicholas and Lugg, 1982). In most systems, particularly with in vitro assays, the direction of the reaction is determined by the relative concentrations of NADP and NADPH (Nicholas and Lugg 1982); however, Abramowitz et al. (1982) found only oxidative activity in homogenate of human fetal lung even in the presence of NADPH. There is one report that the oxygen tension influences the amount of reductase activity in human fibroblasts (Tanswell and Smith 1980).

Early studies on this question indicated that fetal tissues, including the lung, of the human and guinea pig actively converted cortisol to cortisone but not vice versa (Pasqualini et al. 1970a; Pasqualini et al. 1970b). The first study to demonstrate conversion of cortisone to cortisol by cultured lung cells was published by Smith et al. (1973). Monolayer cultures of mixed cells from midgestation human fetal lung converted cortisone to cortisol but there was no significant conversion of cortisol to cortisone. Unter the same incubation conditions, mixed populations of cells from fetal larynx, trachea and esophagus, as well as two populations of skin fibroblasts, showed no ability to convert cortisone to cortisol but did support some metabolism of cortisol to cortisone. The possible physiologic significance of the steroid metabolism was indicated by the finding that both cortisol and cortisone stimulated the growth rate of the lung cells.

Subsequent studies with human tissue have established that lung fibroblasts actively generate cortisol. Cultures derived from lung mesenchymal cells and fibroblasts of fetal and adult lung, respectively, were found to be approximately ten times more active in reduction of cortisone than fibroblasts cultured from skin of the same individuals (Aronson et al. 1983). A similar level of conversion occurs in established lung fibroblast lines (WI-38 and IMR-90), and cortisone is equivalent to cortisol in stimulating growth of WI-38 cells (Aronson et al. 1983; Kondo et al. 1983).

A different picture of corticosteroid metabolism by human fetal lung arose from the study by Murphy et al. (1978). Samples of tissue were obtained at hysterotomy and autopsy, minced and incubated in saline at 37 °C with [^{3}H] cortisol or [^{3}H] cortisone. With samples from first and second trimester abortions, the conversion rate of cortisol to cortisone was 5–25 times greater than the reductive reaction. This finding was supported by the presence of more cortisone than cortisol in lung tissue. With tissue from anencephalic infants who delivered nearer term, conversion was somewhat less but still predominantly oxidative. There was little metabolic activity in either direction found in postmortem tissue from liveborn infants dying of RDS and prematurity, possibly reflecting technical problems in the assay with damaged and hemorrhagic tissue. These results with lung tissue in vitro agree with in vivo perfusion data (Pasqualini et al. 1970a) but are in contrast with the findings in cultured fibroblasts.

To address this discrepancy for human tissue, a subsequent study by Abramovitz et al. (1982) compared corticosteroid metabolism in mixed cell monolayer cultures, explants in culture, and homogenates of lung tissue from 9–13 weeks gestation human fetuses. In both the monolayer and the explant cultures, metabolism was initially primarily oxidative. With continued time in culture, cortisone to cortisol conversion increased in both systems (Fig. 4.13). This change in corticosteroid conversion was associated with fibroblast outgrowth in the explant cultures and overgrowth in monolayer cultures. In assays with lung homogenates, only oxidative activity was detected. Rapid metabolism of cortisol has also been observed with explants from second trimester human lung (Ballard, unpublished data). These results imply that lung fibroblasts exhibit reductive activity while other cell types exhibit predominantly oxidative activity. Presumably, metabolism by whole lung tissue primarily reflects enzyme activity in nonfibroblastic cells. Of note, the human cell line A-549, which may have derived from the Type II cell, converts corti-

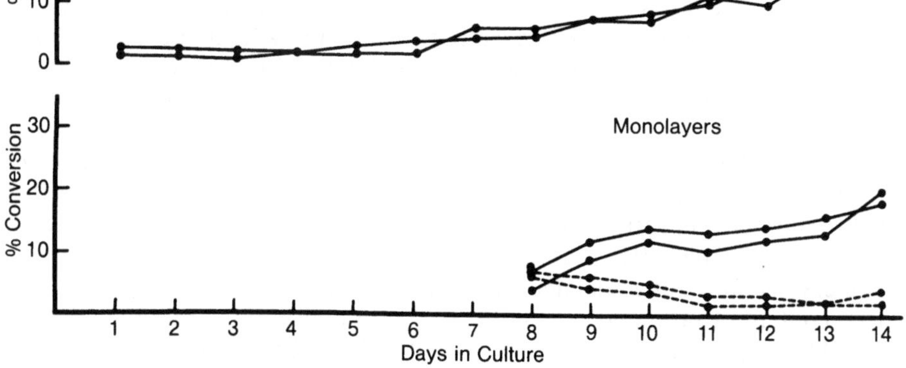

Fig. 4.13. Interconversion of cortisone and cortisol by human fetal lung in culture. Lung tissue from human abortuses of 9–13 weeks gestation was cultured as explants (*upper set* of curves) or as monolayers prepared by treatment with trypsin (*lower set* of curves). The percent conversion of tritiated steroid (36 nM) per 24 h is shown. From Abramovitz et al. (1982), by permission

sol to cortisone but not vice versa. Consistent with this finding, cortisol produced a modest stimulation of choline incorporation into PC, whereas cortisone at the same concentration was inactive (Smith 1977). One interpretation of the human data is that two different enzymes, catalyzing metabolism in opposite directions, are found in fibroblasts vs. other pulmonary cell types. Recent evidence suggests that independent but closely associated enzymes catalyze the the oxidative and reductive reactions in the liver (Lakshmi and Monder 1985). Additional information, including data on the relative biologic potency of cortisone and cortisol, are required to fully define the role of cortisone:cortisol interconversion in maturation of the human lung.

There is a good agreement in the literature regarding the direction of the dehydrogenase reaction and its biologic role in lung of rat and rabbit. In fetuses of these species, conversion is primarily from cortisone to cortisol in assay systems using cultured fibroblasts (Smith and Giroud 1975), lung minces (Tye and Burton 1980; Nicholas et al. 1978; Giannopolous 1974), organ culture (Ballard et al. 1984), homogenates (Torday et al. 1976; Brooks et al. 1977; Nicholas and Lugg 1982; Smith et al. 1982), and perfusion of isolated lung (Nicholas and Kim 1975; Torday et al. 1976). In adult rabbit lung, the major metabolic pathway for corticosteroid is conversion of cortisone to cortisol with little reverse activity and little formation of either tetrahydrocortisol or tetrahydrocortisone. By contrast, formation of the tetrahydro compounds is the major pathway in liver tissue (Brooks et al. 1977). Although little oxidation of corticosteroid occurs in the perfused lung, both reduction and oxidation of the 11-position occur in lung homogenates and microsome preparations depending on the relative concentrations of NADPH and NADP, respectively (Nicholas and Lugg, 1982). If the reaction is equally reversible in vivo, then the direction may be determined by the relative concentrations of the two cofactors. The very active pentose-phosphate shunt in lung tissue, as a source of NADPH, is consistent with the high level of reductive activity which has been observed in these species.

In both the rat and rabbit, the capacity of the fetal lung to form cortisol from cortisone increases during late gestation (Torday et al. 1976; Smith and Giroud 1975; Nicholas et al. 1978; Smith et al. 1982). In the study shown in Fig. 4.14, for example, reductive activity per gram weight increases about 4-fold during the last week of gestation in the fetal rabbit. This change is temporally associated with the increase in rate of choline incorporation into total lung lipids. In the fetal rat, corticosteroid 11-reductase activity, expressed per milligram protein, increases in an exponential manner about 6-fold between days 18 and 21 of gestation. Differentiation of rat lung occurs rapidly on the last two days of this period. When 11-ketoprogesterone was injected into fetal rats on day 17, the ratio of circulating 11-dehydrocorticosterone:corticosterone increased and was associated with both increased fetal lung weight and reduced content of saturated PC (Smith 1978). In addition to other possible effects, 11-ketoprogesterone inhibits reductase activity (Nicholas and Lugg 1982). Although levels of steroids in fetal lung were not determined, these results would be consistent with inhibition of corticosterone production within fetal lung by 11-ketoprogesterone with delayed pulmonary maturation.

The factors responsible for the developmental increase in cortisol produc-

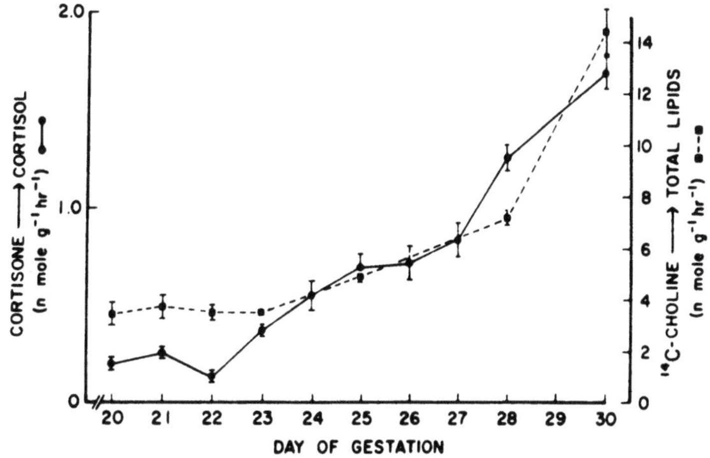

Fig. 4.14. Comparison of cortisol production and choline incorporation by fetal rabbit lung during the third trimester of gestation. Values are mean ± SE of 6–9 samples. Data from Nicholas et al. (1978), by permission

tion by the lung are uncertain. There is progressively less stimulation of reductase activity during gestation with addition of NADPH cofactor to lung homogenates (Torday et al. 1976). This finding would be consistent with an increasing supply of endogenous NADPH during development as one stimulus of reductase activity. It has been proposed that increasing levels of glucocorticoids in the fetal lung during late gestation lead to enhanced glycogenolysis with increased flux of glucose through the hexose-monophosphate shunt; this would increase the production of NADPH and enhance reductive activity (Smith et al. 1982).

Steroid dehydrogenase may also be under hormonal regulation. In monolayer cultures of human fetal lung cells, conversion of cortisone to cortisol was stimulated by the presence of pharmacologic levels (5.5 μM) of cortisol (Smith et al. 1973). This effect was studied in more detail with several lines of fibroblast cultures derived from human lung. Addition of cortisol for 16 h stimulated the conversion of cortisone to cortisol by 20–180 % in four cell lines; in each case, the half-maximal effect was observed between approximately 50–100 nM (Aronson et al. 1983), suggesting a physiologically relevant process. Administration of betamethasone to pregnant rats was found to stimulate cortisone to cortisol conversion by fetal lung, but not by fetal liver, and to cause precocious depletion of lung glycogen (Smith et al. 1982). In contrast with these results, one study reports no effect of glucocorticoid treatment either in vivo or in culture on cortisol production by fetal rabbit lung (Ballard et al. 1984).

Perhaps the strongest evidence for the physiologic significance of cortisone-cortisol conversion comes from binding studies. Incubation of fetal rabbit lung in vitro with [^{3}H] cortisone results in the appearance of [^{3}H] cortisol in the nuclei (Giannopoulos 1974; Ballard et al. 1984). The data of Fig. 4.15 show the time course for binding of cortisone and cortisol to cytoplasmic re-

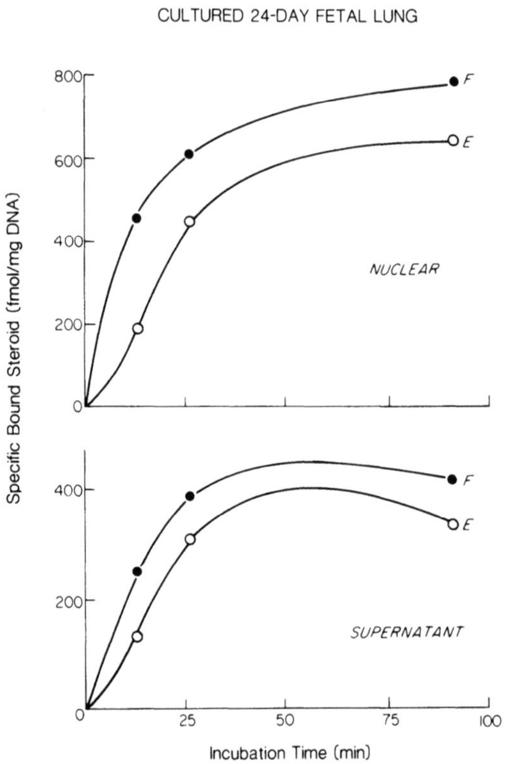

Fig. 4.15. Time course for cortisol and cortisone binding in nuclear and cytoplasmic fractions of fetal rabbit lung. Tissue from 24-day fetal rabbit in organ culture was incubated with [^{3}H]cortisol or [^{3}H]cortisone at 24 nM concentration for the times indicated. Data from Ballard et al. (1984), by permission

ceptor and nuclear localization of receptor-steroid complex. There is an initial lag in binding of cortisone, presumably reflecting conversion to cortisol, and then a similar time course as for cortisol. At equilibrium, the level of binding with the two steroids at equimolar concentrations are comparable. In dose response studies, the K_D for cortisone binding within nuclei of lung cells is similar to that found for cortisol (Ballard et al. 1984). Furthermore, cortisone is nearly as potent as cortisol in stimulating PC synthesis by both monolayers and organ cultures of fetal rabbit lung (Torday et al. 1975; Gross et al. 1983).

Thus, the available information indicates that cortisone is a physiologically active glucocorticoid, through its conversion to cortisol, for the fetal lung of rodents. Since both total and free concentrations of circulating cortisol decrease during gestation in the rabbit, cortisone may actually be the major endogenous glucocorticoid influencing fetal lung in late gestation for this species. Fetal lung might also constitute a source of cortisol for other tissues. Cortisol produced from cortisone within the lung is accumulated within pulmonary cells but a majority is returned to the circulation (in the case of perfusion studies) or diffuses into the medium in culture experiments. During early fetal life the contribution of the lung to circulating cortisol would be limited by the relatively low pulmonary blood flow. However, since both blood flow to the lung and 11-β-hydroxysteroid reductase activity increase in late gestation, the output of cortisol could become physiologically important near term (Smith 1978).

4.4 Clinical Evidence

Endogenous corticosteroids may be important for terminal differentiation in many tissues prior to birth. According to this concept, as reviewed by Liggins (1976), the process of initiation of labor, and stress to the fetus associated with rupture of membranes, infection, or possibly medical intervention in the case of the human, stimulate synthesis of corticosteroids which accelerate maturation in a variety of tissues in preparation for birth. In some species, but not in man, the rise in plasma corticoids precedes and actually initiates the onset of labor. This developmental role for endogenous glucocorticoids would obviously be of particular importance with preterm delivery when accelerated maturation would increase the chances for infant survival.

A number of studies have measured corticosteroid concentrations in human cord blood looking for an association with various prepartum factors. This subject has been recently reviewed by Murphy (1983). She points out the difficulties in assessing these data which are influenced by numerous factors including whether arterial or venous blood was assayed, the duration of labor, the mode of delivery, the amount of maternal pain, the type of anesthesia and the gestational age. Since cortisol crosses the placenta, maternal levels can influence concentrations in cord blood. This relationship is illustrated by the significant correlation between simultaneous maternal and fetal plasma cortisol levels during parturition (Ohrlander et al. 1976). These investigators obtained blood from the fetal scalp early in the course of spontaneous labor or with the induction of labor, again at full dilatation, and subsequently in cord blood. Both maternal and fetal cortisol concentrations rose during the course of labor and delivery; however, the relative contribution of the maternal and fetal adrenal to the rise of fetal cortisol is unclear. Most studies have found higher cord levels of total and free cortisol in infants of spontaneous onset vaginal delivery versus elective cesarean section without labor. Although higher concentrations generally occur in both umbilical venous and arterial blood with vaginal delivery, the possible contribution of maternal corticosteroid is also likely in this situation. Following premature rupture of the membranes, an increase in amniotic fluid cortisol with time has been reported (Cohen et al. 1976). Cortisol levels in cord blood are also higher in infants delivered after prolonged rupture of membranes versus those with a shorter duration (Bauer et al. 1974).

There is general agreement that the incidence of RDS is lower in infants delivered after labor versus those of cesarean section without labor (Farrell and Avery 1975). The possible effect of prolonged rupture of membranes on incidence of RDS remains controversial (Taeusch and Tulchinsky 1980). Other chronically stressful conditions of pregnancy, such as severe diabetes, chronic bleeding, severe preeclampsia and Rh isoimmunization, are associated with accelerated maturation of the amniotic fluid L/S ratio and phosphatidylglycerol content (Gluck and Kulovich 1973; Bustos et al. 1979). Since cord levels of cortisol are higher for infants of pregnancies with labor and prolonged rupture of membranes than in those without these conditions, it seems likely that *chronic* stress in utero would also elevate fetal cortisol. The relative contribution of the maternal and fetal adrenal to increasing fetal cortisol concentrations in these various situations is not established. Nevertheless, there does appear to be an association between higher fetal cortisol and greater lung maturity in premature infants.

RDS occurs more commonly in males, and there appears to be a developmental lag for males in both the L/S ratio and cortisol concentration in amniotic fluid (Torday et al. 1981). Other indirect clinical evidence for the role of corticosteroids includes the observations that RDS is associated with a larger thymus at birth (Fletcher et al. 1979) and smaller adrenals at postmortem examination (Naeye et al. 1971). Whereas the size of the thymus likely reflects cortisol concentrations in utero, postmortem adrenal size could result from the stress of RDS, rather than being a pre-existing condition.

The relationship between plasma cortisol concentration and occurrence of RDS has been investigated to test the hypothesis that RDS is associated with a relative glucocorticoid deficiency. Information from four studies suggests a trend toward lower cortisol in those infants who develop RDS (Table 4.6). Interpretation of these data is complicated by differences in mean gestational ages and by the difficulty of controlling for the many other variables that can effect the cortisol level at birth. Nevertheless, the data support the concept that endogenous glucocorticoids are related to lung maturity in the human.

Liveborn infants with congenital absence of the adrenals, unresponsiveness to ACTH, or anencephaly (often with adrenocortical hypoplasia) do not usually develop RDS. However, such infants are generally born at term or after term and thus may have had sufficient time for adequate lung development despite low cortisol levels. Indeed, Naeye et al. (1971) noted fewer lamellar bodies in type II cells of the lungs from anencephalic infants.

It is generally observed that survivors of RDS begin their recovery 2–3 days after birth irrespective of gestational age. This has led to the suggestion that the postnatal increase in cortisol levels associated with RDS (Baden et al. 1972; Reynolds 1973; Ballard et al. 1975) induces surfactant production. The time interval is similar to that necessary for clinical benefit after prenatal corticosteroid treatment and the levels of plasma glucocorticoid activity occurring with RDS are comparable with those achieved with betamethasone. Such levels are calculated to be sufficient for a near optimal effect in the lung (discussed in Chap. 6). Indeed, in one study, *postnatal* administration of hy-

Table 4.6. Cortisol concentrations in cord blood of premature infants with and without RDS

Study	Gestational age (weeks)			Cortisol (μg/dl)[a]		P
	No RDS	(range)	RDS	No RDS	RDS	
Murphy 1974	33.2		31.6	4.7±0.9 (21)	2.4±0.4 (22)	<0.05
Sybulski & Maughan 1976	34.7		32.0	5.6±0.4 (67)	4.0±0.8 (23)	<0.1
Gluckman et al. 1978		(32-35.5)		10.9±0.8 (23)	8.3±1.4 (17)	<0.1
Hauth et al. 1978	33.7	(30-35)	32.2	8.4±1.1 (48)	7.6±0.2 (27)	NS

[a] The number of infants is shown in parentheses

drocortisone to infants with RDS did not improve the clinical course or outcome (Baden et al. 1972). However, delivery and/or RDS also increase concentrations of other hormones (including thyroid hormones and catecholamines). Thus, resolution of RDS could be influenced by several hormones or might even be independent of hormonal action.

4.5 Summary and Conclusion

The evidence supporting a role for endogenous corticosteroids in lung differentiation is substantial. Glucocorticoid receptors are present in lung, and physiologic concentrations of administered corticosteroids evoke responses. In many species, there is a close temporal association between fetal lung maturation and the concentration of free corticosteroid. The possible causal relationship between circulating corticoids and the maturational process is supported by the strong correlations between the degree of lung maturity and cortisol concentration in individual animals such as the sheep. The effect of ablation procedures, particularly in the fetal sheep, have established that an intact pituitary is required for development of a normally mature lung by term. These various findings have led to the concept that endogenous corticosteroids influence the timing of terminal lung development. This proposed role for glucocorticoids in fetal lung is supported by observations that many other tissues are responsive to glucocorticoids during fetal and neonatal development. Thus, increasing availability of corticosteroid near term would act to prepare the fetus for extrauterine life. In the pregnancy complicated by premature labor or other stressful situations, a precocious rise in circulating corticosteroids would accelerate maturation in preparation for premature delivery. According to this hypothesis, prenatal administration of corticosteroids mimics the normal action of endogenous hormone.

There are species differences in the process by which more endogenous glucocorticoid becomes available during normal fetal development. In sheep and primates, both total and free concentrations of cortisol increase near term secondary to increased output by the fetal adrenal. In the rat and mouse, adrenal corticosteroid production decreases near term, but plasma concentrations of free corticosterone rise as a result of the rapid decline in plasma CBG. Neither of these mechanisms appear to operate in the rabbit, where free cortisol decreases during the third trimester. In this species increased conversion of cortisone to cortisol and increasing intracellular concentrations of glucocorticoid receptor may be important mechanisms underlying the glucocorticoid influence in the lung.

Considerable evidence suggests that endogenous corticosteroids, acutely elevated by stress, can cause precocious pulmonary maturation in utero. This effect has been observed repeatedly in the fetal rabbit, and clinical data for stressful pregnancies are consistent. During labor and delivery in the human, maternal cortisol rises and contributes to the fetal pool. Thus, corticosteroid from the mother may have a role in preparing the fetus for birth, particularly with preterm delivery. The mediation of glucocorticoid action by receptor indicates that the fetal lung is responsive to physiologic concentrations of corticosteroid. It is not yet known, however, whether other stress-induced hormones participate in accelerating maturation. Indeed, more recent information indicates the complexity of hormonal involvement. In the study with hypophysectomized fetal sheep, for example, infusion of ACTH, but not cortisol, stimulated surfactant concentration. One interpretation of these results has been the possible role of adrenal medullary products in lung maturation. In addition, it is clear that thyroid hormones, as discussed in Chap. 7, also influence the rate of lung maturation, probably in concert with corticosteroids. The involvement of other endogenous hormones is less certain but certainly possible. Thus considerable data support the concept that there is multi-hormonal regulation of lung maturation in vivo. While endogenous corticosteroids may be an important stimulus to accelerating pulmonary maturation, their effectiveness in different individuals and at different points in gestation may be determined by the overall hormonal milieu.

It might have been anticipated that studies with fetal lung in culture would help to define the role of endogenous corticoids. Quite the opposite situation has developed, since conflicting results have been obtained under different culture conditions. Monolayer cultures of dispersed lung cells appear to require the presence of glucocorticoids in order to increase PC synthetic capacity. By contrast, explants of lung from three species display increasing PC synthetic rates and/or morphologic changes in cultures maintained without hormones and little or no serum. These conflicting observations raise questions about the effects of different culture conditions and about the parameters which are routinely used to assess maturity. It could be argued that organ cultures more closely mimic the in vivo situation than monolayer cultures because intercellular relationships are maintained. On the other hand, explants are more susceptible to problems with diffusion of nutrients and oxygen to the cells. Also, the overproliferation of type II cells with organ culture compared with in vivo raises concern about transposing results to the situation in vivo. The existence of a serum factor which inhibits lung development in utero could explain in part the maturation of lung in organ culture without added glucocorticoids. One apparent conclusion arising from these data is that spatial interrelationships between different pulmonary cell types are an important factor in differentiation of the epithelium.

It is obvious that more experiments regarding the role of endogenous glucocorticoids are needed. For example, the effect of fetal adrenalectomy (with and without thyroidectomy) and various replacement regimens would be of considerable interest. Continued studies of cultured lung in the absence and presence of various hormones should include careful morphologic and morphometric evaluation to further define the changes. Information in this area of investigation will not only help determine normal regulatory mechanism, but may lead to improved treatment regimens for prevention of RDS.

References

Abramovitz M, Branchaud CL, Murphy BEP (1982) Cortisol-cortisone interconversion in human fetal lung: Contrasting results using explant and monolayer cultures suggest that 11 beta-hydroxysteroid dehydrogenase (EC 1.1.1.146) comprises two enzymes. J Clin Endocrinol Metab 54:563

Alescio T, Dani AM (1972) Hydrocortisone increased glycogen deposition and its dependence on tissue interactions in mouse embryonic lung developed in vitro. J Embryol Exp Morphol 27:155

Alexander DP, Britton HG, James VHT, Nixon DA, Parker RA, Wintour EM, Wright RD (1968) Steroid secretion by the adrenal gland of foetal and neonatal sheep. J Endocrinol 40:1

Alexander DP, Britton HG, Nixon DA, Ratcliffe JG, Redstone D (1973) Corticotrophin and cortisol concentrations in the plasma of the chronically catheterized sheep fetus. Biol Neonate 23:184

Aronson JF, McClaskey JW, Cristofalo VJ (1983) Human fetal lung fibroblasts: observations on origin and stability in culture. Mech Aging Dev 21:229

Aronson JF (1984) Demonstration of lung Type II cell differentiation by polarized light microscopy. Devel Biol 101:1

Baden M, Bauer CR, Colle E, Klein G, Taeusch HW, Stern L (1972) A controlled trial of hydrocortisone therapy in infants with respiratory distress syndrome. Pediatrics 50:526

Ballard PL, Granberg P, Ballard RA (1975) Glucocorticoid levels in maternal and cord serum after prenatal betamethasone therapy to prevent respiratory distress syndrome. J Clin Invest 56:1548

Ballard PL, Gluckman PD, Brehier A, Kitterman JA, Kaplan SL, Rudolph AM, Grumbach MM (1978) Failure to detect an effect of prolactin on pulmonary surfactant and adrenal steroids in fetal sheep and rabbits. J Clin Invest 62:879

Ballard PL (1979a) Glucocorticoids and differentiation. In: Baxter JD, Rousseau GG (ed), Glucocorticoid Hormone Action, Monographs on Endocrinology Vol 12, Springer, Berlin, Heidelberg, New York, pp 493–513

Ballard PL (1979b) Delivery and transport of glucocorticoids to target cells. In: Baxter JD, Rousseau GG (ed), Glucocorticoid Hormone Action, Monographs on Endocrinology Vol 12, Springer, Berlin, Heidelberg, New York, pp 25–48

Ballard PL, Benson BJ, Brehier A, Carter JP, Kriz BM, Jorgensen EC (1980) Transplacental stimulation of lung development in the fetal rabbit by 3,5-dimethyl-3'-isopropyl-L-thyronine. J Clin Invest 65:1407

Ballard PL (1982a) Hormonal aspects of fetal lung development. In: Farrell PM (ed), Lung Development: Biological and Clinical Perspectives, Vol II, Neonatal Respiratory Distress, Academic Press, New York, pp 205–253

Ballard PL, Kitterman JA, Bland RD, Clyman RI, Gluckman PD, Platzker CG, Kaplan SL, Grumbach MM (1982b) Ontogeny and regulation of corticosteroid binding globulin capacity in plasma of fetal and newborn lambs. Endocrinology 110:359

Ballard PL, Klein AH, Fisher DA (1983) Thyroid hormones and plasma corticosteroid binding globulin capacity in fetal and newborn lambs. Endocrinology 113:1197

Ballard PL, Ballard RA, Gonzales LK, Hümmelink R, Wilson CM, Gross I (1984) Corticosteroid binding by fetal rat and rabbit lung in organ culture. J Steroid Biochem 21:117

Barr HA, Lugg MA, Nicholas TE (1980) Cortisone and cortisol in maternal and fetal blood and in amniotic fluid during the final ten days of gestation in the rabbit. Biol Neonate 38:214

Bassett JM, Thorburn GD (1969) Foetal plasma corticosteroids and the initiation of parturition in sheep. J Endocrinol 44:285

Bassett JM, Thorburn GD (1973) Circulating levels of progesterone and corticosteroids in the pregnant ewe and its fetus. In: The Endocrinology of Pregnancy and Parturition. Experimental Studies in Sheep, Pierrepoint CG (ed), Alpha Omega Alpha Publishing, Cardiff, pp 126–140

Bauer CR, Stern L, Colle E (1974) Prolonged rupture of membranes associated with a decreased incidence of respiratory distress syndrome. Pediatrics 53:7

Beamer N, Hagemenas FC, Kittinger GW (1972) Protein binding of cortisol in the Rhesus monkey *(Macaca mulatta).* Endocrinology 90:325

Bernal AL, Flint APF, Anderson ABM, Turnbull AC (1980) 11-beta-hydroxysteroid dehydrogenase activity (E.C. 1.1.1.146) in human placenta and decidua. J Steroid Biochem 13:1081

Bernal AL, Anderson ABM, Turnbull AC (1982) The lack of influence of labor on human placental 11-β-hydroxysteroid dehydrogenase activity. J Clin Endocrinol Metab 54:1251
Blackburn WR, Travers H, Potter DM (1972) The role of the pitutiary-adrenal-thyroid axes in lung differentiation. I. Studies of the cytology and physical properties of anencephalic fetal rat lung. Lab Invest 26:306
Blackburn WR, Kelly JS, Dickman PS, Travers H, Lopata MA, Rhodea RA (1973) The role of the pituitary-adrenal-thyroid axes in lung differentiation. II. Biochemical studies of developing lung in anencephalic fetal rats. Lab Invest 28:352
Bland RD (1972) Cord-blood total protein levels as a screening aid for idiopathic respiratory-distress syndrome. N Engl J Med 287:9
Bourbon J, Jost A (1982) Control of glycogen metabolism in the developing fetal lung. Pediatr Res 16:50
Boyden EA (1976) The development of the lung in the Pig-tail monkey (*Macaca nemestrina*, L.). Anat Rec 186:15
Brooks SM, Sholiton LJ, Wessel JJ, Taylor B (1977) Cortisol metabolism by the lung. Chest 71 (Suppl):275S
Bro-Rasmussen F, Buus O, Trolle D (1962) Ratio cortisone/cortisol in mother and infant at birth. Acta Endocrinol Copenh 40:579
Buckingham S, Avery ME (1962) Time of appearance of lung surfactant in the foetal mouse. Nature 193:688
Bustos R, Kulovich MV, Gluck L, Gabbe SG, Evertson L, Vargas C, Lowenberg E (1979) Significance of phosphatidylglycerol in amniotic fluid in complicated pregnancies. Am J Obstet Gynecol 133:899
Carr BR, Parker Jr CR, Madden JD, MacDonald PC, Porter JC (1981) Maternal plasma adrenocorticotropin and cortisol relationships throughout human pregnancy. Am J Obstet Gynecol 139:416
Carson GD, Bolla JD, Challis JRG (1979) The availability of cortisol in amniotic fluid to the fetus and chorionic and amniotic membranes. Endocrinology 104:1053
Challis JRG, Patrick JE, Cross J, Workewych JV, Manchester E, Power S (1981) Short-term fluctuations in the concentration of cortisol and progesterone in fetal plasma, maternal plasma, and amniotic and allantoic fluids from sheep during late pregnancy. Can J Physiol Pharmacol 59:261
Challis JRG, Manchester EL, Mitchell BF, Patrick JE (1982) Activation of adrenal function in fetal sheep by the infusion of adrenocorticotropin to the fetus in utero. Biol Reprod 27:1026
Challis JRG, Mitchell BR, Lye SJ (1984) Activation of fetal adrenal function. J Dev Physiol 6:93
Chen JM (1954) The cultivation in fluid medium of organized liver, pancreas, and other tissue of foetal rats. Exp Cell Res 7:518
Chiswick ML, Ahmed A, Jack PMB, Milner RDG (1973) Control of fetal lung development in the rabbit. Arch Dis Child 48:709
Clements JA, Tooley WH (1977) Kinetics of surface-active material in the fetal lung. In: Hodson WA (ed), Development of the Lung, Marcel Dekker, New York, pp 349–366
Cohen W, Fencl MdeM, Tulchinsky D (1976) Amniotic fluid cortisol after premature rupture of membranes. J Pediatr 88:1007
Comline RS, Nathanielsz PW, Paisey RB, Silver M (1970) Cortisol turnover in the sheep foetus immediately prior to parturition. J Physiol (London) 210:141
Crone RK, Davies P, Liggins GC, Reid L (1983) The effects of hypophysectomy, thyroidectomy, and postoperative infusion of cortisol or adrenocorticotrophin on the structure of the ovine fetal lung. J Dev Physiol 5:281
Dalle M, Giry J, Gay M, Delost P (1978) Perinatal changes in plasma and adrenal corticosterone and aldosterone concentrations in the mouse. J Endocrinol 76:303
Dalle M, Delost P (1980) Maturation of glucocorticosteroid activity in the foetal guinea-pig during the end of gestation. Reprod Nutr Develop 20:331
De Courcy C, Gray CH, Lunnon JB (1952) Adrenal cortical hormones in human placenta "●" Nature 170:494
Dupouy JP, Coffigny H, Magre S (1975) Maternal and foetal corticosterone levels during pregnancy in rats. J Endocrinol 65:347
Dvorak M (1972) Adrenocrotical function in fetal, neonatal and young pigs. J Endocrinol 54:473

Epstein MF, Farrell PM (1975) The choline incorporation pathway: Primary mechanism for de novo lecithin synthesis in the fetal primate lung. Pediatr Res 9:658
Erenberg A, Rhodes ML, Weinstein MM, Kennedy RL (1979) The effect of fetal thyroidectomy on ovine fetal lung maturation. Pediatr Res 13:230
Fairclough RJ, Liggins GC (1975) Protein binding of plasma cortisol in the foetal lamb near term. J Endocrinol 67:333
Fairclough RJ, Hunter JT, Welch RAS, Payne E (1975) Plasma corticosteroid concentrations in the bovine foetus near term. J Endocrinol 65:139
Farrell PM, Avery ME (1975) Hyaline membrane disease. Am Rev Respir Dis 111:657
Farrell PM, Blackburn WR, Adams AJ (1977) Lung phosphatidylcholine synthesis and choline-phosphotransferase activity in anencephalic rat fetuses with corticosteroid deficiency. Pediatr Res 11:770
Fencl M deM, Tulchinsky D (1975) Total cortisol in amniotic fluid and fetal lung maturation. N Engl J Med 292:133
Fencl M deM, Osathanondh R, Tulchinsky D (1976) Plasma cortisol and cortisone in pregnancies with normal and anencephalic fetuses. J Clin Endocrinol Metab 43:80
Fencl M deM, Koos B, Tulchinsky D (1980a) Origin of corticosteroids in amniotic fluid. J Clin Endocrinol Metab 50:431
Fencl M deM, Stillman RJ, Cohen J, Tulchinsky D (1980b) Direct evidence of sudden rise in fetal corticoids late in human gestation. Nature 287:225
Fletcher BD, Masson M, Lisbona A, Riggs T, Papgeourgiou AN (1979) Thymic response to endogenous and exogenous steroids in premature newborn infants. J Pediatr 95:111
Funkhouser JD, Hughes ER, Peterson RDA (1976) An organ culture system for study of fetal lung development. Biochem Biophys Res Commun 70:630
Gewolb IH, Hobbins JC, Tan SY (1977) Amniotic fluid cortisol as an index of fetal lung maturity. Obstet Gynecol 49:462
Giannopoulos G (1974) Uptake and metabolism of cortisone and cortisol by the fetal rabbit lung. Steroids 23:845
Giannopoulos G, Jackson K, Tulchinsky D (1982) Glucocorticoid metabolism in human placenta, decidua, myometrium and fetal membranes. J Steroid Biochem 17:371
Giroud CJP (1971) Aspects of corticosteroid biogenesis and metabolism during the perinatal period. Clin Obstet Gynecol 14:745
Glickman JA, Carson DG, Challis JRG (1979) Differential effects of synthetic adrenocorticotrophin$_{1-24}$ and alpha-melanocyte-stimulating hormone on adrenal function in human and sheep fetuses. Endocrinology 104:34
Glickman JA, Challis JRG (1980) The changing response pattern of sheep fetal adrenal cells throughout the course of gestation. Endocrinology 106:1371
Gluck L, Kulovich MV (1973) Lecithin/sphingomyelin ratios in amniotic fluid in normal and abnormal pregnancy. Am J Obstet Gynecol 115:539
Gluck L, Chez RA, Kulovich MV, Hutchinson DL, Niemann WH (1974) Comparison of phospholipid indicators of fetal lung maturity in the amniotic fluid of the monkey *(Macaca mulatta)* and baboon *(Papio papio)*. Am J Obstet Gynecol 120:524
Gluckman PD, Ballard PL, Kaplan SL, Liggins GC, Grumbach MM (1978) Prolactin in umbilical cord blood and the respiratory distress syndrome. J Pediatr 93:1011
Gonzales LW, Ballard PL, Ertsey R, Williams MC (1985) Hormones and surfactant synthesis in explants of human fetal lung. Pediatr Res, 19:343A (abstract)
Gross I, Walker-Smith GH, Maniscalco WM, Czajka MR, Wilson CM, Rooney SA (1978) An organ culture model for study of biochemical development of fetal rat lung. J Appl Physiol: Respirat Environ Exercise Physiol 45:355
Gross I, Wilson CM (1983) Fetal rat lung maturation: initiation and modulation. J Appl Physiol: Respirat Environ Exercise Physiol 55:1725
Gross I, Ballard PL, Ballard RA, Jones CT, Wilson CM (1983) Corticosteroid stimulation of phosphatidylcholine synthesis in cultured fetal rabbit lung: evidence for de novo protein synthesis mediated by glucocorticoid receptors. Endocrinology 112:829
Hauth JC, Parker CR, MacDonald PC, Porter JC, Johnston JM (1978) A role of fetal prolactin in lung maturation. Obstet Gynecol 51:81
Heifetz A, Snyder JM (1981) The effects of hydrocortisone on the biosynthesis of sulfated glycoconjugates by human fetal lung. J Biol Chem 256:4957

Hennessy DP, Coughlan JP, Hardy KJ, Scoggins BA, Wintour EM (1983) The origin of cortisol in the blood of fetal sheep. J Endocrinol 95:71
Hitchcock KR (1979) Hormones and the lung. I. Thyroid hormones and glucocorticoids in lung development. Anat Rec 194:15
Holt PG, Oliver IT (1968) Plasma corticosterone concentrations in the perinatal rat. Biochem J 108:339
Hümmelink R, Ballard PL (1984) Endogenous corticosteroids and lung maturation in the fetal rabbit. Pediatr Res 18:1395 (abstract)
Jaffe RB, Seron-Ferre M, Parer JT, Lawrence CC (1978) The primate fetal pituitary-adrenal axis in the perinatal period. Am J Obstet Gynecol 131:164
Jones CT (1974) Corticosteroid concentrations in the plasma of fetal and maternal guinea pigs during gestation. Endocrinology 95:1129
Jones CT, Boddy K, Robinson JS (1977a) Changes in the concentration of adrenocorticotrophin and corticosteroid in the plasma of foetal sheep in the latter half of pregnancy, and during labour. J Endocrinol 72:293
Jones CT, Boddy K, Robinson JS, Ratcliffe JG (1977b) Developmental changes in the responses of the adrenal glands of foetal sheep to endogenous adrenocorticotrophin, as indicated by hormone responses to hypoxaemia. J Endocrinol 72:279
Kass EH, Hechter O, Macchi IA, Mou TW (1954) Changes in patterns of corticosteroids in rabbits after prolonged treatment with ACTH. Proc Soc Exper Biol Med 85:583
Kauffman SL (1977) Acceleration of canalicular development in lungs of fetal mice exposed transplacentally to dexamethasone. Lab Invest 36:395.
Kitterman JA, Liggins GC, Campos GA, Clements JA, Forster CS, Lee CH, Creasy RK (1981) Prepartum maturation of the lung in fetal sheep: relation to cortisol. J Appl Physiol: Respirat Environ Exercise Physiol 51:384
Kitterman JA (1984) Fetal lung development. J Develop Physiol 6:67
Kittinger GW (1974) Feto-maternal production and transfer of cortisol in the Rhesus *(Macaca mulatta).* Steroids 23:229
Kling OR, Kotas RV (1975) Endocrine influences on pulmonary maturation and the lecithin/sphinomyelin ratio in the fetal baboon. Am J Obstet Gynecol 121:664
Koerner DR (1966) 11 beta-hydroxysteroid dehydrogenase of lung and testis. Endocrinology 79:935
Kondo H, Kasuga H, Noumura T (1983) Effects of various steroids on in vitro lifespan and cell growth of human fetal lung fibroblasts (WI-38). Mech Aging Dev 21:335
Kotas RV (1973) Accelerated pulmonary surfactant after intrauterine infection in the fetal rabbit. Pediatrics 51:655
Kotas RV, Farrell PM, Ulane RE, Chez RA (1977) Fetal rhesus monkey lung development: lobar differences and discordances between stability and distensibility. J Appl Physiol: Respirat Environ Exercise Physiol 43:92
Lakshmi V, Monder C (1985) Evidence for independent 11-oxidase and 11-reductase activities of 11-β-hydroxysteroid dehydrogenase: enzyme latency, phase transitions and lipid requirements. Endocrinology 116:552
Lefebvre Y, Chapdelaine A, Bolte E (1970) Effects of labor on plasma dehydroepiandrosterone sulfate and cortisol. Gynec Invest 1:57
Leong MKH, Murphy BEP (1976) Cortisol levels in maternal venous and umbilical cord arterial and venous serum at vaginal delivery. Am J Obstet Gynecol 124:471
Levitz M, Jansen V, Dancis J (1978) The transfer and metabolism of corticosteroids in the perfused human placenta. Am J Obstet Gynecol 132:363
Liggins GC (1969) Premature parturition after infusion of corticotrophin or cortisol into foetal lambs. J Endocrinol 42:323
Liggins GC (1976) Adrenocortical-related maturational events in the fetus. Am J Obstet Gynecol 126:931
Liggins GC, Fairclough RJ, Grieves SA, Forster CS, Knox BS (1977) Parturition in sheep. In: Knight J, O'Connor M (eds), The Fetus and Birth, Ciba Foundation Symposium No. 47, p.5
Liggins GC, Kitterman JA, Campos GA, Clements JA, Forster CS, Lee CC, Creasy RK (1981a) Pulmonary maturation in the hypophysectomized ovine fetus. Differential responses to adrenocorticotrophin and cortisol. J Develop Physiol (Oxford) 3:1

Liggins GC, Vilos GA, Campos GA, Kitterman JA, Lee CH (1981b) The effect of spinal cord transection on lung development in fetal sheep. J Develop Physiol (Oxford) 3:267
Llanos AJ, Ramachandran J, Creasy RK, Rudolph AM, Seron-Ferre M (1979) Alpha-melanocyte-stimulating hormone and adrenocorticotropin in the regulation of glucocorticoid secretion during the perinatal period in sheep. Endocrinology 105:613
Longmuir KJ, Snyder JM, Mendelson CR, Johnston JM (1981) Phospholipid composition of lamellar bodies formed by fetal rabbit lung type II cells in organ culture. Arch Biochem Biophys 212:491
Lugg MA, Nicholas TE (1983) Transfer of ^{3}H-cortisone and ^{3}H-cortisol between the amniotic, allantoic, and fetal blood compartments in the rabbit at day 25 of gestation. Biol Neonate 44:42
Magyar DM, Devaskar J, Fridshal D, Buster JE, Nathanielsz PW (1980a) Responsiveness and maximum secretory capacity of isolated fetal lamb adrenocortical cells throughout the last third of gestation. Endocrinology 107:1582
Magyar DM, Fridshal D, Elsner CW, Glatz T, Eliot J, Klein AH, Lowe KC, Buster JE, Nathanielsz PW (1980b) Time-trend analysis of plasma cortisol concentrations in the fetal sheep in relation to parturition. Endocrinology 107:155
Magyar DM, Elsner CW, Fridshal D, Eliot J, Klein A, Glatz T, Lowe KC, Nathanielsz PW, Buster JE (1981) Time-trend analysis of plasma 11-deoxycorticosterone, corticosterone, cortisol, and aldosterone in fetal and maternal sheep during the last 18 days of gestation. J Ster Biochem 14:1091
Martin CE, Cake MH, Hartmann PE, Cook IF (1977) Relationship between foetal corticosteroids, maternal progesterone and parturition in the rat. Acta Endocrinol 84:167
Mendelson CR, Johnston JM, MacDonald PC, Snyder JM (1981) Multihormonal regulation of surfactant synthesis by human fetal lung in vitro. J Clin Endocrinol Metab 53:307
Mescher EJ, Platzker ACG, Ballard PL, Kitterman JA, Clements JA, Tooley WH (1975) Ontogeny of tracheal fluid, pulmonary surfactant, and plasma corticoids in the the fetal lamb. J Appl Physiol 39:1017
Meyrick B, Bearn JG, Cobb AG, Monkhouse CR, Reid L (1975) The effect of in utero decapitation on the morphologic development of the fetal rabbit lung. J Anat 119:517
Migeon CJ, Bertrand J, Gemzell CA (1961) The transplacental passage of various steroid hormones in mid-pregnancy. Rec Prog Horm Res 17:207
Minor RR (1979) Organ cultures of embryonic lung tissues. J Pediatr 94:910
Mitchell BF, Seron-Ferre M, Hess DL, Jaffe RB (1981) Cortisol production and metabolism in the late gestation Rhesus monkey fetus. Endocrinology 108:916
Mitchell BF, Seron-Ferre M, Jaffe RB (1982) Cortisol-cortisone interrelationship in the late gestation Rhesus monkey fetus in utero. Endocrinology 111:1837
Mulay S, Giannopoulos G, Solomon S (1973) Corticosteroid levels in the mother and fetus of the rabbit during gestation. Endocrinology 93:1342
Murphy BEP (1974) Cortisol and cortisone levels in the cord blood at delivery of infants with and without the respiratory distress syndrome. Am J Obstet Gynecol 119:1112
Murphy BEP, Patrick J, Denton RL (1975) Cortisol in amniotic fluid during human gestation. J Clin Endocrinol Metab 40:164
Murphy BEP (1977) Chorionic membrane as an extra-adrenal source of foetal cortisol in human amniotic fluid. Nature 266:179
Murphy BEP (1978) Conjugated glucocorticoids in amniotic fluid and fetal lung maturation. J Clin Endocrinol Metab 47:212
Murphy BEP, Vedady D, Patchell M, Hyde M (1978) Cortisol production and inactivation by the human lung during gestation and infancy. J Clin Endocrinol Metab 47:243
Murphy BEP (1981) Ontogeny of cortisol-cortisone interconversion in human tissues: A role for cortisone in human fetal development. J Steroid Biochem 14:811
Murphy BEP (1982a) The absorption by the human fetus of intra-amniotically injected cortisol. J Steroid Biochem 16:415
Murphy BEP (1982b) Human fetal serum cortisol levels related to gestational age: Evidence of a midgestational fall and a steep late gestational rise, independent of sex or mode of delivery. Am J Obstet Gynecol 144:276
Murphy BEP (1983) Human fetal serum cortisol levels at delivery. A review. Endocrine Rev 4:150
Naeye RL, Harcke HT, Blanc WA (1971) Adrenal gland structure and the development of hyaline membrane disease. Pediatrics 47:650

Nathanielsz PW, Comline RS, Silver M, Paisey RB (1972) Cortisol metabolism in the fetal and neonatal sheep. J Reprod Fert (Suppl) 16:39
Nelson GH, Eguchi K, McPherson JC (1976) Effect of gestational age, dexamethasone and metopirone on lecithin concentration in fetal lung tissue and amniotic fluid in rats and guinea pigs. Gynecol Invest 7:337
Nicholas TE, Kim PA (1975) The metabolism of ^{3}H-cortisone and ^{3}H-cortisol by the isolated perfused rat and guinea pig lungs. Steroids 25:387
Nicholas TE, Johnson RG, Lugg MA, Kim PA (1978) Pulmonary phospholipid biosynthesis and the ability of the fetal rabbit lung to reduce cortisone to cortisol during the final ten days of gestation. Life Sci 22:1517
Nicholas TE, Lugg MA (1982) The physiological significance of 11 beta-hydroxysteroid dehydrogenase in the rat lung. J Steroid Biochem 17:113
Oakey RE (1974) Serum cortisol binding capacity and cortisol concentration in the pregnant baboon and its fetus during gestation. Endocrinology 97:1024
Ohrlander S, Gennser G, Eneroth P (1976) Plasma cortisol levels in human fetus during parturition. Obstet Gynecol 48:381
Okazaki T, Johnston JM, Snyder JM (1982) Morphogenesis of the lamellar body in fetal lung tissue in vitro. Biochim Biophys Acta 712:283
Osinski PA (1960) Steroid 11-beta-ol dehydrogenase in human placenta. Nature 187:777
Paisey RB, Nathanielsz PW (1971) Plasma cortisol levels in the newborn lamb from birth to 30 days. J Endocrinol 50:701
Palmer S, Morgan TE, Prueitt JL, Murphy JH, Hodson WA (1977) Lung development in the fetal primate, *Macaca nemestrina.* II. Pressure-volume and phospholipid changes. Pediatr Res 11:1057
Pasqualini JR, CostaNovaes S, Ito Y, Nguyen BL (1970a) Reciprocal cortisol-cortisone conversions in the total tissue and subcellular fractions of foetal and adult guinea pig liver. J Steroid Biochem 1:341
Pasqualini JR, Nguyen BL, Uhrich F, Wiqvist N, Diczfalusy E (1970b) Cortisol and cortisone metabolism in the human foeto-placental unit at mid-gestation. J Steroid Biochem 1:209
Patrick JE, Challis JRG, Johnson P, Robinson JS, Thorburn GC (1976) Cortisol in amniotic fluid of Rhesus monkeys. J Endocrinol 68:161
Perelman RH, Engle MJ, Kemnitz JW, Kotas RV, Farrell PM (1982) Biochemical and physiological development of fetal Rhesus lung. J Appl Physiol Respirat Environ Exercise Physiol 53:230
Platzker ACG, Kitterman JA, Mescher EJ, Clements JA, Tooley WH (1975) Surfactant in the lung and tracheal fluid of the fetal lamb and acceleration of its appearance by dexamethasone. Pediatrics 56:554
Platzker ACG, Lew CD, Ballard PL, Landing B, Freshman K, Lewis A (1976) Delayed secretion of pulmonary surfactant into tracheal fluid in fetal lambs with hydranencephaly. Clin Res 24:198A (Abst.)
Prueitt JL, Palmer S, Standaert TA, Luchtel DL, Murphy JH, Hodson WA (1979) Lung development in the fetal primate *Macaca nemestrina.* III. HMD. Pediatr Res 13:654
Randall GCB (1983) Changes in the concentrations of corticosteroids in the blood of fetal pigs and their dams during late gestation and labor. Biol Reprod 29:1077
Reynolds JW (1973) Serum total corticoid and cortisol levels in premature infants with respiratory distress syndrome. Pediatrics 51:884
Robert MF, Bator AT, Taeusch HW Jr (1975) Pulmonary pressure-volume relationships after corticotropin (ACTH) and saline injections in fetal rabbits. Pediatr Res 9:760
Roebuck MM, Jones CT, Holland D, Silman R (1980) In vitro effects of high molecular weight forms of ACTH on the fetal sheep adrenal. Nature 284:616
Rooney SA, Gobran I, Wai-Lee TS, Nardone LL, Motoyama EK (1976) Studies on pulmonary surfactant. Effects of cortisol administration to fetal rabbits on lung phospholipid content, composition and biosynthesis. Biochim Biophys Acta 450:121
Rooney SA, Gobran LI, Marino PA, Maniscalco WM, Gross I (1979) Effects of betamethasone on phospholipid content, composition and biosynthesis in fetal rabbit lung. Biochim Biophys Acta 572:64
Rose JC, Meis PJ, Urban RB, Greiss FC Jr (1982) In vivo evidence for increased adrenal sensitivity to adrenocorticotropin-(1–24) in the lamb fetus late in gestation. Endocrinology 111:80

Russell BJ, Nugent L, Chernick V (1974) Effects of steroids on the enzymatic pathways of lecithin production in fetal rabbits. Biol Neonate 24:306

Savu L, Nunez E, Jayle M-F (1977) Corticosterone binding by mouse sera during foetal and postnatal development. Acta Endocrinol 84:177

Schindler AE, (1982) Hormones in amniotic fluid. Monographs on Endocrinol Vol 21, Springer, Berlin, Heidelberg, New York

Seron-Ferre M, Rose JC, Parer JT, Foster DB, Jaffe RB (1978a) In vivo regulation of the fetal Rhesus monkey adrenal gland. Endocrinology 103:368

Seron-Ferre M, Lawrence CC, Siiteri PK, Jaffe RB (1978b) Steroid production by definitive and fetal zones of the human fetal adrenal gland. J Clin Endocrinol Metab 47:603

Siiteri TK, Murai JT, Hammond GL, Nisker JA, Raymoure WJ, Kuhn RW (1982) The serum transport of steroid hormones. Rec Prog Horm Res 38:457

Simpson LL, Tanswell AK, Joneja MG (1985) Epithelial cell differentiation in organotypic cultures of fetal rat lung. Am J Anat 172:31

Sivakumaran T, Duncan ML, Effer SB, Younglai EV (1975) Relationship between cortisol and lecithin/sphingomyelin ratios in human amniotic fluid. Am J Obstet Gynecol 122:291

Smith BT, Torday JS, Giroud JP (1973) The growth promoting effect of cortisol on human fetal lung cells. Steroids 22:515

Smith BT, Torday JS, Giroud CJP (1974) Evidence for different gestation-dependent effects of cortisol on cultured fetal lung cells. J Clin Invest 53:1518

Smith BT, Giroud CJP (1975) Effects of cortisol on serially propogated fibroblast cell cultures derived from the rabbit fetal lung and skin. Can J Physiol Pharmacol 53:1037

Smith BT (1977) Cell line A549: A model system for the study of alveolar type II cell function. Am Rev Respir Dis 115:285

Smith BT, Worthington D, Maloney HA (1977a) Fetal lung maturation. III. The amniotic fluid cortisol/sortisone ratio in preterm human delivery and the risk of respiratory distress syndrome. Obstet Gynecol 49:527

Smith BT, Worthington D, Piercy WN (1977b) The relationship of cortisol and cortisone to saturated lecithin concentration in ovine amniotic fluid and fetal lung liquid. Endocrinology 101:104

Smith BT (1978) The role of pulmonary corticosteroid 11-reductase activity in lung maturation in the fetal rat. Pediatr Res 12:12

Smith BT (1979) Prevention of hyaline membrane disease. An attempt to mimic a physiologic process. In: Moss (ed), Pediatrics Update. Elsevier-North Holland, New York, pp. 151–167

Smith BT, Tanswell AK, Minshall D, Bogues WN, Vreeken E (1982) Influence of corticosteroids on glycogen content and steroid 11-reductase activity in lung and liver of the fetal and newborn rat. Biol Neonate 42:201

Smith ID, Shearman RP (1974a) Fetal plasma steroids in relation to parturition. I. The effect of gestational age upon umbilical plasma corticosteroid levels following vaginal delivery. J Obstet Gynaecol Br Comm 81:11

Smith ID, Shearman RP (1974b) Fetal plasma steroids in relation to parturition. II. The effect of gestational age upon umbilical plasma corticosteroids following hysterotomy and caesarean section. J Obstet Gynaecol Br Comm 81:16

Snyder JM, Johnston JM, Mendelson CR (1981a) Differentiation of type II cells of human fetal lung in vitro. Cell & Tissue Research 220:17

Snyder JM, Johnston JM, Mendelson CR (1981b) The effect of cortisol on rabbit fetal lung maturation in vitro. Dev Biol 85:129

Sorokin S (1961) A study of development in organ cultures of mammalian lungs. Dev Biol 3:60

Stahlman MT, Gray ME (1978) Anatomical development and maturation of the lungs. Clin Perinatol 5:181

Stryker JL, Dziuk PJ (1975) Effects of fetal decapitation on fetal development, parturition and lactation in pigs. J Animal Sci 40:282

Sundell HW, Tsiantos H, Relier JP, Dolanski E, Victorine L, Otten A, Strott C, Orth D, Chytil F, Stahlman M (1973) Prevention of HMD with ACTH infusion in fetal lambs. Pediatr Res 7:407

Sundell HW, Gray ME, Relier JP, Kovar IZ, Catterton WZ, Swift LL, Stahlman MT (1979) The effects of ACTH in lung maturation in fetal lambs. Am J Pathol 97:393

Sybulski S, Maughan GB (1976) Relationship between cortisol levels in umbilical cord plasma

and development of the respiratory distress syndrome in premature newborn infants. Am J Obstet Gynecol 125:239
Taeusch HW, Avery ME (1977) Regulation of pulmonary alveolar development in late gestation and the perinatal period. In: Hodson WA (ed), Development of the Lung, Marcel Dekker, Inc., New York, pp 399–418
Taeusch HW, Tulchinsky D (1980) Obstetric factors affecting risk of respiratory distress syndrome. Mead Johnson Symp, Perinat Dev Med 15:48
Tan SY, Gewolb IH, Hobbins JC (1976) Unconjugated cortisol in human amniotic fluid: Relationship to lecithin/ sphingomyelin ratio. J Clin Endocrinol Metab 43:412
Tanswell AK, Worthington D, Smith BT (1977) Human amniotic membrane corticosteroid 11-oxidoreductase activity. J Clin Endocrinol Metab 45:721
Tanswell AK, Smith BT (1978) The relationship of amniotic membrane 11-oxidoreductase activity to lung maturation in the human fetus. Pediatr Res 12:957
Tanswell AK, Smith BT (1980) Influence of oxygen tension and cortisol environment upon growth and cortisone conversion to cortisol by cultured human fetal lung fibroblasts. Biol Neonate 37:32
Tanswell AK, Joneja MG, Lindsay J, Vreeken E (1983a) Differentiation-arrested rat fetal lung in primary monolayer cell culture. I. Development of a differentiation-arrested and growth-supporting culture system using carbon-stripped bovine fetal calf serum. Exp Lung Research 5:37
Tanswell AK, Joneja MG, Vreeken E, Lindsay J (1983b) Differentiation-arrested rat fetal lung in primary monolayer cell culture. II. Dexamethasone, triiodothyronine, and insulin effects on different gestational age cultures. Exp Lung Res 5:49
Thorburn GD, Nicol DH, Bassett JM, Shutt D, Cox RI (1972) Parturition in the goat and sheep: changes in corticosteroids, progesterone, oestrogens and prostaglandin F. J Reprod Fert (Suppl) 16:61
Torday JS, Smith BT, Giroud CJP (1975) The rabbit fetal lung as a glucocorticoid target issue. Endocrinology 96:1462
Torday JS, Olson EB Jr, First NL (1976) Production of cortisol from cortisone by the isolated, perfused fetal rabbit lung. Steroids 27:869
Torday JS (1980) Glucocorticoid dependence of fetal lung maturation in vitro. Endocrinology 107:839
Torday JS, Nielson HC, Fencl M deM, Avery ME (1981) Sex differences in human fetal lung maturation. Am Dev Respir Dis 123:205
Tye LM, Burton AF (1979) Variation in the pattern of metabolism of corticosteroids in fetal mouse tissues. Life Sci 26:35
Van Baelen H, Vandoren G, De Moor P (1977) Concentration of transcortin in the pregnant rat and its foetuses. J Endocrinol 75:427
Vidyasagur D, Chernick V (1975) Effect of metopirone on the synthesis of lung surfactant in does and fetal rabbits. Biol Neonate 27:1
Vilos GA, Challis JRG, Lye SJ, Possmayer F, Harding PG (1983) Accelerated prepartum maturation of the fetal sheep lung with physiological doses of adrenocorticotrophin. J Dev Physiol 5:341
Vilos GA, Challis JRG, Lye SJ, Possmayer F, Harding PG (1985) Metopirone inhibits the maturational effect of ACTH in ovine lung even in the presence of exogenous corticosteroids. In: Jones CT, Nathanielsz PW (eds), Physiologic Development of the Fetus and Newborn, Academic Press, London (in press)
Wigglesworth JS, Desai R (1979) Effects on lung growth of cervical cord section in the rabbit fetus. Early Hum Dev 3:51
Winters AJ, Oliver C, Colston C, MacDonald PC, Porter JC (1974) Plasma ACTH levels in the human fetus and neonate as related to age and parturition. J Clin Endocrinol Metab 39:269
Wintour EM, Brown EH, Denton DA, Hardy KJ, McDougall JG, Oddie CJ, Whipp GT (1975) The ontogeny and regulation of corticosteroid secretion by the ovine foetal adrenal. Acta Endocrinol 79:301
Zsolnai B, Gyevai A (1984) Induction of lamellar body synthesis by corticosteroids in first-trimester human fetal lungs. Gynecol Obstet Invest 17:258

5 Antenatal Glucocorticoid Therapy: Clinical Effects

"When meditating over a disease, I never think of finding a remedy for it, but instead a means of preventing it."
Louis Pasteur, 1884

5.1 Respiratory Distress Syndrome

Any discussion of either therapeutic or preventive measures for a given disease must first describe the illness, its occurrence and severity, and the magnitude of the problem it presents to the public health. Respiratory distress syndrome (RDS), or hyaline membrane disease (HMD), is a clinical syndrome occuring primarily in preterm infants and characterized by increasing respiratory distress which persists at least 48 h and improves spontaneously, usually with recovery at around 72 h of age. Clinically, these infants have grunting, nasal flaring, retractions, and tachypnea associated with cyanosis; chest radiographic findings are consistent with diffuse atelectasis; arterial blood gases show hypoxia and hypercarbia in the absence of therapy.

5.1.1 Occurrence

Farrell and Wood (1976) reviewed the contribution of RDS (and HMD) to neonatal mortality in 1976. They point out that, for the years 1968 to 1973, the National Center for Health Statistics reported HMD and RDS as the cause of death in 54,064 infants, or an estimated 9,110 ± 560 per year. In an additional 24% of infant deaths for this period, RDS/HMD was a contributing factor; therefore, RDS was related to approximately 12,000 infant deaths per year, or 20% of all neonatal deaths. The contribution of RDS to neonatal mortality peaked in 1974, and then declined during the years 1975–1978.

However, Perelman and Farrell (1982) note that, in spite of the general decline in neonatal mortality rate during these years, there was marked variation in this decrease associated with both gestational age and geographic location within the U.S. In addition, prior to the early 1970's, the age of death in those infants who expired from RDS was within the first 72 to 96 h of life. However, death from RDS and its complications in the late 1970's and early 1980's has occurred later after birth, with a significant proportion of deaths now falling outside the newborn period (first 28 days of life), and well into the first year of life.

The actual *incidence* of RDS in the U.S. is somewhat difficult to define. Farrell and Avery (1975) calculated from data available in 1975 that the incidence of HMD in infants weighing less than 2500 g was 14%. Assuming a national live birth rate of 3.5×10^6 per year, and an associated frequency of premature births of 8%, they estimated that the minimal incidence of RDS in the U.S. was 40,000 cases/year. Incidence is clearly inversely related to birth weight and gestational age. Usher et al. (1971) described an incidence of HMD in infants of 29 to 30 weeks gestation of up to 65%. In infants born vaginally, the incidence fell at 31 to 32 weeks gestation to 38%, and to 20% at 33 to 34 weeks; the incidence was less than 2% after 37 weeks gestation. Usher and coworkers also found that the incidence was significantly higher among infants born by cesarean section between 31 and 38 weeks gestation than among infants born vaginally. Since this work was published, therapeutic approaches to perinatal care of the preterm infant have become more vigorous. Improved resuscitation and treatment of smaller and smaller infants has changed the incidence and characteristics of occurrence.

We reviewed the incidence of RDS in 1982–1983 for inborn infants at Mount Zion Hospital and Medical Center in San Francisco, where glucocorticoids are used routinely, when not contraindicated, between 26 and 34 weeks gestation. For infants weighing 750 to 1250 g (26 to 30 weeks gestation), 1251–1750 g (30 to 34 weeks gestation), and 1751–2500 g, the incidence of RDS was 54 %, 11 % and less than 2 %, respectively. There were no deaths attributable to RDS in infants weighing more than 1250 g during this time, and only 1 death in an infant between 1000 g and 1250 g (5%) ascribable to RDS. Obviously, while RDS remains an important clinical problem requiring substantial therapeutic intervention, it need not be a major cause of death, even in small preterm infants.

5.1.2 Pathophysiology

It is questionable whether the diagnosis of RDS in infants under 1250 g represents the same clinical syndrome described in larger preterm infants. Avery and Mead (1959) first described the deficiency of surface-active material in HMD (see Chap. 1). In their review of HMD, Farrell and Avery (1975) stated that "... HMD occurs as a consequence of the relative inability of the lung to synthesize and/or secrete surfactant in amounts sufficient for respiratory adaption." While this cleary remains the essential aspect of RDS for larger infants, it now seems likely that multiple physiological variables contribute to cause respiratory distress experienced by smaller infants. These variables include:

Lung Structure. Development of lung acini is closely related to gestational age. At 26 weeks gestation, alveoli are not present, the walls of alveolar ducts are relatively thick, and airway compliance is high. Gas exchange is inefficient at this age, even if surfactant is present. By 34 weeks gestation, however, early alveolar saccules have appeared, with increased surface area and decreased distance for gas diffusion. (See Chap. 1.) At this more mature age, respiratory distress is more likely to result from surfactant deficiency than from structural immaturity *per se*.

In addition, lung development is clearly influenced by genetic background, and, just as other aspects of development occur on a timetable subject to individual variation, newborns from different families mature their lungs at different gestational ages. It is a common clinical observation that once a family has had an infant with RDS, subsequent infants born at the same gestational age are much more likely to suffer from RDS than would be expected for the general population.

Lung Liquid. Rapid clearance of lung fluid into the circulation at the time of delivery is essential for successful etablishment of ventilation. Under normal circumstances, production of lung liquid ceases, and resorption begins, during normal, term labor (discussed in Chap. 8). This process is often delayed and less efficient in the preterm infant. In particular, asphyxia and hypoxia, which frequently accompany preterm birth, will delay resorption of lung fluid and thereby aggravate respiratory distress in the very low-birthweight infant.

Pulmonary Blood Flow. Adequate blood flow throughout the pulmonary vessels is essential for both normal gas exchange and delivery of oxygen and nutrients to the lung for its metabolic functions. During fetal development, there is increasing muscularization of the pulmonary arterial vessels, and, accordingly, changes in vessel reactivity to oxygen and pH. Abnormalities of either blood volume (in particular, hypovolemia) or flow (vasoconstriction or shunts, as through a patent ductus arteriosus) have a marked effect on neonatal respiratory function. The very premature infant is at greater risk for these abnormalities than the older infant.

Birth Asphyxia. It is well known that preterm infants suffering from birth asphyxia are among those most likely to develop RDS. Animal studies have demonstrated that asphyxia has multiple effects on pulmonary blood flow, cellular metabolism, lung water clearance, and the synthesis and release of surfactant.

Ventilation at Birth. Appropriate physiological expansion of the lungs at birth stimulates both release of surface active material and clearance of lung water. Inadequate expansion often leads to progressive atelectasis and subsequent lung damage, whereas overdistention, e.g., mechanical ventilation, may also disrupt the epithelial lining of terminal airways, leading to leakage of fluid and proteins into the airspaces. With an unstable chest wall and weak respiratory musculature, the very small infant often is unable to maintain normal ventilation at birth.

Thus, each of the above factors may be involved, along with a deficiency of surfactant, in the respiratory distress of premature infants. Deficiency of surfactant and inadequate respiratory effort diminish the infant's ability to expand its lungs and to maintain aeration on deflation, which in turn prevents the normal transition from the fetal to neonatal circulation. The persistence of right-to-left shunting, often exacerbated by a patent ductus arteriosus, interferes with clearance of lung water. A consequence of these events is increased hypoxia and acidosis, which increase pulmonary vascular resistance and decrease surfactant production, leading to continuation of the "vicious cycle" of RDS. In examining the overall impact of prenatal glucocorticoids on infant morbidity and mortality, it is therefore important to consider not only effects of therapy on the incidence of RDS but also possible effects of other conditions contributing to morbidity in the preterm infant.

5.2 Prevention of RDS: Factors Influencing Efficacy of Therapy

Liggins and Howie (1972) reported the first clinical trial of the use of antepartum glucocorticoid therapy for the prevention of RDS in premature infants. During the period from 1969 to 1974, they carried out two trials of prenatal glucocorticoid therapy. Results of the first trial were reported in the initial publication of the therapeutic benefit of glucocorticoids (1972). A second trial, with double the dose of betamethasone, ended in 1974. Table 5.1 shows the combined data from the two trials (Howie and Liggins 1982). In these trials, 1,068 mothers were entered into a double-blind, randomized controlled study. The number of mothers with diabetes, Rh immunization, or major placentae previa were small, and no significant differences for incidence of RDS between treated and control groups were evident. There were 821 women who presented with unplanned preterm labor: 411 treated mothers (with 443 infants) and 410 control mothers (with 441 infants). The study showed a significant decrease in RDS and perinatal (primarily neonatal) deaths in the treated infants, compared to control infants. There was no significant effect of betamethasone on infants who were delivered less than 24 h after the first dose of glucocorticoid or more than 7 days after therapy was initiated. Overall, there was a decrease in incidence in RDS from 23.7% in controls to 8.8% in treated infants. They also reported (Table 5.1) that the greatest benefit from glucocorticoid therapy was in the group of infants of less than 32 weeks gestation, with some continued significant benefit up to 34 weeks, and no benefit in infants of more than 34 weeks gestation.

Since that time, numerous reports of both nonrandomized, retrospective studies and carefully controlled, prospective, double-blind studies of prenatal glucocorticoid therapy have appeared. Table 5.2 presents a review of the major studies in the English literature. These studies have uniformly confirmed the benefits of glucocorticoids in reducing the incidence of RDS in preterm infants. From this body of work, there has emerged considerable information about factors which influence the efficacy of glucocorticoid therapy. These are summarized in Table 5.3.

Table 5.1. Incidence of RDS by gestational age in the study of Howie and Liggins (1982). Data are for infants delivered 24 h to 7 days after entry into the trial

Gestational age at delivery (weeks)	Betamethasone treated		Control		p
	RDS/N	(%)	RDS/N	(%)	
< 30	10/36	(27.8)	15/26	(51.7)	< 0.04
30–32	2/23	(8.7)	14/25	(56.0)	< 0.001
32–34	0/50	(0.0)	4/31	(12.9)	< 0.04
34	4/73	(5.5)	4/74	(5.4)	NS
All infants	16/182	(8.8)	37/156	(23.7)	< 0.001

Table 5.2. Clinical studies of prenatal glucocorticoid therapy

Investigator	Type of study	Number – mothers/ infants	Drug	Less RDS	Less severe RDS	Less mortality	ROM effect	Toco-lytic effect	Gest. age or wt. group	Other
Liggins & Howie 1972; Howie & Liggins 1982	Prospective Blind	821/884	Beta	Yes	Yes	Yes	No	No	Mean weights near 2100 g	No difference with double dose. No difference in infection
Fargier et al. 1974	Retrospective	461/492 (34 Rx)	Beta	Yes	NE	Yes	NE	No	Mean weight 1900–2000 g	
Bureau et al. 1975	Retrospective	112/112	Beta	Trend	NE	No	NE	NE	25–32 weeks	
Kennedy 1976	Retrospective Paired	82/82	Beta	Yes	NE	Trend	NE	NE	27–34 weeks	No difference in infection. Follow-up OK after 3 years
Caspi et al. 1976	Retrospective	117/131	Dex	Yes	NE	Yes	No	No	Mean weight 1650–1730 g	Increased L/S ratio with therapy. No effect on infection
Dluholucky et al. 1976	Prospective "Random"	?/105	Hydro	Yes	NE	Yes	No	NE	Mean weights 1550–1700 g	No effect in 24 h
Thornfeldt et al. 1978	Retrospective Paired	?/511	Dex	Yes	NE	NE	NE	NE	Effective All weights examined	No difference with different dosages
Osler et al. 1978	Retrospective "controls"	111/120 160	Beta/ Pheno-barbital	Yes	NE	Yes	NE	NE	2500 g	160 "controls" not concurrent
Block et al. 1977	Prospective Blind	142/150	Beta/ MP	Yes No	NE NE	Trend Trend	Yes	NE		No effect of time of therapy to delivery
Morrison et al. 1978	Prospective Blind	126/126	Hydro	Yes	Yes	Trend	NE	NE	32 weeks	No effect on infection. Trend to lower RDS at 18 h therapy
Ballard et al. 1979	Retrospective	220/252	Beta	Yes	Yes	Yes	No	No	750–1750 g (mean, 1300)	No effect on infection
Papageorgiou et al. 1979	Prospective Blind	104/146	Beta	Yes	Yes	Yes	No	NE	27–34 weeks (mean 1881 vs.1601)	Less effect in male Hypoglycemia in Rx. No effect on infection

Continued

Table 5.2. (contd.)

Investigator	Type of study	Number – mothers/ infants	Drug	Less RDS	Less severe RDS	Less mortality	ROM effect	Toco-lytic effect	Gest. age or wt. group	Other
Taeusch et al. 1979	Prospective Blind	122/127	Dex	Yes	Yes	Yes	No	NE	Mean wt 1650 g	Increased maternal infection with PROM. No effect admission to delivery time
Young et al. 1980	"Matched controls"	300/312	Dex	Yes	Yes	Yes	No	NE	28–32 weeks	Increased infection in Rx with PROM
Doran et al. 1980	Prospective Blind	137/144	Beta	Yes	Yes	Yes	No	No		Less RDS in whole group; trend in 24–32 weeks
Caspi et al. 1980	Retrospective	218/259	Dex	Yes	NE	No	No	No	28–32 weeks	Increased RDS in any group with low Apgar score
Schutte et al. 1980	Prospective Blind	212/259	Beta	Yes	Yes	No	±	No	Mean ages 30–31 weeks	Increased RDS in infants born <12 h or>3 weeks after admission
Garite et al. 1981	"Random" with PROM	160/159	Beta	Trend 30 weeks	No	No	NE	NE	28–34 weeks	Increased infection with Beta + PROM
Collab. 1981	Prospective Blind	661/720	Dex	Yes	NE	No	Yes	NE	28–35 weeks	No effect in twins. Effect decreased in male. Decreased hospital stay. No difference in infection.
Kuhn et al. 1982	Prospective "Random"	355/355[a]	Beta	Yes	NE	Yes	Yes	No		Beta + ROM + female = best. Increased infection with cerclage. Increased infection in male 27–30 weeks.
Schmidt et al. 1984	Prospective Blind	92/97	Beta MP Hydro	Yes	Yes	No	No	NE	Mean weight 1660 g	Increased maternal infection with Hydro. No effect on neonatal infection.

[a] Excluded second twin Beta, betamethasone; Dex, dexamethasone; Hydro, hydrocortisone; MP, methylprednisolone; ROM, rupture of membranes; PROM,

Table 5.3. Factors affecting efficacy of prenatal glucocorticoid therapy

I. Clear effect established:	III. Insufficient evidence of effect
a) Gestational age	a) Maternal diabetes
b) Therapeutic agent, treatment interval and dose	b) Rhesus sensitization
c) Interval from exposure to delivery	c) Cesarean section
II. Probable effect	d) Tocolytics
a) Gender and racial origin	e) Toxemia
b) Asphyxia	
c) Multiple birth	
d) Prolonged rupture of membranes	

5.2.1 Effect Established

5.2.1.1 Gestational Age

Since the incidence of RDS in untreated infants is related to gestational age, it must be a major consideration in assessing the efficacy of steroid therapy. In the New Zealand studies (Liggins and Howie 1972; Howie and Liggins 1982), there is no statistically significant response to betamethasone among infants over 34 weeks gestation. The incidence of RDS in both treated and untreated infants at this gestational age was 5.5%. All other studies have similarly failed to demonstrate an effect after 34 weeks gestation. This finding probably reflects the low incidence of RDS at this gestation in most populations. Accordingly, a very large number of women and infants would need to be treated (the majority unnecessarily) before any significant difference in incidence of RDS would be detectable. The effect of glucocorticoids after 34 weeks is of limited interest, because of the low incidence of RDS and the relative ease with which the disease can be managed in these older infants. After 34 weeks gestation, glucocorticoids are most commonly considered in situations where delivery of an infant with immature lungs is required for medical reasons (e.g., maternal carcinoma, diabetes). To date, there is only anecdotal evidence for efficacy in such cases.

The lower end of the age spectrum at which infants respond to glucocorticoids has been a matter of greater controversy. Howie and Liggins (1982) found the greatest response in infants of 30 to 32 weeks gestation: an incidence of 56% and 8.7% in control and treated infants, respectively. In the group of infants of less than 30 weeks gestation, the reducation in RDS was from 57.7% to 27.8% (Table 5.1). Ballard et al. (1979) examined the incidence of RDS by weight groups. They found that the effectiveness of glucocorticoids was most pronounced for infants between 750 g and 1250 g (26 to 30 weeks gestation). There was no apparent benefit of glucocorticoids in a small group of infants under 750 g (less than 26 weeks gestation), and Kuhn et al. (1982) reported similar findings. Most of the other studies contain relatively few infants of very low birth weight. In the U.S. National Collaborative Study (1981), for example, of the single infants entered in the study, there were only 10 treated and 16 untreated infants of less than 30 weeks gestation.

The apparent ineffectiveness of therapy among infants (less than) 26 weeks is not unexpected, since, before this gestational age, the structural maturity of the lung plays a central part in lung function. Thus, although glucocorticoids do affect lung structure in animals (see Chap. 2), it is unlikely that a few days of exposure could adequately stimulate acinar development in the extremely immature human lung. In addition, a concern has been voiced that use of glucocorticoids before 26 weeks gestation may be associated with the live birth of some infants who survive initially because of accelerated pulmonary development but subsequently die from other complications of the tiny premature. Examination of the effect of treatment on the very small preterm infant clearly needs further delineation.

5.2.1.2 Therapeutic Agent, Treatment Interval and Dose

Betamethasone. In their original trial, Liggins and Howie (1972) used Celestone Soluspan, a combination of short-acting betamethasone phosphate (6 mg) and longer-acting betamethasone acetate (6 mg). In the second trial the dose of Celestone was doubled. No difference in the results of therapy was found. Ballard et al. (unpublished data) found no difference in the incidence of RDS when the 2 doses of betamethasone were given at intervals of 12, 18, or 24 h; however, there was a trend toward lower incidence of RDS among infants born less than 48 h after initiation of treatment if steroid had been administered at 12-h intervals.

Dexamethasone. Several studies have used dexamethasone, given at 4-h to 6-h intervals, in a dose considered to be equivalent to the "Liggins dose" of betamethasone. Dexamethasone has a potency similar to that of betamethasone (Chap. 6). Use of the phosphate form of dexamethasone, which has a shorter t½ than the acetate form, has required more frequent administration than for Celestone. The efficacy of dexamethasone appears similar to that of betamethasone, although the two agents have not been directly compared in any one study.

Hydrocortisone. Hydrocortisone has been used at doses of 100 to 500 mg per injection, and may also be effective in preventing RDS when administered prenatally (Dluholocky et al. 1976; Morrison et al. 1978; Whitt et al. 1976; Ballard and Liggins 1982). However, efficacy and optimal dosage schedule have not been etablished.

On the other hand, Baden et al. (1972) administered hydrocortisone after birth to infants who developed RDS and found no effect on either mortality or morbidity of RDS. Witt et al. (1976) compared betamethasone with hydrocortisone; however, the drugs were given to only 14 women, 7 in each group, and no assessment could be made of the incidence of RDS. They found that 1,000 mg of hydrocortisone administered intravenously, compared with 12 mg of betamethasone, produced a more dramatic, rapid fall in maternal estriol levels. They suggested that this observation also applied to maturational effects in the fetal lung.

In a small series of patients, Schmidt et al. (1984) found no effect of treatment with 250 mg of hydrocortisone administered in 2 doses 24 h apart. The lack of effect in this study is probably due to the length of the treatment interval, since hydrocortisone is cleared rapidly from both the maternal and fetal circulations (see Chap. 6). In cultured lung, at least, glucocorticoid effects are reversible and thus influenced by the duration of exposure (Chap. 3).

The various regimes used in studies of prenatal hydrocortisone treatment, and the levels of plasma glucocorticoid activity achieved in the fetus are summarized in Table 6.7. In light of animal studies demonstrating that growth and development are adversely affected by prolonged exposure to high doses of glucocorticoids (Chap. 2), regimens employing higher doses of hydrocortisone are not recommended. Moreover, there is no evidence that higher doses of corticosteroid are more effective than the standard dose of betamethasone.

Methylprednisolone. Two studies (Block et al. 1977; Schmidt et al. 1984) have compared the effect of methylprednisolone with betamethasone: Schmidt et al. evaluated hydrocortisone (250 mg q 24 h) as well. Both studies used 125 mg of methylprednisolone, given in 2 doses 24 h apart. In each case there was no reduction in the incidence of RDS by methylprednisolone, whereas betamethasone was effective. The failure of methylprednisolone to decrease RDS in these studies may be a result of its rapid clearance from the fetus (see Chap. 6).

5.2.1.3 Interval from Initiation of Therapy to Birth

Liggins and Howie (1972) originally reported no evidence of efficacy in infants whose mothers delivered less than 24 h after initiation of glucocorticoid therapy. Others (Table 5.2) have concurred that effectiveness is limited to infants who are delivered at least 24 h to 48 h after initiation of therapy. The lag between treatment and clinical response is consistent with the time course of glucocorticoid effects in animals and in culture and reflects the requirement for *de novo* synthesis of proteins (Chap. 2 and 3). Untreated preterm infants born with RDS respond with a rise in endogenous cortisol, a response which may be considered part of the normal "emergency" mechanism of the preterm infant for accelerating surfactant production. This response probably explains, at least in part, the well-known rapid improvement and recovery from RDS which occurs 48–72 h after birth. Even though the occurrence of RDS is not decreased with less than 24 h of therapy, it is possible that in utero exposure to corticosteroid accelerates "spontaneous recovery" and thereby reduces morbidity from RDS.

There is less information available regarding the outer limit of the treatment-delivery interval. In several studies (Table 5.2), treatment was apparently effective among infants who were delivered as long as 7–10 days after the first dose of corticosteroid. The only data regarding longer exposure (Howie and Liggins 1982; U.S. National Collaborative Study 1981) indicate no benefit for infants delivered more than 7–20 days and more than 7 days after the first treatment, respectively. In the New Zealand trial, there were 12 infants who were treated at less than 32 weeks gestation and more than 7 days prior to delivery. RDS occurred in 6 (50%) of these infants, compared with 29 of 51 (56.9%) of control infants and 12 of 59 (20.3%) of infants treated 1–7 days (Liggins, 1975). The apparent lack of effect after 7 to 10 days is most likely explained by "de-induction" of the enzyme systems involved in increasing surfactant production (Chap. 3). In the studies by Caspi et al. (1976) and

Schutte (1981), the incidence of RDS remained low in infants treated weekly for a 3-week period, compared with controls.

5.2.2 Probable Effect on Efficacy

5.2.2.1 Gender and Racial Origin

Taeusch and Tulchinsky (1979) were the first to suggest a difference in the efficacy of prenatal dexamethasone dependent upon gender. There have been additional reports (Ballard et al. 1980; Papageorgiou et al. 1981; U.S. National Collaborative Study 1981) indicating that the male disadvantage in incidence of RDS extends to glucocorticoid responsiveness as well (Table 5.4). This effect, however, is not clear-cut, and obviously varies in different populations. Howie (1984) has been unable to find a male disadvantage in effect of prenatal glucocorticoid therapy, and, in fact, reports that males in New Zealand may respond somewhat better than females. Although the incidence of RDS was slightly higher in males of the control population at all ages, the incidence of RDS in treated males compared with females was lower at less than 30 weeks and 30–32 weeks (21.1 vs. 35.3, 0.0 vs. 15.4, respectively). In a study conducted in Melbourne, Australia, Kuhn et al. (1982) also found a trend toward better responsiveness among males at 27-30 weeks. The U.S. National Collaborative Study (1981) reported that the gender effect applied equally to infants of different racial backgrounds; there was also a suggestion that non-white (Hispanic, North American Indian and "others") female infants had a greater response to prenatal therapy than white females. Clearly, a combination of genetically determined factors influences both the normal occurrence of RDS and responsiveness to prenatal steroid treatment.

5.2.2.2 Asphyxia

The significant role of asphyxia in the development of RDS has long been appreciated (Farrell and Avery 1975). Several investigators have attempted to ex-

Table 5.4. Influence of gender in corticosteroid therapy

Study	Gestational age/ mean birth weight (g)	Incidence of RDS in treated infants				P
		Male	(%)	Female	(%)	
Ballard et al. 1980	750-1750 (1332)	11/31	(35.5)	3/25	(12)	0.03
Papageorgiou et al. 1981	900-2600 (1680)	14/48	(29.1)	4/46	(8.7)	0.02
U.S. National Collab. Study 1981	26-37 weeks (2042)	24/161	(14.9)	7/146	(4.8)	0.01
Caspi et al. 1980	28-36 weeks (32.5)	12/128	(9.4)	11/131	(8.4)	NS
Kuhn et al. 1982	27-33 weeks	7/76	(9.2)	9/56	(16.1)	NS
Howie 1984	28-34 weeks	6/95	(6.3)	10/87	(11.5)	NS

amine this effect in studies of the efficacy of glucocorticoids. Quirk et al. (1979) reported on the outcome of a group of preterm infants delivered with careful attention to advoiding intrapartum hypoxia and providing an atraumatic delivery. Glucocorticoids were given at the discretion of the physicians managing the cases. Weights of treated vs. untreated infants were similar (1540 g vs. 1528 g, mean weights, respectively). There was no difference between the treated and untreated infants in either the incidence of RDS (16.4% vs. 16.1%) or survival (88% vs. 87%). However, it was noted that the overall incidence of RDS in the base population at their institution during the study period was 27–33%, raising a question concerning the selection of patients for the study.

Caspi et al. (1980) examined the incidence of RDS in 259 preterm infants whose mothers had received antepartum dexamethasone therapy. The mean Apgar score was lower in infants who developed RDS than in those without RDS. Caspi (1980) also found a higher incidence of RDS in treated infants who were born by vaginal breech (15.4%), cesarean section (14.6%), or multiple births (16.0%) than those experiencing vaginal vertex delivery (6.8%), and considered this effect to be due in part to more asphyxia. Papageoiou et al. (1979) found no difference between treated and control infants in 1-min Apgar scores, however, scores were higher in treated infants at 5 minutes. They suggested that these infants were more easily resuscitated because of their greater lung maturity.

Schutte et al. (1980) pointed out that there was an increased incidence of RDS in any goup of preterm infants delivered less than 12 h after admission, suggesting intrapartum clinical instability. Taeusch (1979) et al., however, could not confirm this finding and found rather that the decreased incidence of RDS with time after admission was restricted to the steroid-treated group. Apparently, no single therapeutic maneuver, such as the administration of betamethasone to the mother, can completely compensate for the variety of factors which contribute to perinatal asphyxia and, in turn, RDS. Thus, studies examining the effect of betamethasone on infant outcome must also consider the factors leading to asphyxia.

5.2.2.3 Multiple Birth

The second of twins is known to be more likely to suffer from RDS (Farrell and Avery 1975). This has, in general, been considered to be related to the high likelihood of asphyxia with the second twin (Rokos et al. 1968; Hobel et al. 1972; Martin et al. 1974; Worthington and Smith 1978). In their group of infants exposed to dexamethasone, Caspi et al. (1980) noted a difference in incidence of RDS in cases of multiple birth (16%), compared with singleton births (6%). They also found that the incidence of RDS in the first-delivered infant of multiple births was 8.8%, compared with 22% in subsequent infants born second, third, or fourth. In this study, dexamethasone was administered to all women in premature labor; therefore, it was impossible to determine whether asphyxia alone was responsible for the higher incidence of RDS, or whether glucocorticoids are less effective for twins.

In the U.S. National Collaborative Study (Collaborative Study Group, 1981), in the incidence of RDS was higher in twins than in singletons, whether they were in the placebo (38.5 % vs. 16.1 %) or in the stereoid-treated group (41.7 % vs. 10 %). Although the numbers in the twin subgroup study are small, the results are consistent with those of Caspi et al. (1980). The authors speculate that steroid pharmacokinetics might be different in multiple pregnancies; they did not examine the question of whether the effect might be due to asphyxia of the second twin.

5.2.2.4 Prolonged Rupture of Membranes

In the early 1970's, a number of investigators (Yoon and Harper 1973; Richardson et al. 1973; Bauer et al. 1974; Berkowitz et al. 1976) reported decreased incidence of RDS associated with prolonged rupture of membranes (greater than 24 h, in general). However, Jones et al. (1975) in reviewing 16,458 births in Denver over a 12-year period, could find no protective effect of prolonged rupture of membranes in prevention of RDS. The controversy concerning a protective effect of rupture of membranes has still not been settled. Of the 21 studies of prenatal glucocorticoid treatment reviewed in Table 5.2, 13 studies examined the influence of prolonged rupture of membranes on RDS incidence. Of these, only three demonstrated any reduction in RDS which could be attributed to prolonged rupture of membranes (Block et al. 1977; U.S. Collaborative Study 1981; Kuhn et al. 1982).

In attempting to answer this question, Garite et al. (1981) conducted a prospective, randomized study involving patients with prolonged premature rupture of membranes between the 28th and 34th weeks of pregnancy. They divided the patients into two groups: one group received glucocorticoids and had "active management of labor", including delivery 48 h following initiation of therapy. A nontreated group was managed by the "expectant approach" and allowed to deliver by spontaneous labor or by cesarean section when chorioamnionitis or fetal distress developed. In this study, there was no demonstrated benefit of glucocorticoids on the incidence or severity (mechanical ventilation for more than 24 h) of RDS, and there was an increase in maternal infection in the actively managed group. However, there was a trend toward decreased incidence of RDS among infants of 28–32 weeks gestation who received corticosteroids: 6 of 24 (25%) vs. 10 of 21 (48%) in the untreated group. Since treated mothers were managed "actively" in ways different from the untreated mothers, it is difficult to distinguish the effect of glucocorticoids alone. The mean duration of rupture of membranes in the two groups was not statistically different, although there was a trend toward earlier delivery of the active management group.

Kuhn et al. (1982) has, perhaps, the most convincing data for a protective effect of ruptured membranes. They assessed the effect of prolonged rupture of membranes in association with glucocorticoids in 469 patients admitted before 34 weeks gestation (see Table 5.5). Steroid treatment reduced the incidence of RDS from 42% to 26% ($p < 0.05$) in those without prolonged ruptured membranes and from 25% to 7% in infants with prolonged rupture ($p < 0.02$). When examined separately within the steroid and control groups, the presence of prolonged rupture reduced the incidence of RDS in both control (42% vs. 25%, $p < 0.02$) and steroid-treated infants (26% vs. 7%, $p < 0.01$).

Table 5.5. Incidence of severe RDS with prolonged rupture of membranes (Kuhn et al. 1982)

	Steroidtherapy RDS/N (%)		Controls RDS/N (%)		p
No prolonged rupture of membranes	25/95	(26 %)	46/100	(42 %)	< 0.05
Prolonged rupture of membranes	4/55	(7 %)	24/95	(25 %)	< 0.02
	p < 0.01		p < 0.02		

A number of other investigators, however, (see Table 5.2) have been unable to demonstrate any beneficial effect of membrane rupture in addition to the steroid effect. Obviously, this effect is not a consistent finding and is difficult to quantify. It would appear that, while prolonged rupture of membranes may indeed aid in accelerating fetal lung maturity in some patients who are not experiencing infection, this circumstance does not substitute for the beneficial effect of glucocorticoids. Management of women with ruptured membranes should always be expectant, combined with close monitoring for signs of maternal or fetal infection or fetal distress.

5.2.3 Insufficient Evidence Regarding Efficacy

5.2.3.1 Maternal Diabetes

It has been appreciated for some time that infants of diabetic mothers have an increased incidence of RDS (Usher et al. 1971; Robert et al. 1976; see also Chap. 9). Robert et al. (1976), for example, reported that respiratory distress was 5.6 times as likely to develop in infants of diabetic mothers as in infants of nondiabetic mothers at 32–38.5 weeks gestation ($p < 0.00001$). In addition, a significant percentage of infants of diabetic mothers with "mature" L/S ratios will develop RDS; additional markers of lung maturity, such as phosphatidylglycerol levels and substantially higher L/S ratios are required for accurate prediction of lung maturation (Lowensohn and Gabbe 1979; Kulovich and Gluck 1979; Kulovich et al. 1979). The mechanism of these changes in the amniotic fluid lipid profile is not understood; however, Draisey et al. (1977) found that amniotic-fluid, immunoreactive-insulin concentrations were inversely correlated with lecithin concentrations.

A number of studies evaluating glucocorticoids have excluded diabetic women from the trials. Even in those series in which they were included (Howie and Liggins 1982), the number of diabetic patients was too small to determine reliably whether or not glucocorticoids affected the incidence of RDS. Steroid administration to the diabetic mother is known to increase insulin requirements and thus complicate the management of diabetes (Baxter and Rousseau 1979). In women whose diabetes is very difficult to control, steroid therapy is probably contraindicated for this reason. Otherwise, use of glucocorticoids should follow recommendations similar to those for other infants.

5.2.3.2 Rhesus Sensitization

In the New Zealand study (Howie and Liggins 1982), there were 59 women entered who had Rh-isoimmunization, an insufficient number for demonstration of a corticosteroid effect on the incidence of RDS. Caritis et al. (1977) treated 6 women, delivering at less than 32 weeks gestation, who had severe Rh-sensitization and L/S ratios of less than 1.5:1. Only one of the 7 infants had mild RDS, and all survived. They noted that, in these cases, there was a marked decrease in the delta optical density (OD) at 450 in the amniotic fluid following treatment. Anderson and Cordero (1980) reported a similar change in the OD in 5 women at 32–34 weeks gestation who were treated with a large dose of hydrocortisone (1 g q 8 h×4). Two of these women were delivered at term; 2 of 3 infants who were delivered prematurely had RDS but survived. The mechanism for the decrease in OD of the treated women is not understood. These investigators propose that the change may represent an immunosuppressant effect of corticosteroids due to either (a) decreased anti-Rh antibody levels or (b) decreased red-cell antigen-antibody affinity with decreased red-cell destruction. Another possible mechanism might be either decreased excretion (in lung fluid) or increased clearance of bilirubin from amniotic fluid; in this situation there would be no benefit to the fetus with regard to red-cell hemolysis. This effect of corticosteroids in erythroblastic infants deserves further investigation. It is also an effect of which the obstetrician must be aware.

5.2.3.3 Cesarean Section

There is an increased incidence of RDS in infants born by cesarean section without preceding labor (see Chap. 8). The factors involved in this effect are likely multiple and probably include endogenous levels of corticoids and catecholamines. Delivery by cesarean section may also influence the response to glucocorticoid therapy. Caspi et al. (1980) reported a somewhat higher incidence of RDS among treated infants born by cesarean section (14.6%) versus vaginal vertex delivery (6.8%); however, these differences were not statistically significant. Vaginal *breech* delivery was also associated with more RDS (15.4%). The 5-min Apgar score was significantly lower in both breech and section deliveries versus vaginal vertex births. However, Papageorgiou et al. (1981), in their study reporting a gender difference in response to glucocorticoids, found no apparent effect of cesarean section vs. vaginal delivery on the incidence of RDS (30.3% vs. 29.7% for male infants and 14.2% vs. 6.2% for female infants, respectively).

5.2.3.4 Tocolytics

In all of the studies of prenatal glucocorticoid, some tocolytic agent has been used to delay delivery. Since there have been a few reports of a beneficial effect of β-adrenergic agents on the incidence of RDS (Kero et al. 1973; Boog et al. 1975 and summarized in Table 8.5), it is important to evaluate the effect of the tocolytic agent, whether it be ethanol, a betamimetic agent, or magnesium sulfate, on the incidence of RDS. Eight of the 21 studies reported in Table 5.2 examined the effect of tocolytics on the incidence of RDS. None found a beneficial effect of tocolytics distinct from the effect of delaying labor and allowing longer exposure to corticosteroids.

5.2.3.5 Toxemia (Hypertension/Edema/Proteinuria Syndromes)

Liggins and Howie (1972), in their initial study, reported findings on 89 mothers (who delivered 90 infants) who had severe hypertension/edema/proteinuria syndromes. Although there was a decreased incidence of RDS in the treated group when compared with the controls (8.6% vs. 30%, $p < 0.05$), there were more fetal deaths in the betamethasone-treated infants than in the controls (25.5% vs. 7%). This finding, although statistically not significant, caused Liggins as well as other investigators and clinicians to proceed with great caution in treating women with hypertension/proteinuria syndrome. On further review, however, Howie and Liggins (1982) found that the excessive fetal death rate was due to a random difference in population selection, since the severity of pre-eclampsia in the treated and control mothers was not comparable. The betamethasone-treated group had much more severe toxemia, with earlier onset and a longer interval between onset and delivery. In fact, all of the fetal deaths in the betamethasone treated group occurred in women who had proteinuria of more than 2 g per day for at least 14 days. Subsequent management by the New Zealand group, as well as by other perinatal groups, has not allowed such delay in delivery of women with toxemia of this severity, and there have been no further reports of increased fetal death.

Two additional studies (Nochimson and Petrie 1979; Ricke et al. 1980) have addressed the question of safety of corticosteroids in pregnancy-induced hypertension. In both studies, women of 27 to 34 weeks gestation were initially stabilized on intravenous magnesium sulfate, and the fetus was evaluated by ocytocin challenge test (OCT). If the test showed a reactive fetus, the mother was considered a candidate for glucocorticoid therapy. Betamethasone was administered, the fetus and mother were monitored continuously, and the infants were delivered if there was any evidence of fetal or maternal deterioration. In Nochimson and Petrie's study (1979), women with a diastolic blood pressure of more than 110 to 120 mm Hg for more than 12–24 h were delivered, regardless of exposure time to glucocorticoids.

Table 5.6 reviews their findings. In the 45 treated mothers in the two studies, there was only one fetal death. No adverse neonatal or maternal findings,

Table 5.6. Glucocorticoids in hypertension-proteinuria syndromes outcome in treated infants

	n	Fetal death		RDS		Liveborn survived	
		#	%	#	%	#	%
Liggins & Howie (1972)[a]	47	12	25.5	3	8.6	44	94
Nochimson and Petrie (1979)[b]	21	1	4.8	5	25	18	85
Ricke et al. (1980)[b]	25	0	0	6[c]	25	22	88

[a] Women with severe toxemia (2 gm protein/day 14 days)
[b] Continuous fetal monitoring
[c] RDS mild to moderate

such as further increase in blood pressure, infection, or abnormal wound healing, were found. One woman developed pulmonary edema while receiving magnesium sulfate and betamethasone (Ricke et al. 1980). This complication has previously been reported in women receiving betamimetic tocolytics, with or without concurrent glucocorticoid therapy (Robertson et al. 1981). The incidence of RDS in both studies was 25%. There were no control groups, however, so it is impossible to evaluate whether glucocorticoids were effective in lowering the incidence of RDS in these patients. In the study by Ricke et al. (1980), however, 15 of the 17 women of more than 30 weeks gestation had an amniocentesis, and the L/S ratio was less than 2:1 in each case. Of these, 13 had an L/S ratio of less than 1.5:1, predicting a higher likelihood of RDS than the observed 25%. They also note that, when RDS did occur, it was only of mild to moderate severity.

It is now clear that glucocorticoids may be used safely in women with hypertension/proteinuria syndrome, provided there is careful continuous monitoring of both maternal and fetal condition. Further data are needed to establish efficacy in this situation.

5.2.4 Summary and Recommendations

Table 5.7 presents the current understanding of the indications and contraindications for use of glucocorticoids for the prevention of RDS, as well as

Table 5.7. Guidelines for glucocorticoid administration for prevention of RDS

Indications

1. Threatened premature delivery between 27 and 34 weeks gestation (if dates are in doubt, may give as early as 26 weeks gestation)
2. Threatened premature delivery after 34 weeks if studies show immature fetal lungs (LS ratio, shake test, etc.)

Contraindications

1. Fetal distress
2. Amnionitis
3. Severe maternal bleeding or significant fetal blood loss
4. Gestational age less than 26 weeks unless family fully informed and wishes to take risk of tiny premature
5. Gestational age more than 34 weeks unless amniotic fluid shows immature lungs

Premature rupture of membranes without labor

1. Assess possibility of amnionitis in mother
   If present:
   Deliver infant – do not give glucocorticoids
2. If no sign of amnionitis:
   a) Obtain cervical cultures
   b) Give glucocorticoid

Ruptured membranes and mother in labor – cervical dilation less than 4-5 cm

1. May give tocolytics for 24 h to provide at least 24 h exposure to glucocorticoid
2. Discontinue tocolytics after 24 h
3. Monitor mother for signs of amnionitis
4. Deliver infant if signs of maternal infection appear

Table 5.8. Glucocorticoids of established efficacy

A.	Liggins & Howie 1972 Form: Celestone Soluspan (betamethasone acetate 6 mg and betamethasone phosphate 6 mg) Dose: 12 mg, IM. Repeat once either 12 or 24 h after first dose
B.	Taeusch et al. 1979 Form: Dexamethasone Dose: 4 mg, IM, q 8 h × 6
C.	U.S. National Collaborative Study 1981 Form: Dexamethasone Dose: 5 mg, IM, q 12 h × 4
Repeat Course in 7-10 days:	
If:	
	1. Premature delivery still threatens 2. Amniotic fluid indices still show immature lungs 3. Gestational age still less than 32 weeks
Maximum number of courses recommended 3	

guidelines for their use in premature rupture of the membranes. Table 5.8 summarizes the different types of glucocorticoids, dosages, and treatment intervals for which efficacy in preventing RDS has been established.

5.3 Other Effects of Therapy

5.3.1 L/S Ratio

Liggins and Howie (1972) determined L/S ratios on amniotic fluid of some of the women in their study, and concluded that there was no detectable effect of betamethasone therapy. Spellacy et al. (1973) later reported a greater rise in the L/S ratio 2 weeks after dexamethasone injections than in uninjected control pregnancies. Subsequently there have been a number of investigations of this issue (reviewed by Morrison et al. (1977)); there are approximately equal numbers of studies reporting an increase in L/S ratio as those finding no change. Arias et al. (1979) examined both saturated PC and the L/S ratio in amniotic fluid; they found a slight, but significant, increase in L/S ratio (1.49 ± 0.21 vs. 1.09 ± 0.29). In addition, 12 betamethasone-injected patients had an increase in saturated PC within 14 days following treatment, compared with no change in 6 untreated women ($p = 0.016$). Caspi et al. (1975) measured the effect of dexamethasone on amniotic fluid L/S ratio in 15 women at 34 weeks gestation or less. They found an increase in L/S ratio to mature levels in 12 patients. However, the interval for re-examining fluid ranged from 24 h to 11 days after therapy. The only infant of the 12 who developed RDS was a 1240-g second twin delivered at 30 weeks gestation who had a post-treatment L/S ratio of 1.4:1.

Farrell et al. (1983), reporting for the U.S. National Collaborative Study, found no significant difference in amniotic fluid L/S ratios measured 1 week after treatment in a group of 25 dexamethasone-treated pregnancies (increase of 0.94), compared with 20 control pregnancies (increase of 0.57, NS). However, the analysis is complicated by the fact that the average gestational age of the fetuses being studied was 32.9 weeks, a period when L/S ratios are normally rising. There was a lower incidence of RDS in the 25 infants exposed to dexamethasone in utero (4% vs. 10% in the control group of 20 infants). The authors also presented more specific data from 17 pregnancies in the treated group. Again, the mean gestational age was 32.5 weeks, and the average interval between amniocenteses was 6.8 days. A significant increase after treatment was noted in the amount of PC and in saturated PC, although phosphatidylglycerol could not be detected in either pre- or post-treatment samples. They noted, however, that the L/S ratio in this group of patients *was* predictive of which infants would develop RDS. In the 12 infants who did not develop RDS, the ratio was 4.56 ± 1.05, significantly higher than in the 5 infants who developed RDS (L/S ratio 1.83 ± 0.27, $p < 0.03$). Nevertheless, they conclude that current tests routinely used to assess fetal lung maturity do not provide a reliable means for detection of fetal pulmonary responses to prenatal glucocorticoid administration and that repeat amniocentesis should not be done for this purpose.

The reasons that amniotic fluid tests fail as accurate predictors of accelerated lung maturity after glucocorticoid treatment are probably several-fold. First, as mentioned earlier, most studies have involved gestations of mean age of 32–33 weeks, a time when lung maturation is normally occurring in untreated fetuses. A glucocorticoid effect on the L/S ratio might be easier to demonstrate in younger fetuses. However, amniocentesis usually is not done because it is assumed that, before 30 weeks gestation, the likelihood of fetal lung immaturity is very high, and the procedure is not justified. Second, the volume of the amniotic fluid pool is known to vary widely. This introduces variability into values for the L/S ratio, particularly among women in premature labor with leaking membranes, and may obscure changes in surfactant secretion induced by corticosteroids. Third, the amount of increased surfactant production induced by corticosteroid may be insufficient to substantially alter the surfactant concentration measured in amniotic fluid, although still sufficient to improve alveolar stability and prevent RDS. Finally, it is possible that much of the (assumed) increased surfactant production stimulated by glucocorticoid is only released with lung inflation at the time of birth.

5.3.2 Risks and Benefits

Although RDS continues to be a a major disease of the preterm infant, its relative contribution to mortality and morbidity has decreased markedly during the past 15 years, while other problems of the preterm infant have emerged as clinically important. In evaluating the overall impact of therapy, it is therefore necessary to examine *all* of the beneficial effects of prenatal corticosteroids, as well as known and possible risks.

5.3.2.1 Potential Risks

Taeusch (1975) reviewed the potential toxicity of prenatal glucocorticoid therapy, and others (Gluck 1976; Ballard and Ballard 1979; Crowley 1981; Depp et al. 1980) have deliberated risk vs. benefit considerations. Studies in rats and rabbits have led to concerns in the areas of infection, growth – both of the lung specifically and general somatic growth – neurological development, immunological competency, metabolic and hormonal disturbances, and placental function (reviewed in Chap. 2). All of these concerns have been addressed in the human, with the following findings in mother and fetus.

1) Maternal

Increased Infection in the Presence of PROM. Taeusch et al. (1979) and Young et al. (1980), using dexamethasone, and Garite et al. (1981), using betamethasone, found an increased incidence of infection in mothers with prolonged rupture of membranes. Schmidt et al. (1984) found increased infection in women who delivered vaginally after treatment with hydrocortisone but *not* after betamethasone or methylprednisolone. While other authors have not found a similar increase, it is clear that treated women must be monitored for signs of infection.
Metabolic Disturbances in Diabetics. It is well known that glucocorticoid administration is associated with increased difficulty of management of glucose homeostasis in the diabetic (Usher et al. 1971; Robert et al. 1976), and therefore glucocorticoids may be contraindicated in some women with severe diabetes.
Pulmonary Edema. There have been several reports of women in preterm labor who receive tocolytics, either beta-mimetic agents or magnesium sulfate, who have developed pulmonary edema. In their series, Robertson et al. (1981) found that only 50 % of the women had received glucocorticoid with a similar number developing the syndrome after receiving only beta-mimetic agents. Since tocolytics are routinely used in conjunction with corticosteroids, pulmonary edema may be considered as an indirect associated risk of glucocorticoid therapy.

2) Infant

Infection. Although there has been considerable concern about possible increased incidence of neonatal infection, none of the investigators (see Table 5.2) who has examined this question has found a significant increase in infection, and in several studies there was an apparent decrease.
Metabolic Disturbances. One study (Papageorgiou et al. 1979) reported an increased incidence of transient hypoglycemia in the first hour after birth. Other investigators have not confirmed this finding, and no clinical significance of this measurement has been described. The same group, however, reported a tendency toward hypocalcemia in the *placebo* group, possibly because those infants were, in general, sicker.
Immunologic Function. Since glucocorticoids are well known to affect immune responses, there has naturally been concern that administration of prenatal glucocorticoids might affect the fetal and subsequently even the adult immune system. Table 5.9 reviews the studies to date addressing this topic.

Table 5.9. Immunologic evaluation of infants exposed to prenatal glucocorticoid

Granberg et al. 1975	No difference in IgM in treated vs, control preterm infants without RDS
Cederqvist et al. 1978	No difference in IgA, IgA_1, IgA_2, IgM in treated vs control infants; Questionable decrease in IgG with betamethasone; No decrease in IgG with dexamethasone
Ryhanen et al. 1980	No difference in lymphocyte count; ANAE% of lymphs; normal ANAE response at 6 days. Normal response to PHA, PWM stimulation
Fletcher et al. 1979	Thymic size decreased in normal preterms without RDS; same after betamethasone
Howie 1984	No difference at 7 years of age in immunoglobulins, lymphocyte percentages or PHA response
Case reports (see text)	Benign leukemoid reaction associated with prenatal glucorticoids in 7 preterm infants (6 females)

ANAE, Acid alphanaphthyl acetate esterase; PHA, Phytohemagglutinin; PMW, Pokeweed mitogen

Granberg et al. (1975) reported that there was no difference in IgM concentrations at birth in a group of 10 preterm infants who received prenatal glucocorticoids, vs. 10 healthy untreated infants. Cederqvist et al. (1978) looked at the effect of prenatal dexamethasone or betamethasone on immunoglobulin levels. They studied IgA, IgM and IgG classes and IgA_1 and IgA_2 subclasses in cord blood and anmiotic fluid following administration of glucocorticoid, and combined data from studies done in Finland and Sweden. They found no difference in IgA, IgA_1, IgA_2 or IgM concentrations in cord serum in treated infants compared with controls. Interestingly, they did find a significantly decreased level of IgG compared to controls in the group of 10 infants whose mothers received betamethasone, although there was no depression of IgG level in the dexamethasone-treated infants. They also noted that, in cases where there was premature rupture of membranes, treated fetuses responded with accelerated synthesis of either IgA or IgM, as would be expected in normal infants.

Ryhanen et al. (1980) examined the effect of glucocorticoid therapy on neonatal cell-mediated immunity in a small group of infants (6 treated, 4 controls). These infants were studied using blood leucocyte count, the relative and absolute amount of acid alpha-naphthal acetate esterase (ANAE)-positive cells and the lymphocyte response to both phytohemagglutinin (PHA) and poke-weed mitogen (PWM)-stimulation. They found no difference in the increase in the number of lymphocytes and ANAE-positive cells during the first week of life in the two groups, and concluded that neonatal peripheral blood leucocyte function does not appear to be disturbed by short-term prenatal dexamethasone therapy.

Fletcher et al. (1979) compared thymic size, measured on radiographs as the cardiothymic-thoracic (CT/T) ratio, for groups of treated infants and control infants with and without RDS. They found that healthy preterm infants had a CT/T ratio of 0.35. The 19 patients treated prenatally with betamethasone had a mean ratio of 0.37, which was significantly lower than that of the

12 placebo-treated infants, who had a mean ratio of 0.41. In addition, they noted that the infants without RDS showed a significantly lower CT/T ratio than newborns with RDS, whether or not they had received glucocorticoids. They suggested that perhaps smaller thymic size, reflecting elevated fetal plasma corticoids, is an indicator of lung maturation.

There has been interest in the effect of prenatal glucocorticoids on neutrophilic leukocytosis. Wong and Taeusch (1978) reported that during steroid treatment, mothers had a 25% increase in total WBC, with a 40% increase in neutrophil count and a 35% decrease in lymphocyte count.

There have also been several case reports (Bielawski et al 1978; Otero et al. 1981; Anday and Harris 1982) of leukemoid reaction in preterm infants associated with antenatal glucocorticoid therapy. White cell counts in these cases were well outside the normal range (9,000 to 30,000 per microliter) for the first week of life, ranging from 42,500 to 112,000. All of the infants were evaluated for other possible causes of their leukocytosis, but no cases of infection were found. All had a benign clinical course and white cell levels returned to normal levels by approximately 1 week of age. It is interesting that 6 of the 7 infants reported were females.

Other possible immunological consequences of prenatal glucocorticoid therapy later in life will be reviewed in the section on Follow-up (Sect. 5.4).

5.3.2.2 Established Benefits

1) Decreased Patent Ductus Arteriosus

Patent ductus arteriosus (PDA) is a major cause of morbidity in small preterm infants. Two groups (Clyman et al. 1981a; Waffarn et al. 1983) have reported that prenatal glucocorticoids reduce the incidence of PDA in prematures (Table 5.10). Clyman reported an incidence of clinically significant PDA in 34% in untreated infants, compared to 18% among glucocorticoid-treated infants. Waffarn et al. (1983) found a decrease from 44% to 6.5% in infants under 2000 g. The long-term follow-up study from the U.S National Collaborative Study (1984) also found less PDA in treated infants. It might be argued that betamethasone decreases the incidence of PDA by reducing the inci-

Table 5.10. Prenatal glucocorticoid therapy and patent ductus arteriosus

Study	Birthweight range (control vs. treated)	Incidence of PDA	
		Betamethasone therapy	Untreated
Clyman et al. 1981a	500-1300 g (1138 vs. 1128)	19/104 (18 %)	36/107 (34 %)[a]
Waffarn et al. 1983	< 2 000 g (mean 1408 vs. 1640)	1/15 (6.5 %)	14/32 (44 %)[b]

[a] $p < 0.002$
[b] $p < 0.01$

dence of RDS. However, Clyman etal. (1981 a) point out that, in their study, betamethasone appeared to reduce the incidence of PDA by 24 h after therapy, although there was no apparent effect of therapy on the incidence of RDS until more than 48 h. Moreover, although prevention of RDS appeared to be more effective in females, prevention of PDA with betamethasone was more effective in males; PDA occurred in 38% of untreated males vs. 11% in the treated group ($p < 0.01$), whereas there was no difference in PDA incidence between treated and untreated female infants. Since administration of glucocorticoid to the premature fetal lamb matures responsiveness of the ductus arteriosus to prostaglandins, Clyman et al. (1981 b) suggest that treated infants are less sensitive to the prostaglandins which maintain ductal patency. These clinical observations on PDA are also supported by data on glucocorticoid effects in rats (Momma et al. 1981).

A reduction in the occurrence of PDA may have a major impact on neonatal morbidity. Infants without a significant shunt and the associated increase in pulmonary and decrease in systemic blood flow require less ventilatory assistance, are easier to feed, experience less necrotizing enterocolitis (Kitterman 1975), and do not require either indomethacin (with its potential renal problems) or surgery for ductal closure. The effect of glucocorticoids on the ductus probably contributes to decreased severity of RDS, as well as decreased overall morbidity among treated infants.

2) Decreased Intracranial Hemorrhage

In their initial report, Liggins and Howie (1972) examined the incidence of intracranial hemorrhage in liveborn preterm infants who died within 24 h to 7 days after entry into the trial. They found hemorrhage in 2 (1.7%) of the treated infants, compared with 11 (11.1%) of the control infants ($p < 0.01$). Taeusch et al. (1979) diagnosed intracranial hemorrhage (pre-CT scanning) in four of the 65 placebo-treated infants (all died) and in none of the 30 treated infants in their study. Clark et al. (1981) also found that prenatal treatment with betamethasone was one of the most significant preventive factors associated with decreased incidence of intracranial hemorrhage in infants born in a perinatal center (12%) vs. outborn, transported infants (56%); 65% of the inborn infants received betamethasone, compared with only 8% of outborn ($p < 0.001$).

3) Decreased Severity of RDS

Of the 21 studies reviewed in Table 5.2, 10 evaluated the clinical course of RDS which occurred, and 9 of these reported decreased severity of RDS in infants exposed to prenatal glucocorticoid treatment (Table 5.11). Papageorgiou et al. (1979) found that only one of 29 treated infants (3.4%) was diagnosed clinically as having moderate or severe RDS, compared with 11 of 32 (34.3%) of the control infants ($p < 0.05$). Taeusch et al. (1979) reported severe RDS in only 1 of 30 infants whose mothers received a course of steroids, compared with 11 (including 4 deaths from RDS) of 65 mothers who received at least 1 dose of placebo ($p = 0.05$). Ballard et al. (1979) found that 18.2% of treated compared with 69% of untreated infants required more than 24 h of greater than 50% inspired oxygen concentrations ($p < 0.025$).

Table 5.11. Severity of RDS after prenatal glucocorticoids

Study	Finding	Incidence		p
		Treated (%)	Controls (%)	
Papageorgiou et al. 1979	Decrease in moderate-severe RDS	3.4	34.3	0.05
Taeusch et al. 1979	Decrease in severe RDS	3.3	17 (4 deaths)	0.05
Ballard et al. 1979	Decrease in O_2 requirement (> 24 h in 50 % O_2)	18.2	69	0.025
Young et al. 1980	Decrease in severe RDS	10	34	0.001

The effect of glucocorticoids on the severity of RDS may reflect partial but inadequate stimulation of surfactant production in some infants. Although RDS occurs in such cases, it is milder than it would be without treatment. An alternative or additional mechanism contributing to decreased severity might be earlier or more efficient clearance of lung water at birth. Since glucocorticoids induce the beta-adrenergic receptor in the lung, and secretion of lung water appears to be under beta-adrenergic control (see Chap. 8), it is tempting to speculate that treated infants would have more compliant lungs at birth. This would result in less asphyxia, easier resuscitation, and less need for high pressures and oxygen tensions for ventilation. Although no study has been large enough to examine definitively the impact of glucocorticoid therapy on chronic lung disease, the decreased severity of RDS in treated infants may be associated with reduced morbidity from chronic lung disease, one of the major problems still facing the preterm infant.

4) Decreased Necrotizing Enterocolitis

Bauer et al. (1984) reported from the U.S. National Collaborative Study that there was a significantly decreased incidence of necrotizing enterocolitis in infants receiving treatment. Necrotizing enterocolitis occurred in 6 of 307 (2%) of the steroid-treated group, compared with 21 of 297 (7.1%) of the placebo-treated group ($p = 0.002$). They examined the incidence of necrotizing enterocolitis within groups stratified by a number of different conditions, including race, sex, gestational age, birthweight, prolonged rupture of membranes, incidence of pre-eclampsia, requirement for resuscitation, and intubation. They also compared the incidence of necrotizing enterocolitis for infants with and without sepsis, PDA, hypertensive episodes, bleeding, RDS, hypocalcemia and congenital heart disease. In all of these situations, the incidence of necrotizing enterocolitis was significantly decreased in steroid-treated groups. They found that the best predictors of necrotizing enterocolitis occurrence were sepsis, intubation, and use of umbilical artery catheters. It is of interest that the incidence of necrotizing enterocolitis in infants with sepsis, was 35% in the placebo group (7 of 20 infants) and 0% (0 of 13 infants) in the steroid-treated group.

There is ample animal evidence (reviewed by Ballard 1979) of glucocorticoid induction of enzyme systems in the developing intestine. Therefore, it is

Table 5.12. Effect of prenatal glucocorticoid therapy on cost of hospitalization (Collaborative group on Antenatal Steroid Therapy 1981; Avery 1984)

Decreased length of stay	3.5 days/infant
Number of infants in study	342
Reduction in hospital days	$3.5 \times 342 = 1\,197$
Average cost ICN/day (1984)	$ 1,200
Cost saving for infants in study	$ 1,436,400
Cost saving if 25 % of 40,000 infants/yr With RDS were treated Prenatally	$ 42 Million/yr

not surprising that prenatal glucocorticoid therapy might also accelerate maturation of the preterm intestine, providing a protective effect against necrotizing enterocolitis in these infants.

5) Decreased Length of Hospital Stay and Cost

Two studies (Collaborative Study 1981; Johnson et al. 1981) have specifically examined the effect of prenatal glucocorticoids on the length of stay and cost of hospital care as indices of morbidity. The collaborative study (1981) found a significant decrease in mean length of stay from 25 days in the placebo group to 21.4 days in the treated group. In addition, there was a decrease in postdischarge emergency room visits among treated infants. Johnson et al. (1981) examined these factors in their institution during 1979. They found significantly increased survival in 750–1250 g infants with *no* difference in cost or length of stay. However, for infants of 1250–1750 g birthweight, treatment was associated with a significant decrease in cost.

Table 5.12 presents calculations on the potential impact of glucocorticoid therapy on the national cost of providing care for preterm infants.

5.3.3 Other Observations

5.3.3.1 Retinopathy of Prematurity

Another continuing area of concern for morbidity among preterm infants is retinopathy of prematurity. A number of studies have looked at factors associated with an increased incidence of retinopathy of prematurity in the preterm infant. There are at present no data relating to a possible effect of prenatal glucocorticoids on incidence of retinopathy of prematurity.

5.3.3.2 Skin

It has been suggested from clinical observations that glucocorticoids might accelerate maturation of the skin of the premature infant. A maturational effect on the skin would be of benefit, since its integrity and ability to prevent both insensible water loss and infection become major limiting factors in survival.

5.3.3.3 Fetal Breathing

Patrick et al. (1981) studied fetal breathing movements in 6 women who received exogenous glucocorticoids during their pregnancy. They were studied initially while receiving prednisone for their own illness and then one week later on an equivalent dose of dexamethasone (which crosses the placenta in greater amounts). They found no difference in fetal breathing movements when comparing the prednisone-treated with the dexamethasone-treated group. They did find more breathing movements following meals and in the late evening following glucocorticoid administration. The authors suggest that maternal glucocorticoid concentrations may influence patterns of fetal breathing.

5.4 Follow-up After Glucocorticoid Therapy

The outcome of low-birthweight infants, in general, and those with RDS, in particular, has been reviewed recently by Lipper et al. (1981), Samaroff (1980), Stewart and Reynolds, (1974), Stewart et al. (1977, 1981), Brann and Volpe (1980), and Farrell (1982). The pulmonary outcome of these infants has been studied by Heldt et al. (1980), and Maclusky et al. (1984). It is relatively well established that the group of infants who suffer from RDS do have some significant problems in long-term outcome (Drorbaugh et al. 1975; Fisch et al. 1975; Fitzhardinge et al. 1976; Moore 1976; Kampner 1978a, b; Pape 1978). However, since most infants with RDS are preterm and require a variety of therapeutic interventions, it is impossible to separate the impact of RDS alone from that of prematurity or the therapies used. The outcome for infants who were exposed to glucocorticoids in utero must be considered against this background of concern about both the neurodevelopmental and pulmonary outcome of preterm infants.

5.4.1 General Growth and Development

MacArthur et al. (1981) published the first comprehensive report of the cognitive and psychosocial development of 4-year-old children whose mothers had been treated antenatally with betamethasone. He reported follow-up of 258 children from the original Liggins and Howie study (1972). Because of increased survival among treated infants, they note that the treated group was weighted with a greater number of less mature subjects, as well as with more boys (with a statistically significant lower birth weight, i.e., 322.8 g less than control boys). The groups, however, were well matched in terms of ethnic origin, maternal age, educational level, parental occupation, number of siblings and position of the subject within the family. The information they obtained on these infants included (1) Stanford-Binet I.Q. and Peabody Picture Vocabulary Tests, (2) Frostig developmental test of visual perception, (3) Vineland Social Maturity Scale, (4) tape recordings of speech samples, (5) general assessment of the developmental history from birth, and (6) an assessment of environmental factors that might have influenced outcome. They also obtained parent questionnaires to ascertain general health and well-being of the children. They found no difference between treated and control infants in any of these areas, despite the expectation that the lower birth weight and shorter gestation of the treated group might have been expected to depress the results of this group on several of the variables irrespective of any effects of treatment. They also reported the interesting finding from the parental questionnaire that more mothers of control girls (34.6 %) than of betamethasone-treated girls (10.5 %) felt there had been feeding problems after taking their infants home from the hospital ($p < 0.001$). In addition fewer of the mothers of treated girls (36.3 %) than of control girls (50 %) saw them as being particularly vulnerable to illness during the first four years of life. This held true for the entire group of subjects as well (29.5 %, compared with 44.7 % of controls, $p < 0.002$).

Two hundred fifty of the same children were further evaluated by Mac Arthur et al. (1982) at a mean age of 6 years, 2 months, when they had attended school in New Zealand for at least one year (139 treated, 111 controls). Tests of cognitive development were given: (1) The Illinois Test of Psycholinguistic Abilities, (2) the Peabody Picture Vocabulary Test, (3) Raven's Colored Progressive Matrices, and (4) Bender Motor-Visual Gestalt Test. In addition, general physical and mental development were assessed, and evaluation of school progress by both teacher and parent interviews, rating systems, language skills, and speech development were evaluated. Again, in spite of the generally lower weight and gestational age of the treated infants, no differences in most of the areas were found between treated and control groups. There was, however, a small but statistically significant lower mean score on the Raven Matrices (the visual perceptual test). This effect was found only in the treated boys who, as noted earlier, were significantly smaller at birth than the control infants. The possible significance of this isolated finding is unclear, but may warrant further evaluation.

They also found that betamethasone-treated girls were taller and somewhat heavier than their matched controls, and, in addition, were reported as having fewer behavioral problems and better motor coordination. There were no differences in incidence of neurological abnormalities, general medical problems or ophthalmological abnormalities between the two groups.

The Collaborative Group on Antenatal Steroid Therapy in the U.S. (1984) has now accummulated follow-up evaluations during the first three years of life. These were carried out on 406 of the 646 surviving infants in that study. They evaluated the infants by Dubowitz evaluation for gestational age, and growth was monitored with standard growth curves. Newborn neurological assessment was done at 40 weeks using a modified Prechtl examination, and standard neurological evaluations were done at 9, 18 and 36-month visits. They found no difference in head circumference or neurological abnormalities between the two groups. They did find that infants in the treated group had approximately 3 % greater growth in weight and length than controls ($p = 0.05$) at 18 and 36 months of age.

Developmental assessments included the mental developmental index (MDI) and psychomotor index (PDI) of the Bayley Scales of Infant Development at 9 and 18-month visits, and McCarthy Scales of Children's Abilities at the 36 month examination. They also evaluated socioeconomic status and social support systems by a questionnaire which was specifically developed for the study, allowing them to categorize families into three levels: upper quartile, middle two quartiles, or lower quartile. There were no differences in developmental outcome between control and treated children in any of these scales. Over all, the only differences found were more respiratory complications reported in the placebo-group by parent questionnaire at the 18-month visit (3.5 % vs. 0.5 % in the treated group, $p = 0.002$) and a slight excess of heart murmurs in the placebo group at 36 months (11.2 % compared with 5.6 %, $p = 0.04$). In this study, there was no difference in outcome found between males and females or racial groups in treated versus untreated groups; however, they found the expected, progressively lowering effect of lower socioeconomic status on the MDI, and PDI scales of Bayley Developmental assessments and the DCI of the McCarthy Index.

These studies present comprehensive outcome data from two large, well-controlled prospective studies of prenatal betamethasone administration. However, both studies report outcome for relatively mature, large infants. In the New Zealand study, the mean weight was 2,226 g for the treated and 2,402 g for the untreated group, and in the Collaborative Study, the mean weight of the placebo group was 1,893 g, compared with 1,896 g in the treated group. In the New Zealand study, only 22 infants weighed less than 1,250 g. In the Collaborative Study, there were only 10 treated and 16 untreated infants entered at less than 30 weeks gestation. The findings with these large infants may not necessarily apply to the smaller, more vulnerable preterm infants.

Ballard et al. (1981, 1983, 1985) have recently reported on neurological and developmental outcome for infants weighing less than 1,250 g at birth. A group of 96 children were tested at 4½ to 10 years of age; 36 were exposed to betamethasone in utero and 60 were not. Since some of the infants were trans-

Table 5.13. Developmental follow-up evaluations after prenatal glucocorticoid administration

I. New Zealand study	
4 years 3 months (MacArthur et al. 1981)	
Stanford Binet I. Q.	
Peabody picture vocabulary tests	
Frostig developmental test of visual perception	
Vineland social maturity scale	
Recordings of speech	
6 years 2 months (MacArthur et al. 1982)	
Illinois test of psycholinguistic abilities	
Peabody picture vocabulary test	
Bender motor-visual "gestalt" test	
II. Collaborative Study Group 1984 – term, 9, 18, 36 months	
Prechtl exam	40 weeks
Neurological exam	9, 18, 36 months
Bayley MDI/PDI	9, 18 months
McCarthy	36 months
III. San Francisco study – birthweight < 1250 g	
4½ years to 10 years (Ballard et al. 1985)	
Neurological assessment	
McCarthy scales of children's abilities	
Wechsler preschool and primary scales	
Wechsler intelligence scale for children – revised	

ported to the nursery after birth, the two groups were divided into inborn and outborn infants. This study found that 94 % of the treated and 92 % of the untreated infants were neurologically normal or had only mild abnormalities. There was also no difference between the groups in median GCI for preschool children, on the McCarthy Scales (1970) or preschool I. Q. on the WISC-R (Wechsler, 1974) for schoolage children. Table 5.13 summarizes the developmental evaluations which have been done.

5.4.2 Lung Development

Wong et al. (1982) examined thoracic gas volume, dynamic pulmonary compliance and airway resistance at one year of age in 15 infants weighing less than 1,500 g at birth. None of these infants had respiratory distress; however, seven had received prenatal dexamethasone. They found no difference between these two groups, and, in addition found that the values correlated well with previous studies done on infants weighing more than 1,500 g at birth. Howie (1984) also reported on pulmonary function testing, including vital capacity, specific airway resistance, functional residual capacity, and carbonmonoxide removal. They found no difference between treated and control infants or in comparison with predicted values for older children.

5.4.3 Immunological Development

As mentioned previously (Sec. 5.3) the possibility of either a short- or long-term effect on immunological competence has been of great concern to those administering prenatal glucocorticoids. Studies in the newborn period have not revealed any immunologic effects (discussed in Sect. 5.3.2.1).

Howie (1984) reported on immune function of 40 children from their study at age 7 years. They found no difference in immunoglobulin levels, percentages or distribution of lymphocyte types or PHA response. To date, the only finding of concern is that of Gunn et al. (1981), who reported 5-year follow-up on a group of infants who were treated *post*natally with high doses of hydrocortisone after they developed RDS. (These infants were initially also reported by Fitzhardinge et al. (1974) as having some minor neurological abnormalities at 1 year of age.) Compared with a control group, there was no difference in several measures of immunological competence, including lymphocyte count, immunoglobulin levels, diphtheria and tetanus titers, complement levels and cell-mediated immunity as measured by intradermal delayed skin tests. They did, however, find a difference in the percentage of T-lymphocytes in steroid-treated patients (53 % compared with 69 % in untreated infants, $p < 0.0005$). In some patients, the decreased percentage of T-lymphocytes was associated with higher percentages of cells with C-3 receptors (20.1 %) than observed in adult or control groups (10.4 % and 13.8 %, respectively, $p < 0.0025$). No differences were observed in the percentage of cells with surface immunoglobulins or Fc receptors. Finally, they reported a greater number of infections in the treated (8/11) compared with the control group (2/7).

The relevance of the findings of Gunn et al. (1981) for *pre*natal glucocorticoid therapy is uncertain. All of the infants in this series received steroids postnatally and had blood levels of cortisol in excess of 100 g/dl for more than 48 h, compared with levels of 30 g/dl in placebo-treated infants. The Estimated maximal level of plasma unbound glucocorticoid in the hydrocortisone treated infants was 300 times greater than normal (Table 6.7). Nevertheless, further follow-up studies on T-cell function are clearly indicated in treated infants, particularly for those in whom a leukemoid reaction was reported at the time of birth.

5.5 Summary

From the foregoing discussion, it is clear that administration of prenatal glucocorticoids not only decreases the incidence and severity of RDS, but, in addition, has numerous other beneficial effects for the premature infant. There has been a healthy skepticism and concern about possible deleterious effects of prenatal glucocorticoids. On the other hand, there has been at times, perhaps, an excessive pride in the capabilities of modern neonatal intensive care. The lesson implicit in the following quotation, from 1936, may well still apply in the "modern" era of neonatal prophylactic and supportive care.

Table 5.14. Risk vs. benefit analysis of prenatal glucocorticoid therapy

Risks
Possible increased risk of infection in mothers with prolonged rupture of membranes (Taeusch et al. 1979; Young et al. 1980; Garite et al. 1981; Schmidt et al. 1984)
Disturbs glucose homeostasis in diabetic mothers (Baxter & Rousseau 1979)
Possible impact on T-cell development (with postnatal treatment) (Gunn et al. 1981)
Questionable effect on visual perception in boys (MacArthur et al. 1982)
No Difference
Infection in infants (Liggins & Howie 1972; Kennedy 1976; Caspi et al. 1976; Morrison et al. 1978; Ballard et al. 1979; Papageorgiou et al. 1979; Kuhn et al. 1982; Schmidt et al. 1984)
Growth: Height, weight, head circumference; neurological development; cognitive development (MacArthur et al. 1981, 1982; Collab. Study Group 1984; Ballard 1985)
Development of very low-birthweight-infants (Ballard 1985)
Lung mechanics and growth (Howie 1984)
Retrolental fibroplasia or vision (Howie 1984)
Benefits
Improved survival[a]
Decreased incidence of RDS[a]
Decreased severity of RDS[a]
Decreased incidence of significant patent ductus arteriosus (Clyman et al. 1981; Waffarn et al. 1983)
Decreased incidence of intracranial hemorrhage (Liggins and Howie 1972; Taeusch et al. 1979; Clark et al. 1981)
Decreased incidence of necrotizing enterocolitis (Bauer et al. 1984)
Decreased hospital costs (Johnson et al. 1981; Collab. Study Group 1981)
Decreased hospital stay (Johnson et al. 1981; Collab. Study Group 1981)
Decreased respiratory complications at 18 months of age (Collab. Study Group 1984)
Decreased incidence of murmurs at 36 months of age (Collab. Study Group 1984)
Improved feeding of females after discharge (MacArthur et al. 1981)
Decreased susceptibility to illness during first 4 years (MacArthur et al. 1981)

[a] Detailed in Table 5.2

"General mortality and morbidity rates give very little help in assessing the value of special forms of treatment, since, where nursing skill is of a high standard, such rates are already remarkably low. Indeed, the experience of the past few years ... suggests that in expert hands the prognosis for the premature baby is remarkably good." A. Moncrieff (1936)

Despite the major improvements in neonatal intensive care since 1936, there remain many very significant problems in providing care for the small preterm infant which are costly, both financially and with regard to emotional stress for the families. It is therefore appropriate to summarize the current status of our knowledge of the risk versus the benefits of prenatal glucocorticoid therapy (see Table 5.14) and to examine the influence of glucocorticoids on the important variables for survival of the preterm infant discussed in the Introduction.

Lung Structure. There is ample evidence that prenatal glucocorticoids, in addition to their effects on surfactant production, accelerate maturation of lung structure and improve alveolarization and pulmonary compliance (Chap. 1), factors important to the small preterm infant. No risks related to lung growth, development or function have been found; however, the established benefit of glucocorticoids, in addition to decreased incidence of RDS and decreased mortality, include decreased severity of RDS (Table 5.11) when it does occur and decreased respiratory complications up to 18 months of age (National Collaborative Study 1984).

Lung Liquid. Due to their maturational effect in animals on lung structure and on beta-adrenergic receptor concentration, glucocorticoids would be expected to improve the preterm infant's ability to clear lung fluid at birth (Chap. 8), decreasing the need for resuscitation and contributing to decreased severity of RDS.

Pulmonary Blood Flow. Although little is known about the effect of glucocorticoids on the development of the pulmonary vasculature, certainly after birth, pulmonary blood flow is affected by flow through the patent ductus arteriosus. By decreasing sensitivity of the ductus to prostaglandins (Clyman et al. 1981b) and reducing the incidence of patent ductus arteriousus (Clyman et al. 1981a; Waffarn 1983), glucocorticoids enhance the infant's ability to normalize pulmonary blood flow more rapidly.

Birth Asphyxia. In treated preterm infants with accelerated maturation of surfactant and possibly of lung fluid clearance, the infant is better able to deal with complications occurring during delivery, and therefore sustains less exposure to birth asphyxia. The benefits related to this include improved survival and decreased incidence of intracranial hemorrhage (Liggins and Howie 1972; Taeusch et al. 1979; Clark et al. 1981). Along with decreased incidence of PDA, decreased asphyxia probably contributes to the decreased incidence of necrotizing enterocolitis found in treated infants (Bauer et al. 1984).

Ventilation at Birth. The greater availability of surfactant and improved clearance of lung liquid in treated infants increases lung compliance and functional lung volume. This makes the initial ventilation of preterm infants easier, reducing the need for high concentrations of oxygen and high pressures for mechanical ventilation which are associated with numerous complications. These factors ultimately contribute to the decreased hospital stay and cost for these infants (Johnson et al. 1981; Avery 1984), as well as the decreased susceptibility to illness (MacArthur et al. 1981).

"When evidence is accummulated according to careful prospective studies and statistically significant incidence of benefit without recognized toxicity is found, good medical care dictates acting on that evidence. The failure to do so is costly in terms of morbidity and, I believe, constitutes poor practice."

Mary Ellen Avery, 1984

References

Anday EK, Harris MC (1982) Leukemoid reaction associated with antenatal dexamethasone administration. J Pediatr 101:614

Anderson CW, Cordero L (1980) Changes in amniotic fluid optical density at 450 mu in Rh-sensitized patients after maternal hydrocortisone treatment. Am J Obstet Gynecol 137:820

Arias F, Pineda J, Johnson LW (1979) Changes in human amniotic fluid lecithin/sphingomyelin ratio and dipalmitoyl lecithin associated with maternal betamethasone therapy. Am J Obstet Gynecol 133:894

Avery ME, Mead J (1959) Surface properties in relation to atelectasis and hyaline membrane disease. Am J Dis Child 133:517

Avery ME (1984) The argument for prenatal administration of dexamethasone to prevent respiratory distress syndrome. J Pediatr 104:240

Baden M, Bauer CB, Colle E, Klein G, Taeusch HW Jr, Stern L (1972) A controlled trial of hydrocortisone therapy in infants with respiratory distress syndrome. Pediatrics 50:526

Ballard PL (1979) Glucocorticoids and differentiation. In: Monographs on Endocrinology, Vol 12: Glucocorticoid Hormone Action, Baxter JD, Rousseau GG (eds), Springer, Berlin, Heidelberg, New York, pp 493–515

Ballard PL, Ballard RA (1979) Corticosteroids and respiratory distress syndrome: Status 1979. Pediatrics 63:163

Ballard PL, Ballard RA, Granberg JP, Sniderman S, Gluckman PD, Kaplan SL, Grumbach MM (1980) Fetal sex and prenatal betamethasone therapy. J Pediatr 97:451

Ballard PL, Granberg P, Ballard RA (1975) Glucocorticoid levels in maternal and cord serum after prenatal dexamethasone therapy to prevent respiratory distress syndrome. J Clin Invest 56:1548

Ballard PL, Liggins GC (1982) Glucocorticoid activity in cord serum: Comparison of hydrocortisone and betamethasone regimens. J Pediatr 101:468

Ballard RA, Ballard PL, Granberg JP, Sniderman S (1979) Prenatal administration of betamethasone for prevention of respiratory distress syndrome. J Pediatr 94:97

Ballard RA, Clark C, Clyman RI, Dekle M, Leonard CH, Roth RS, Sehring S, Sniderman S (1981) Follow-up of preterm infants after prenatal betamethasone. Pediatr Res 15:648

Ballard, RA, Leonard CH, Piecuch R, Clyman RI, Lang MD (1983) Long-term outcome after prenatal glucocorticoid therapy. J Calif Perinatal Assoc 3:21

Ballard RA, Leonard CH, Piecuch R, Lang M, Behle M (1985) Long-term outcome after prenatal glucocorticoid therapy. Clin Res 135A

Bauer CR, Morrison JC, Poole WK, Korones SP, Boehm, JJ, Rigatto H, Zachman RO (1984) Decreased incidence of necrotizing enterocolitis after prenatal glucocorticoid therapy. Pediatrics 73:682

Bauer CR, Stein L, Colle E (1974) Prolonged rupture of membranes associated with a decreased incidence of respiratory distress syndrome. Pediatrics 73:7

Baxter JD, Rousseau GG (1979) Glucocorticoid hormone action: An overview. In: Baxter JD,

Rousseau GG (eds) Glucocorticoid Hormone Action. Springer, Berlin, Heidelberg, New York, pp. 1–24
Berkowitz RL, Bonta BW, Warshaw JE (1976) The relationship between premature rupture of the membranes and the respiratory distress syndrome. Am J Obstet Gynecol 124:712
Bielawski D, Hiatt IM, Hegyi T (1978) Betamethasone-induced leukemoid reaction in pre-term infant. Lancet 1:219
Block M, Kling O, Crosby W (1977) Antenatal glucocorticoid therapy for the prevention of respiratory distress syndrome in the premature infant. Obstet Gynecol 50:186
Boog G, Ben Brahim M, Gandar R (1975) Beta-mimetic drugs and possible prevention of respiratory distress syndrome. Br J Obstet Gynecol 82:285
Brann AW, Volpe JJ (eds) (1980) Neonatal Neurological Assessment and Outcome. Report of 77th Ross Conference on Pediatric Research, Ross Laboratories, Columbus, OH 43216.
Bureau M, Stocker J, Deleon A, Lalonde A, Desjardins P (1975) Utilisation de la betamethasone dans la prevention du syndrome de detresse respiratoire du nouveau-ne premature. L'Union Medicale du Canada 104:99
Caritis SN, Mueller-Heubach E, Edelstone, DI (1977) Effect of betamethasone on analysis of amniotic fluid in the rhesus-sensitized pregnancy. Amer J Obstet Gynecol 127:529
Caspi E, Schreyer P, Weinraub Z, Bukovsky I, Tamir I (1975) Changes in amniotic fluid lecithin-sphingomyelin ratio following maternal dexamethasone administration. Am J Obstet Gynecol 122:327
Caspi E, Schreyer P, Reif R, Goldberg M (1980) An analysis of the factors associated with respiratory distress syndrome in premature infants whose mothers had been given dexamethasone therapy. Br J Obstet Gynecol 87:808
Caspi E, Schreyer P, Weinraub Z, Reif R, Levi I, Mundel G (1976) Prevention of the respiratory distress syndrome in premature infants by antepartum glucocorticoid therapy Br J Obstet Gynaecol 83:187
Cederqvist LL, Ylikorkala O, Ekelund L, Tuimala R, Litwin SD (1978) Fetal immunoglobulin production following prenatal glucocorticoid treatment. Obstet Gynecol 52:539
Clark CE, Clyman RI, Roth RS, Sniderman SH, Lane B, Ballard RA (1981) Risk factor analysis of intraventricular hemorrhage in low-birth-weight infants J Pediatr 99:625
Clyman RI, Ballard PL, Sniderman S, Ballard RA, Roth R, Heymann MA, Granberg JP (1981a) Prenatal administration of betamethasone for prevention of patent ductus arteriosus. J Pediatr 98:123
Clyman RI, Mauray F, Roman C, Rudolph AM, Heymann MA (1981b) Glucocorticoids alter the sensitivity of the lamb ductus arteriosus to prostaglandin E_2. J Pediatr 98:126
Collaborative Group on Antenatal Steroid Therapy (1981) Effect of antenatal dexamethasone administration on the prevention of respiratory distress syndrome. Am J Obstet Gynecol 141:276
Collaborative Group on Antenatal Steroid Therapy (1984) Effects of antenatal dexamethasone administration in the infant: Long-term follow-up. J Pediatr 104:259
Crowley P (1981) Corticosteroids in pregnancy: The benefits outweigh the costs (review). Brit J Obstet Gynaecol 1:147
Depp R, Boehm JJ, Nosek JA, Dooley SL, Hobart JM (1980) Antenatal corticosteroids to prevent neonatal respiratory distress syndrome: Risk versus benefit considerations. Am J Obstet Gynecol 137:338
Dluholucky S, Babic J, Taufer I (1976) Reduction of incidence and mortality of respiratory distress syndrome by administration of hydrocortisone to mother. Arch Dis Child 51:420
Doran TA, Swyer P, MacMurray B, Mahon W, Enhorning G, Bernstein A, Falk M, Wood MM (1980) Results of a double-blind controlled study on the use of betamethasone in the prevention of respiratory distress syndrome. Am Obstet Gynecol 136:313
Draisey TF, Gagneja GL, Thibert RJ (1977) Pulmonary surfactant and amniotic fluid insulin. Obstet Gynecol 50:197
Drorbaugh JE, Moore DM, Warram JH, Jr (1975) Association between gestational and environmental events and central nervous system function in 7-year-old children. Pediatrics 56:529
Fargier P, Salle B, Baud, Gagnaire JC, Arnaud P, Magnin P (1974) Prevention du syndrome de detresse respiratoire chez le premature. Noev Presse med 3:1595

Farrell PM, ed. (1982) Lung Development: Biological and Clinical Perspectives: Vol 2. Neonatal Respiratory Distress. New York, Academic Press, pp 155–188
Farrell PM, Avery ME (1975) Hyaline membrane disease. Am Rev Resp Dis 3: 657
Farrell PM, Engle MJ, Zachman RD, Curet LB, Morrison JC, Rao AV, Poole WK Collaborative group on Antenatal Steroid Therapy (1983) Amniotic fluid phospholipids after maternal administration of dexamethasone. Am J Obstet Gynecol 145:484
Farrell PM, Wood RE (1976) Epidemiology of hyaline membrane disease in the United States. Analysis of national mortality statistics. Pediatrics 58:167
Fisch RO, Bihele MK, Millar LD, Engle RR (1975) Physical and mental status at 4 years of age of survivors of the respiratory distress syndrome. J Pediatr 84:497
Fitzhardinge PM, Eisen A, Lejtenyi C, Metrakes K, Ramsay M (1974) Sequelae of early steroid administration to the newborn infant. Pediatrics 53:887
Fitzhardinge PM, Pape K, Arstikaitis M, Boyle M, Ashby S, Rowley A, Netley C, Swyer PR (1976) Mechanical ventilation of infants less than 1,051 gms birthweight: Health, growth and neurologic sequelae. J Pediatr 88:531
Fletcher BD, Masson M, Lisbona A, Riggs T, Papageorgiou AN (1979) Thymic response to endogenous and exogenous steroids in premature newborn infants. J Pediatr 95:111
Garite TJ, Freeman RK, Linzey EM, Braly PS, Dorchester WL (1981) Prospective randomized study of corticosteroids in the management of premature rupture of the membranes and the premature gestation. Am J Obstet Gynecol 141:508
Gluck L (1976) Administration of corticosteroids to induce maturation of fetal lung. Am J Dis Child 130:976
Granberg, P, Ballard RA, Ballard PL, Berman F (1975) Effects of antenatal betamethasone in preterm infants. Pediatr Res 9:396
Gunn T, Reece ER, Metrakos K, Colle E (1981) Depressed T cells following neonatal steroid treatment. Pediatrics 67:61–67
Hack M, Fanaroff AA, Merkatz IR (1979) The low-birth-weight infant. Evaluation of changing outlook. N Engl J Med 301:1162
Heldt GP, McIlroy BM, Hansen TN, Tooley WH (1980) Exercise performance of the survivors of hyaline membrane disease. J. Pediatr 96:995
Hobel FJ, Hyvarimen M, Oh W (1972) Abnormal fetal heart rate patterns and fetal acid-base balance in low-birthweight infants in relation to respiratory distress syndrome. Obstet Gynecol 39:83
Howie, RN (1984) Pharmacological acceleration of lung maturation. In: Ravio K, Hallman N, Kouvalainen K, Valimaki I (ed) *Respiratory Distress Syndrome.* Academic Press, London pp 385–396
Howie RN, Liggins GC (1982) The New Zealand study of antepartum glucocorticoid treatment in lung development. In Farrell PM (ed) Lung Development: Vol II Biological and Clinical Perspectives, pp 255–265
Johnson DE, Munson DP, Thompson TR (1981) Effect of antenatal administration of betamethasone on hospital costs and survival of premature infants. Pediatrics 68:633
Jones MD Jr, Burd LI, Bowes WA Jr, Battaglia FC, Lubchenco LO (1975) Failure of association of premature rupture of membranes with respiratory distress syndrome. N Eng J Med 292:1253
Kampner J (1978a) Long-term prognosis of infants with severe IRDS. I. Neurological and mental outcome. Acta Paediatr Scand 67:61
Kampner J (1978b) Long-term prognosis of infants with severe IRDS. II. Cardio-pulmonary outcome. Acta Paediatr Scand 67:71
Kennedy JL (1976) Clinical experience with betamethasone for the prevention of respiratory distress syndrome. In: Lung Maturation and the Prevention of Hyaline Membrane Disease, Proceedings of the Seventieth Ross Conference on Pediatric Research, Columbus, Ohio, Ross Laboratories, pp 181–184
Kero P, Hirvonan T, Valimaki I (1973) Prenatal and postnatal isoxsuprine and respiratory distress syndrome. Lancet 2:198
Kitterman JA (1975) Effects of intestinal ischemia in necrotizing enterocolitis in the newborn infant. In: Moore TD (ed) Report of the 68th Ross Conference on Pediatric Research, Columbus OH, Ross Laboratories p. 38
Kuhn RJP, Speirs AL, Pepperell RJ, Eggers TR, Doyle LW, Hutchison A (1982) Betamethasone,

albuterol and threatened premature delivery: Benefits and risks. Obstet Gynecol 60:503
Kulovich MV, Gluck L (1979) The lung profile. II Complicated pregnancy. Am J Obstet Gynecol 64
Kulovich MV, Hallman M, Gluck L (1979) The lung profile. I Normal pregnancy. Am J Obstet Gynecol 135:57
Liggins GC, Howie RN (1972) A controlled trial of antepartum glucocorticoid treatment for prevention of the respiratory distress syndrome in premature infants. Pediatrics 50:515
Lipper E, Lee K, Gartner LM, Grellong B (1981) Determinants of neurobehavioral outcome in low-birth-weight infants. Pediatrics 67:502
Lowensohn RI, Gabbe SG (1979) The value of L/S ratios in diabetes. A critical review. Am J Obstet Gynecol 134:702
MacArthur BA, Howie RN, Dezoete JA, Elkins J (1981) Cognitive and psychosocial development of 4-year-old children whose mothers were treated antenatally with betamethasone. Pediatrics 68:638
MacArthur BA, Howie RN, Dezoete JA, Elkins J (1982) School progress and cognitive development of 6-year-old children whose mothers were treated antenatally with betamethasone. Pediatrics 70:99
Maclusky IB, Zarfin J, Pape K, Levison H (1984) Bronchial hyper-reactivity in long-term survivors of the neonatal respiratory distress syndrome. (abst) Pediatr Res 396A
Martin GB Jr, Siassi B, Hon EH (1974) Fetal heart rate pattern and neonatal death in low-birthweight infants. Obstet Gynecol 44:505-510
McCarthy D (1970) McCarthy Scales of Children's Abilities (MCSA). The Psychological Corporation, New York NY
Momma K, Nishihara S, Ota Y (1981) Constriction of the fetal ductus arteriosus by glucocorticoid hormones. Pediatr Res 15:19
Moncrieff A (1936) The value of oestrin for premature babies. Arch Dis Child 11:9
Moore TD (ed) (1976) Iatrogenic problems in neonatal intensive care. In: Report of the 69th Ross Conference in Pediatric Research, Ross Laboratories, Columbus OH
Morrison JC, Whybrew WD, Bucovaz ET, Wiscer WL, Fish SA (1977) The lecithin/sphingomyelin ratio in cases associated with feto-maternal disease. Am J Obstet Gynecol 127:363
Morrison JC, Whybrew WD, Bucovaz ET, Schneider JM (1978) Injection of corticosteroids into mother to prevent neonatal respiratory distress syndrome. Am J Obstet Gynecol 131:358
Nochimson DJ, Petrie RH (1979) Glucocorticoid therapy for the induction of pulmonary maturity in severely hypertensive gravid women. Am J Obstet Gynecol 133:449
Osler M, Faero O, Friis-Hansen B, Trolle D (1978) Prevention of the respiratory distress syndrome (RDS) by antepartum glucocorticoid (betamethasone) therapy combined with phenobarbitone and ritodrine. Dan Med Bull 25:225
Otero L, Conlon C, Reynolds P, Duval-Arnould B, Golden SM (1981) Neonatal leukocytosis associated with prenatal administration of dexamethasone. Pediatrics 68:778
Papageorgiou AN, Colle E, Farri-Kostopoulos E, Gelfand MM (1981) Incidence of respiratory distress syndrome following antenatal betamethasone: Role of sex, type of delivery, and prolonged rupture of membranes. Pediatrics 67:614
Papageorgiou AN, Desgranges MF, Masson M, Colle E, Shatz R, Gelfand MM (1979) The antenatal use of betamethasone in the prevention of respiratory distress syndrome: A controlled double-blind study. Pediatrics 63:73
Pape KE, Biencia RJ, Ashby S, Fitzhardinge PM (1978) The status at two years of low-birthweight infants born in 1974 with birthweight less than 1,000 gm. J Pediatr 92:253
Patrick J, Challis J, Campbell K, Carmichael L, Richardson B, Tevanwerk G (1981) Effects of synthetic glucocorticoid administration on human fetal breathing movements at 34 to 35 weeks' gestational age. Am J Obstet Gynecol 139:324
Perelman RH, Farrell PM (1982) Analysis of causes of neonatal death in the United States with specific emphasis on fatal hyaline membrane disease. Pediatrics 70:570
Quirk JG Jr, Raket RK, Petrie RH, Williams AM (1979) The role of glucocorticoids, unstressful labor, and atraumatic delivery in the prevention of respiratory distress syndrome. Am J Obstet Gynecol 134:768
Richardson CJ, Pomerance JJ, Cunningham M, Gluck L (1973) Hyaline and ruptured – the membrane dilemma. Pediatr Res 7:178

Ricke PS, Elliott JP, Freeman RK (1980) Use of corticosteroids in pregnancy-induced hypertension. Obstet Gynecol 55:206

Robert MF, Neff RK, Hubbell JP, Taeusch HW, Avery ME (1976) Association between maternal diabetes and the respiratory distress syndrome in the newborn. N Eng J Med 294:357

Robertson PA, Herron M, Katz M and Creasy RK (1981) Maternal morbidity associated with isoxsuprine and terbutaline tocolysis. Europ J Obstet Gynec Reprod Bol 11:371

Rokos J, Vaensorn O, Nadhaman R, Avery ME (1968) Hyaline membrane disease in twins. Pediatrics 42:204

Ryhanen P, Kauppila A, Kolvisto M (1980) Unaltered neonatal cell-mediated immunity after prenatal dexamethasone treatment. Obstet Gynecol 56:182

Sameroff AJ (1980) Social and environmental influences on the developing nervous system. In: Braun W, Volpe JJ (eds) Neonatal neurological assessment and outcome. Report of the 77th Ross Conference on Pediatric Research. Ross Laboratories, Columbus OH, p. 65

Schmidt PL, Sims ME, Strassner HT, Paul RH, Mueller E, McCart D (1984) Effect of antepartum glucocorticoid administration upon neonatal respiratory distress syndrome and perinatal infection. Am J Obstet Gynecol 148:178

Schutte MF (1981) Toepassing van betamethason bij de behandeling van dreigende vroeggeboonte. In: Schutte MF (ed) Over de behandeling van dreigende vroeggeboonte. Podopi, Amsterdam, pp. 58–70

Schutte MF, Treffers PE, Koppe JG, Breur W (1980) The influence of betamethasone and orciprenaline on the incidence of respiratory distress syndrome in the newborn after preterm labour. Brit J Obstet Gynaec 87:127

Spellacy WW, Buhi WC, Riggell TC, Holsinger KL (1973) Human amniotic fluid lecithin/sphingomyelin ratio changes with estrogen or glucocorticoid treatment. Am J Obstet Gynecol 115:216

Stewart AL, Reynolds EOR (1974) Improved prognosis for infants of very low birthweight. Pediatrics 54:724

Stewart AL, Reynolds EOR, Libscomb AP (1981) Outcome for infants of very low birthweight: Survey of World literature. Lancet 1:1038

Stewart AL, Turcan DM, Rawlings G, Reynolds EOR (1977) Prognosis for infants weighing 1 000 gm or less at birth. Arch Dis Child 52:97

Taeusch HW Jr (1975) Glucocorticoid prophylaxis for respiratory distress syndrome: A review of potential toxicity. J Pediatr 87:617

Taeusch HW Jr, Tulchinsky D (1979) Obstetric factors affecting risk of respiratory distress syndrome. Perinatal Developmental Symposium on Premature Labor, Vail CO, Mead Johnson, pp. 48–55

Taeusch WH Jr, Frigoletto F, Kitzmiller J, Avery ME, Hehre A, Fromm B, Lawson E, Neff RK (1979) Risk of respiratory distress syndrome after prenatal dexamethasone treatment. Pediatrics 63:64

Thornfeldt RE, Franklin RW, Pickering NA, Thornfeldt CR, Amell G (1978) The effect of glucocorticoids on the maturation of premature lung membranes, preventing the respiratory distress syndrome by glucocorticoids. Am J Obstet Gynecol 131:143

Usher RH, Allen AC and McLean FH (1971) Risk of respiratory distress syndrome related to gestational age, route of delivery and maternal diabetes. Am J Obstet Gynecol 111:826

Waffarn F, Siassi B, Cabal LA, Schmidt PL (1983) Effect of antenatal glucocorticoids on clinical closure of the ductus arteriosus. Am J Dis Child 137:336

Wechsler D (1974) Wechsler Intelligence Scale for Children – Revised. The Psychological Corporation, New York NY

Whitt GG, Buster JE, Killam AP, Scragg WH (1976) A comparison of two glucocorticoid regimens for acceleration of fetal lung maturation in premature labor. Am J Obstet Gynecol 124:479

Wong YL, Beardsmore CS, Silverman M (1982) Antenatal dexamethasone and subsequent lung growth. Arch Dis Child 57:536

Wong YL, Taeusch HW Jr (1978) White blood cell changes and incidence of fever after maternal treatment with glucocorticoids. Pediatr Res 12:501

Worthington D, Smith BT (1978) Relation of amniotic fluid lecithin/sphingomyelin ratio and fetal asphyxia to respiratory distress syndrome in premature infants. Can Med Assoc J 118:1384

Yoon JJ, Harper RG (1973) Observations on the relationship between duration of rupture of the membranes and the development of idiopathic respiratory distress syndrome. Pediatrics 52:162

Young BK, Klein SA, Katz M, Wilson SJ, Douglas GW (1980) Intravenous dexamethasone for prevention of neonatal respiratory distress: A prospective controlled study. Am J Obstet Gynecol 138:203

6 Antenatal Glucocorticoid Therapy: Hormone Concentrations

The use of prenatal glucocorticoid therapy for prevention of RDS has provided opportunities to study serum concentrations of administered hormones in both mother and fetus. Data are available from women treated in the third trimester with betamethasone, dexamethasone, and hydrocortisone. The amount of transplacental passage of these corticosteroids and the kinetics of their appearance and disappearance in the fetal circulation are discussed. In addition, I review the effect of glucocorticoid treatment on various endogenous hormones in both mother and fetus.

6.1 Concentration of Administered Corticosteroids

6.1.1 Betamethasone

The concentration of serum betamethasone has been measured by radioreceptor assay (Ballard et al. 1975a; Ballard et al. 1980), by radioimmunoassay after Sephadex LH-20 column chromatography (Anderson et al. 1977) and by high

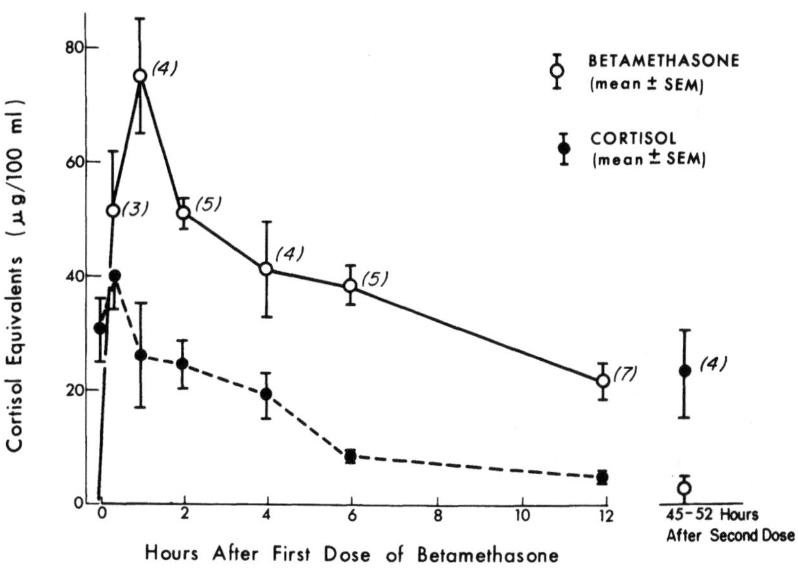

Fig. 6.1. Time course of betamethasone and cortisol concentrations in maternal serum after treatment with 12 mg betamethasone acetate and phosphate. The number of samples is shown in *parentheses.* Reproduced from Ballard et al. (1975a), by permission

pressure liquid chromatography (Petersen et al. 1980). Figure 6.1 shows the time course for serum betamethasone and cortisol after IM injection of a mixture of betamethasone acetate and betamethasone phosphate to women in premature labor. Maximal concentrations of betamethasone were found at 1 h when the level was 105 ng/ml. Based on the affinity of betamethasone for glucocorticoid receptor, this concentration equals 75 μg cortisol equivalents/dl (Ballard et al. 1975b). Following intravenous injection of 8 mg of betamethasone phosphate, the plasma concentration was 65 and 84 ng/ml at 1 h in two patients studied by Petersen et al. (1980). The highest concentration of betamethasone in maternal serum in the series by Anderson et al. (1977) was only 13.3 ng/ml, however the number of hours between injection and sampling is uncertain. When considered in terms of cortisol equivalents, the peak concentrations of glucocorticoid activity in treated maternal serum are about 3 times higher than the endogenous cortisol level during labor.

Betamethasone is cleared from maternal plasma with a $t_{1/2}$ of about 5–6 h (Ballard et al. 1975a; Petersen et al. 1980), similar to the disappearance rate in non-pregnant adults (Meikel and Tyler 1977; Ballard et al. 1975b). Betamethasone was not detected in maternal serum 48 h after the last dose.

The concentration of betamethasone in cord serum of premature infants has been determined after treatment with 12 mg betamethasone acetate and phosphate (Ballard et al. 1975a; Anderson et al. 1977; Ballard et al. 1980), 6 mg betamethasone alcohol (Ballard et al. 1980) and 8 mg betamethasone phosphate (Petersen et al. 1980). Figure 6.2 shows data for infants exposed to the 12 mg regimen. Betamethasone is detected in cord serum as early as 1 h after the dose of steroid to the mother with peak concentrations at 1–2 h of about 20 ng/ml (14 μg cortisol equivalents/dl) for both the 8 and 12 mg doses.

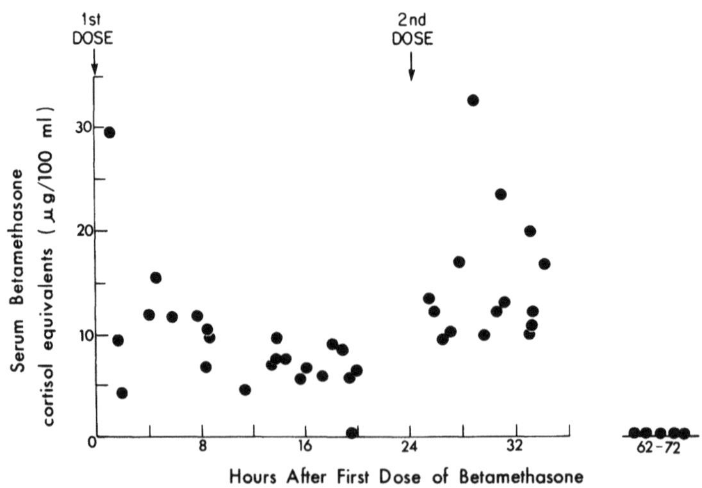

Fig. 6.2. Betamethasone concentration in cord serum of 43 premature infants delivering at various times after maternal treatment with 12 mg betamethasone (acetate plus phosphate). Reproduced from Ballard et al. (1975a), by permission

Clearance of betamethasone appears to be slower in the fetus than in the mother, but the steroid was not detected in fetal serum 2–3 days after the last dose to the mother (Ballard et al. 1975a; Anderson et al. 1977). Betamethasone is also present in amniotic fluid at concentrations similar to those found for umbilical venous blood (Anderson et al. 1977).

Comparisons of betamethasone concentrations in matched maternal and umbilical serum samples indicates there is a substantial maternal/fetal gradient (Ballard et al. 1975a; Anderson et al. 1977; Petersen et al. 1980). The mean cord/maternal plasma concentration ratio was 0.37, 0.66, and 0.28 in these three studies, and the ratio is constant during the first 13–15 h after injection of steroid. For comparison, the fetal/maternal ratio for endogenous cortisol is approximately 0.27 (Ballard et al. 1975a).

6.1.2 Dexamethasone

Dexamethasone has been used for prophylaxis of RDS in several clinical studies and plasma concentrations have been reported (Osathanondath et al. 1977; Kream et al. 1983). In the first study, the mean concentration in maternal plasma was 22 ng/ml 8–11 h after administration of 4 mg of dexamethasone phosphate. In the cord blood of infants delivered by cesarean section of these women, dexamethasone levels were 29 and 26 ng/ml for the umbilical vein and umbilical artery, respectively. The absence of a placental gradient for dexamethasone in this study is in contrast with results for synthetic corticosteroids in other studies. It is possible that these results, obtained with patients at term, reflect a change during gestation in placental transfer or metabolism of dexamethasone.

In the collaborative study, women in premature labor received 5 mg of dexamethasone phosphate every 12 h (Kream et al. 1983). Dexamethasone was assayed in plasma samples by a procedure involving gel filtration (to separate endogenous corticosteroids), paper chromatography (in the case of cord and newborn plasma), and subsequent radioimmunoassay. Comparable results were achieved using high performance liquid chromatography. In 10 maternal samples, the mean concentration of plasma dexamethasone 2 h after injection of 5 mg dexamethasone phosphate was 37 ng/ml (range 22–65). After the last dose, dexamethasone disappeared from maternal plasma with a half-time of about 216 min. In 6 infants delivering less than 12 h after a dose of steroid to their mother, the dexamethasone concentration in umbilical arterial plasma was 6.5 ng/ml (range 3.2–12.5). The highest values of dexamethasone observed in cord plasma were in the range of 16–18 ng/ml (time from last dose to delivery unstated). Dexamethasone was not detected in plasma 24 h after birth of 6 infants who had measurable levels in cord blood. The apparently faster clearance of dexamethasone (3.6 h) than betamethasone (5–6 h) from the maternal circulation may reflect slower hydrolysis of the acetate form of betamethasone and consequently a more sustained release of steroid after injection of the acetate and phosphate mixture.

6.1.3 Methylprednisolone

Plasma concentrations of methylprednisolone were determined in one study (Anderson et al. 1981). Seven women in labor at term received 125 mg of methylprednisolone hemisuccinate intravenously and both maternal and umbilical venous blood specimens were collected at delivery which occurred 27–215 min later. Maternal concentrations of methylprednisolone were greatest at 45 min, when the level was 1,260 ng/ml. Methylprednisolone was cleared from the maternal circulation with a $t_{1/2}$ in the range of 45–75 min, which is considerably faster than observed for dexamethasone or betamethasone. There was a similar time-course for methylprednisolone concentrations in cord blood, and the mean fetal:maternal value was 0.45 (range 0.28–0.73). The mean concentration in cord plasma of 3 samples at 65–80 min exposure was 346 ng/ml (range 251–420). It is evident from this study that methylprednisolone hemisuccinate is rapidly hydrolyzed and transported from mother to fetus in utero.

Methylprednisolone (125 mg q 24 h) has been used in two clinical studies and found ineffective in reducing the incidence of RDS (Block et al. 1977; Schmidt et al. 1984). The pharmacokinetic data suggest that the steroid reached the fetal compartment, although it is conceivable that there is less placental transfer of hormone early in the third trimester than at term. Methylprednisolone has been shown to be an active glucocorticoid for in vitro binding to receptor from human lung (see Table 6.5). In one study with fetal sheep (121 days gestation), however, there was no enhancement of lung maturation after 1 dose (40–80 mg) of methylprednisolone (Taeusch et al. 1972). It is possible that the apparent lack of efficacy of methylprednisolone in both the sheep study and the clinical situation is due to its relatively rapid clearance from the fetal circulation.

6.1.4 Cortisol

The concentration of cortisol was assayed in cord serum of premature infants exposed to maternal treatment with hydrocortisone (Ballard and Liggins 1982). In this clinical trial women in premature labor received 100 mg of hydrocortisone succinate intravenously and the dose was repeated intramuscularly every 8 h (to a total of 400 mg) if delivery had not occurred. Assays were performed on serum from 71 infants of mean gestational age 32.5 wk who delivered at various times after entry into the trial (Fig. 6.3). The highest cortisol concentration occurred shortly after each dose of hydrocortisone, with a progressive decrease thereafter. The highest value observed was 43.8 µg/dl in an infant who delivered 2 h after the third dose. On a semi-logarithmic plot there was a linear relationship between cortisol values and time, from approximately 1–8 h after treatment, independent of the number of doses (Fig. 6.4). By regression analysis the plasma concentration 1 h after injection of hydrocortisone is approximately 32 µg/dl, representing a 3.8-fold increase over the level in untreated infants (8.5 ± 0.2 µg/dl). Hydrocortisone is cleared from the fetal circulation with a $t_{1/2}$ of about 2 h, indicating that nearly all of the steroid is removed from the fetal circulation between doses.

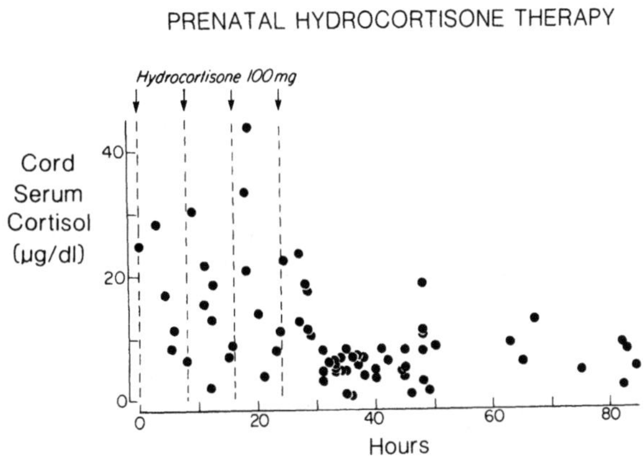

Fig. 6.3. Cortisol concentration in cord serum of 71 premature infants delivering at various times after maternal treatment with 100 mg hydrocortisone sodium succinate. Reproduced from Ballard and Liggins (1982), by permission

In an earlier study, cortisol concentrations were determined after injection of 150 mg hydrocortisone sodium succinate intravenously to women at term. The steroid was given in three doses of 50 mg approximately 10, 6 and 2 h prior to delivery by cesarean section. The mean cortisol concentration in the umbilical circulation of these infants was 18.6 µg/dl compared with 2.5 µg/dl in untreated newborn infants (Simmer et al. 1974). In the mothers at delivery, the cortisol level was 87 µg/dl vs. 27.6 µg/dl in control patients. The elevation of cortisol in the fetal circulation with this treatment regimen at term is consistent with the data for injection of 100 mg hydrocortisone earlier in the third trimester (Ballard and Liggins 1982).

Intra-amniotic injection of hydrocortisone has not been used clinically for prevention of RDS, but Lefebvre et al. (1976) have measured cortisol concentrations after such treatment. Nine women at term received 500 mg of hydro-

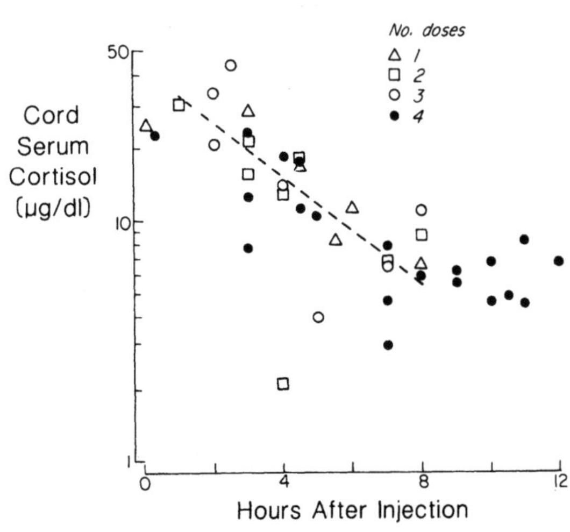

Fig. 6.4. Logarithmic plot of cortisol concentrations in cord serum after hydrocortisone treatment as described in Fig. 6.3. The regression line ($r = 0.81$, $P < 0.001$) indicates a $t_{1/2}$ of 2 h for clearance. Data from Ballard and Liggins (1982)

cortisone sodium succinate intraamniotically 48 h before elective cesarean section. In maternal plasma the corticoid concentration, determined by competitive protein binding assay, was 109 µg/dl (range 44–164 µg/dl) and 33.4 µg/dl (range 26–50 µg/dl) at 24 and 48 h following treatment, respectively, compared with 27.9 µg/dl (range 19–39 µg/dl) before injection. In one case studied in more detail, maternal corticoids increased progressively beginning 4 h after intra-amniotic injection with a peak concentration at 20 h. In cord blood, the mean concentration was 21.3 µg/dl, which is similar to the control values (18.7 µg/dl) using this assay (progesterone and 17α-hydroxyprogesterone were not removed). These findings indicate that some cortisol reaches the maternal circulation 24 h after intra-amniotic injection and is largely cleared by 48 h. Presumably, cortisol concentrations are also transiently elevated in the fetal circulation. Hydrocortisone could reach the fetus through swallowing of amniotic fluid, from the maternal circulation, or via the umbilical circulation after absorption through membrane vasculature (Carson et al. 1979). A possible advantage of this form of glucocorticoid therapy would be the extended period of elevated cortisol concentrations (24–48 h) in the maternal and, presumably, fetal circulations after a single dose. For routine clinical use, however, intramuscular administration of corticosteroid to the mother is a safer, simpler, and a better characterized form of treatment.

6.1.5 Comparison of Regimens

Table 6.1 summarizes the total plasma concentrations of various corticosteroids which have been administered to pregnant women. The data represent approximate maximal circulating concentrations (ng/ml) of administered corticosteroids as estimated from measurements 1–2 h after injection. The different treatment regimens produce a wide range of steroid concentrations in both maternal and fetal circulation expressed as ng steroid/ml plasma. Not

Table 6.1. Plasma concentrations of corticosteroids administered to pregnant women. Peak concentrations represent levels at 1-2 h after IM or IV injection

Steroid injected	Dose (mg)	References	Peak plasma concentrations (ng/ml)		Dose-adjusted peak plasma concentrations (ng/ml/mg injected)	
			Maternal	Fetal	Maternal	Fetal
Betamethasone acetate and phosphate	12	Ballard et al. 1975a; Ballard et al. 1980	105.6	20.1	8.8	1.7
	8	Petersen et al. 1980	75	19.9	9.4	2.5
Methylprednisolone hemisuccinate	125	Anderson et al. 1977	890	346	7.1	2.8
Dexamethasone phosphate	5	Kream et al. 1983	37	≧17	7.4	3.4
Hydrocortisone sodium succinate	100	Ballard & Liggins 1982	-	235	-	2.4
	50	Simmer et al. 1974	594	162	11.9	3.2

surprisingly, the concentration in maternal plasma calculated per mg of steroid injected is similar for the four steroids. This indicates that the volume of distribution is apparently similar for these different preparations. Concentrations in the fetal circulation, calculated per mg dose injected to the mother, range from 1.7 to 3.4 ng/ml/mg. This finding reflects similar passage of these corticosteroids across the placenta from mother to fetus. The major pharmacokinetic difference between these corticosteroids, therefore, is in the clearance rate rather than distribution. In a subsequent section, I discuss the calculated free glucocorticoid activity of fetal plasma with time after various regimens of glucocorticoid therapy.

6.1.6 Maternal-Fetal Distribution

The two major factors influencing placental transfer of corticosteroid are binding to CBG and albumin in the maternal circulation, and metabolism of the steroid in placenta and membranes. Cortisol and prednisolone, but not dexamethasone, betamethasone and methylprednisolone, are bound with high affinity by human CBG (Ballard et al. 1975b). At physiologic concentrations of cortisol, approximately 85 % of the steroid is bound to CBG. At higher concentrations, when CBG binding capacity is saturated, a greater percentage of the cortisol is unbound. By contrast, considerably more dexamethasone and betamethasone remains unbound at all concentrations and available for transfer across the placenta. All four steroids are bound with a similar affinity to albumin, resulting in approximately 40–50 % of the circulating steroid bound to albumin (reviewed in Ballard 1979).

Data regarding the placental transfer of corticosteroids in the human are summarized in Table 6.2 Two of the earlier studies were carried out using tracer doses of radioactive corticosteroid, and the later studies have employed assays after pharmacologic doses as indicated. The concentration of prednisolone in cord serum is 12 % of the maternal value, whether derived from either prednisolone or prednisone. Cord levels of hydrocortisone are about 27 %, compared with 28–37 % for betamethasone. It may be estimated from the data

Table 6.2. Placental transfer of corticosteroids in the human

Steroid preparation	Dose	Concentration in cord plasma[a] (% of maternal)	References
Prednisolone	[^{3}H]	12	Beitens et al. 1972
Prednisone	[^{3}H]	90 (12)[b]	Beitens et al. 1972
Hydrocortisone sodium succinate	150 mg	27	Simmer et al. 1974
	[^{14}C]	27–32	Migeon et al. 1961
Betamethasone acetate plus phosphate	12 mg	37	Ballard et al. 1975
	8 mg	28	Petersen et al. 1980
Dexamethasone phosphate	5 mg	≦ 45	Kream et al. 1983
Methylprednisolone hemisuccinate	125 mg	42	Anderson et al. 1981

[a] Most of the values are derived from data for matched maternal and fetal samples
[b] Prednisolone concentration after administration of prednisone

of Kream et al. (1983) that dexamethasone in cord plasma is no more than 45 % of the maternal value, and a similar value was found for methylprednisolone.

In general, the maternal:fetal distribution is proportional to the unbound concentration of these corticosteroids in plasma. Prednisolone and hydrocortisone are bound by both CBG and albumin, whereas the other steroids are bound only by albumin. Prednisone or prednisolone would therefore be the steroid of choice for preferential treatment of the mother rather than the fetus during pregnancy, whereas the other synthetic steroids would provide a greater fetal exposure for a given dose to the mother. These data are consistent with the observations of most investigators that maternal therapy with prednisone during pregnancy does not produce clinically apparent adrenal insufficiency in the newborn infant (Warrell and Taylor 1968; Schatz et al. 1975).

6.1.7 Placental Metabolism

Human placenta and membranes contain a relatively high concentration of 11β-hydroxysteroid dehydrogenase activity which catalyzes the interconversion of the 11β-hydroxyl and keto group (discussed further in Chap. 4). The ketosteroids have a low affinity for glucocorticoid receptor and as such are biologically inactive (Ballard et al. 1975b). In a study of steroid metabolism by minced human placenta, Blanford and Murphy (1977) found significant conversion of cortisol and prednisolone to cortisone and prednisone, respectively, during 2 h incubation at 37 °C (67.4 and 51.4 %, respectively), while there was little detectable metabolism of both dexamethasone and betamethasone (1.8 and 7.1 %, respectively). Levitz et al. (1978) confirmed the much greater metabolism of cortisol compared with dexamethasone and betamethasone in minces of human placenta. However, using pefusion of the isolated placenta, metabolism of dexamethasone and betamethasone was only slightly less (54 and 47 %, respectively) than for cortisol and prednisolone (73 and 86 %, respectively). The perfusions were carried out in Earl's buffered salt solution with or without 1 % human serum albumin or red blood cells. In these solutions, all of the steroids would be primarily in the unbound form in contrast with the situation in vivo. Although additional studies of placental metabolism are needed, it appears that the somewhat greater placental transfer of betamethasone, dexamethasone and methylprednisolone vs. cortisol and prednisolone reflects a combination of both decreased plasma binding and less placental metabolism.

6.1.8 Time Course Considerations

The efficacy of corticosteroids administered for prenatal therapy is primarily determined by three factors. These are the relative intrinsic glucocorticoid potency, the amount of transfer from mother to fetus, and the clearance rate of administered steroid from the circulation. Data on the last factor are summarized in Table 6.3. Clearance rates in the pregnant women are similar to those for the non-pregnant adult. The plasma half-life of betamethasone, after injection of a mixture of the acetate and phosphate forms, is about 6 h com-

Table 6.3. Clearance of administered corticosteroids from maternal and fetal plasma

Steroid injected	Plasma half-life (h)			References
	Nonpregnant adult	Maternal	Fetal	
Betamethasone acetate and phosphate	3.3[a]	5–6	6–12	Ballard et al. 1975 a Ballard et al. 1975 b Petersen et al. 1980
Dexamethasone phosphate	3.3–5.6	3.6		Meikle and Tyler 1977 Lan & Baxter 1982 Ballard et al. 1975 b Kream et al. 1983
Hydrocortisone sodium succinate	1.5		2	Ballard et al. 1975 b Ballard & Liggins 1982
Methylprednisolone hemisuccinate	3.5	~1	~1	Ballard et al. 1975 b Anderson et al. 1981

[a] Phosphate form alone

pared to 3.6 h for dexamethasone (phosphate) and 1.5 for hydrocortisone (sodium succinate). Less information is available regarding the fetal circulation; however, it appears that the plasma half-life in the fetus is at least as long if not longer than in the maternal circulation.

In designing an optimal treatment regimen with corticosteroids, it is appropriate to consider the half-time of the biologic effect as well as plasma clearance rate. Intuitively, the half-time for the biologic effect should be longer than that for clearance from the plasma. Loss of biologic effect is determined by the rate of dissociation of steroid from receptor in the target cell, the half-times of induced mRNA's and proteins, and plasma clearance rate. The degradation rates for RNA and proteins obviously differ between tissues and for different induced proteins. Meikle and Tyler (1977) estimated the half-time of the biologic effect of corticosteroids on pituitary-adrenal function by determining suppression of plasma corticosterone concentrations. They concluded that the half-time of biologic effect in this system was from 1.5–2 times longer than the half-time for clearance of hydrocortisone, dexamethasone and prednisone from plasma.

The duration of corticosteroid effect in fetal lung in vivo may be estimated from data obtained in cultured fetal rabbit lung. In this system, the half-time for dissociation of receptor-bound steroid from nuclei is 7.2 h for dexamethasone and 1,4 h for cortisol (Ballard et al. 1984). The slower dissociation of dexamethasone is consistent with its higher affinity for receptor. These data provide a minimal estimate for the reversal of glucocorticoid effects in cultured lung and suggest that the half-time for biologic effect in vivo exceeds the clearance half-time from plasma.

6.2 Suppression of Endogenous Cortisol

6.2.1 Maternal

Glucocorticoid therapy decreases the concentration of cortisol in both mother and fetus. With the usual doses of steroid used in prenatal therapy, the maximal decrease in cortisol concentrations is about 60–80 % of untreated values in both fetal and maternal plasma and in amniotic fluid. In the maternal circulation, cortisol concentrations begin to decrease within about 2 h of betamethasone injection and are < 5 μg/dl by 12 h (Fig. 6.1). By 2–3 days after the last injection, cortisol concentrations have returned to the normal range (Ballard et al. 1975a; Liggins and Howie 1972; Maltau et al. 1979; Teramo et al. 1980). The time-course of cortisol suppression is consistent with the kinetics of betamethasone in the maternal circulation.

6.2.2 Fetal

In cord blood, there is a trend toward lower cortisol concentrations within a few hours of the first dose of maternal betamethasone. The mean level for plasma samples collected 6–16 h after injection was 3.7 ± 0.47 μg/dl, which was a significant reduction from the value in untreated infants (8.4 ± 0.44 μg/dl) (Ballard et al. 1980). Fig. 6.5 presents data for cortisol concentrations in 86 premature infants who delivered at various times after the second maternal dose of betamethasone. By regression analysis, the maximal suppression of cortisol compared to the untreated group is 55 % and cortisol returns to the untreated level approximately 7 days after the last dose of 12 mg of betameth-

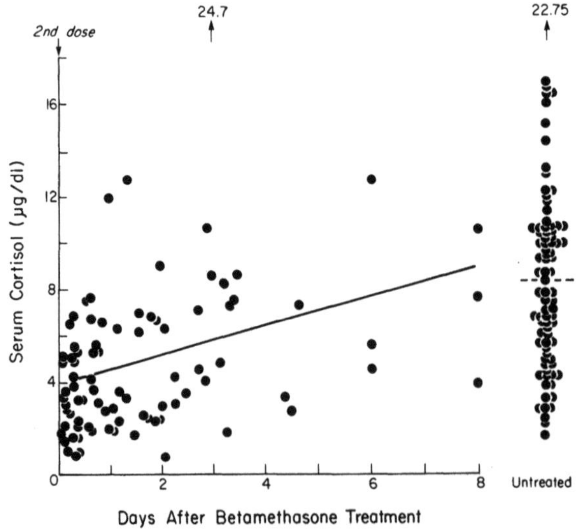

Fig. 6.5. Cortisol levels in cord serum of premature infants delivering at various times after the second dose of 12 mg betamethasone acetate and phosphate. The mean ± SE values for the untreated population is 8.4 ± 0.44 μg/dl. Reproduced from Ballard et al. (1980), by permission

asone (mixture of acetate and phosphate forms). In a separate clinical trial, four maternal injections of 6 mg of betamethasone (alcohol) were given every 12 h. With this regimen, cortisol concentrations in cord serum were lowest at 6–48 h after the first injection (3.6 ± 0.48 μg/dl), and values returned to the untreated level by approximately 6 days (Ballard et al. 1980). After maternal treatment with 12 mg of betamethasone for 3 days, Gennser et al. (1976) found normal cortisol concentrations in cord blood of a group of infants who delivered 6–19 days after the last injection. Similarly, cortisol concentrations in amniotic fluid were low when delivery occurred < 5 days after the last dose of betamethasone and were in the normal range for deliveries occurring 6–19 days after the last injection.

6.2.3 Adrenocortical Responsiveness to Stress

The responsiveness of the pituitary-adrenal axis in treated infants with suppressed cortisol concentrations has been examined. As shown in Table 6.4, treated infants who are stressed by either intrapartum asphyxia or RDS after birth increase their endogenous cortisol concentrations. In response to asphyxia, the increment in cortisol was 4.9 μg/dl for treated infants vs. 7.5 μg/dl for untreated infants. For those infants developing RDS, the increment was 18.4 μg/dl for treated infants and 23.0 μg/dl for untreated babies. The mean time for obtaining maximal cortisol values was 25 and 20.2 h after birth in treated and untreated infants with RDS, respectively. Similar results have been reported by Sybulski (1977) and Kauppila et al. (1978). When treated infants were given $ACTH_{1-24}$ at one day (Ohrlander et al. 1977; Teramo et al. 1980) or at one and four weeks after birth (Nogushi and Reynolds 1978) the increase in plasma cortisol was similar to that in untreated infants. These studies indicate that prenatal therapy with 12 mg of betamethasone for 2 or 3 days does not interfere with the premature infant's adrenocortical response to stress after birth.

Table 6.4. Cortisol concentrations in newborn premature infants stressed by asphyxia or RDS. Data from Ballard et al. (1980)

	Serum cortisol (μg/dl)		p
	Betamethasone-treated infants	Untreated infants	
Intrapartum asphyxia[a]	(n = 14)	(n = 19)	
Level at birth	3.3 ± 0.43	7.3 ± 0.71	< 0.05
Mean level at 1–2 h[b]	8.2 ± 1.23	14.8 ± 1.85	< 0.05
RDS	(n = 13)	(n = 15)	
Level at birth	4.0 ± 0.60	7.0 ± 0.78	< 0.05
Peak level in first 2 days[c]	22.4 ± 3.72	30.0 ± 2.88	NS

[a] Mean ± SE Apgar scores at 1 and 5 min were 1.6 ± 0.3 and 5.2 ± 0.9, respectively, for betamethasone-treated infants, and 1.6 ± 0.2 and 5.6 ± 0.4, respectively, for untreated infants
[b] Mean value for 2–4 determinations
[c] Maximal value found in serial determinations

6.3 Glucocorticoid Activity in Fetal Plasma

6.3.1 Receptor Affinity

The glucocorticoid activity in fetal plasma during treatment can be estimated from data on plasma levels of exogenous corticosteroid and endogenous cortisol (Ballard et al. 1975a, 1980; Ballard and Liggins 1982). In this analysis, plasma concentrations are expressed as cortisol equivalents reflecting the relative affinity of various corticosteroids for binding to glucocorticoid receptor. Data for the relative activity of synthetic and endogenous corticosteroids for binding to receptor are presented in Table 6.5. All of the synthetic glucocorticoids demonstrate a greater affinity for receptor of both hepatoma cells and human fetal lung compared with cortisol. The greater affinity of synthetic corticosteroids is consistent with their greater potency in vivo. Using the conversion factors shown in Table 6.5, the plasma concentration of synthetic corticosteroids can be expressed in terms of cortisol equivalents. These data, combined with endogenous cortisol concentrations, provide an estimate of total plasma glucocorticoid activity.

6.3.2 Calculations

In evaluating the time course of glucocorticoid activity in the fetus after treatment, it was assumed that only the unbound fraction of circulating glucocorticoids is biologically active. In man, approximately 85 % of circulating cortisol is bound to CBG, about 8 % is bound to albumin, and the remainder is unbound. In most studies, biologic activity has been associated only with the unbound fraction (Ballard 1979), although this relationship has not been studied for the fetal lung. The concentration of CBG in the human fetus is about half that found in adult plasma (Ballard 1979), which results in a greater percen-

Table 6.5. Affinity of natural and synthetic corticosteroids for glucocorticoid receptor. Data from Ballard et al. (1975b)

Steroid	Relative activity in radioreceptor assay	
	Hepatoma cell	Human fetal lung
Cortisol	100	100
6α–Methylprednisolone	1740	1190
Dexamethasone	940	710
Betamethasone	710	540
Fluorometholone	640	400
9α–Fluorocortisol	570	350
Triamcinolone acetonide	400	190
Corticosterone	370	85
Prednisolone	230	220
11–Deoxycortisol	23	19
Progesterone	12	11
Prednisone	3	5
Cortisone	2	1

tage of circulating cortisol unbound in fetal vs. maternal circulation. In a study of 83 cord blood specimens, for example, unbound cortisol averaged 22.1 % at a total cortisol concentration of 3 μg/dl (Ballard et al. 1980). Based on the studies of Peets et al. (1969), it is estimated that 47 % of betamethasone is unbound in the cord blood of premature infants. Using the data for concentrations and binding affinities of albumin and CBG, levels of free steroid may be calculated. For dexamethasone and betamethasone only binding to albumin need be considered. Calculation of free cortisol requires the quadratic equation of Tait and Burstein (1964) which includes terms for both albumin and CBG. Calculated values for both free cortisol and free dexamethasone are in good agreement with direct measurements of these steroids (Ballard et al. 1982b; Lan and Baxter 1982).

6.3.3 Time Course

Figure 6.6 compares the estimated time course for unbound glucocorticoid activity in fetal plasma after three different corticosteroid regimens: betamethasone acetate plus phosphate, 2 doses of 12 mg 24 h apart; betamethasone (alcohol), 4 doses of 6 mg at 12-h intervals; hydrocortisone sodium succinate, 4 doses of 100 mg at 8-h intervals. The calculations are based on the data discussed previously for plasma binding and concentrations of total exogenous and endogenous corticosteroids after treatment. The 100 mg dose of hydrocortisone produces higher peak concentrations of unbound glucocorticoid activity than for betamethasone. Since hydrocortisone is cleared more rapidly than betamethasone ($t_{1/2}$ estimated as 2 and 12 h, respectively, for these calculations), there are greater fluctuations in serum glucocorticoid activity with hydrocortisone therapy, with values falling to the untreated level between doses. The total duration of elevated serum glucocorticoid activity is about 32 h with hydrocortisone therapy compared with approximately 60 and 72 h for the 12

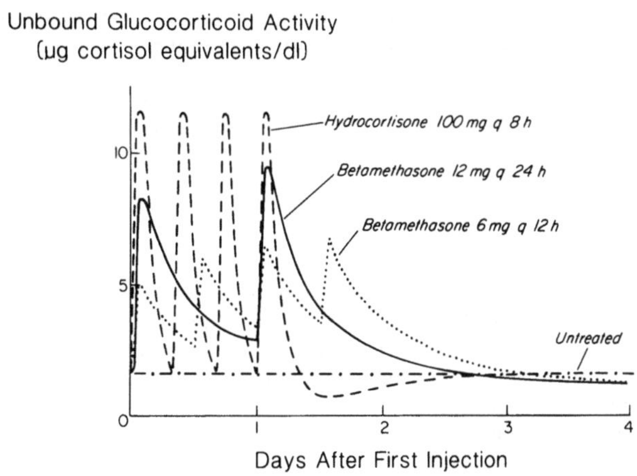

Fig. 6.6. Estimated time courses for unbound glucocorticoid activity in serum of fetuses exposed to maternal therapy with betamethasone or hydrocortisone. The calculations are discussed in the text. Reproduced from Ballard and Liggins (1982), by permission

and 6 mg regimens of betamethasone, respectively. Glucocorticoid activity is below the untreated level for approximately 40 h after the last dose of hydrocortisone due to suppression of endogenous cortisol. The suppression occurs later with betamethasone and remains below the level in untreated infants for approximately 4 days.

6.3.4 Maximal Levels

Table 6.6 compares the maximal concentrations of plasma glucocorticoid activity in untreated premature infants, infants exposed to various regimens of maternal glucocorticoid therapy, and untreated infants who are stressed in the perinatal period. The calculated maximal levels of plasma unbound glucocorticoid activity in treated infants are in the same range as those obtained in untreated infants stressed by intrapartum asphyxia or development of RDS. These regimens of corticosteroid therapy therefore produce plasma levels of glucocorticoid activity in the physiologic stress range. Assuming that the K_D for cortisol binding to glucocorticoid receptor in human fetal lung is approximately 33 nM (Ballard et al. 1978), occupancy of receptor would be 20–50 % in untreated premature infants and increase to approximately 90 % as a maximal value after betamethasone therapy. The increase in occupancy should result in a proportional increase in enzyme induction, based on studies in the rabbit (Gross et al. 1983), and thus elicit a near optimal response in fetal lung.

In other clinical studies, much higher doses of glucocorticoids have been employed. Table 6.7 lists these doses and the estimated plasma concentra-

Table 6.6. Plasma glucocorticoid activity in premature infants exposed to antenatal corticosteroid therapy or stress. All values are from assays in cord blood except for infants with RDS (during first day after birth). Maximal unbound glucocorticoid activities are estimated from measurements of administered corticosteroids (Ballard and Liggins 1982; Ballard et al. 1980; Kream et al. 1983; Ballard et al. 1975a), endogenous cortisol (Ballard and Liggins 1982; Ballard et al. 1980) and CBG binding (Ballard et al. 1975 a; Ballard et al. 1980), and assuming approximately 50% of corticosteroids not bound to CBG are unbound (Peets et al. 1969). Concentrations of synthetic corticosteroids are expressed as cortisol equivalents based on their affinity for human lung receptor (Table 6.5)

Infant group	Dose of steroid to mother	Plasma concentrations (μg cortisol equivalents/dl)	
		Total cortisol	Maximal unbound glucocorticoid activity[a]
Normal untreated	None	8.5	1.6
Hydrocortisone sodium succinate	100 mg q 8h × 4	32.0	11.6
Betamethasone acetate and phosphate	12 mg q 24h × 2	3.8	7.5
Betamethasone alcohol	6 mg q 12h × 4	3.6	5.4
Dexamethasone phosphate	5 mg q 12h × 4	3.6	6.2
Intrapartum asphyxia	None	14.8	4.1
RDS	None	30.0	10.7

[a] Plasma activity, expressed as cortisol equivalents, for endogenous cortisol plus exogenous corticosteroid

Table 6.7 Glucocorticoid levels in infants exposed to higher doses of corticosteroid. Steroids were administered to pregnant women (assumed weight of 60 kg) except in the study of Baden et al. (1972), where newborn premature infants were treated. The unbound plasma glucocorticoid activity was estimated as described for Table 6.6

Steroid administered	Treatment schedule	Dose as cortisol equivalents (mg/kg/24 h)	Estimated maximal unbound glucocorticoid activity in infant plasma (μg cortisol equivalents/dl)	References
None	-	-	1.6	Ballard & Liggins 1982
Methylprednisolone hemisuccinate	125 mg	24.8	207	Anderson et al. 1981
Hydrocortisone	500 mg q 12 h × 5	16.7	59	Morrison et al. 1978
	1000 mg q 8 h × 2-5	50.0	118	Whitt et al. 1976 Elsner et al. 1979 Anderson & Cordero 1980
	1000 mg q 6 h × 4	67.7	135	Zuspan et al. 1977
	15 mg/kg q 12 h × 2	30	550	Baden et al. 1972

tions of glucocorticoid activity which would be achieved in the fetus. Because of the relatively slow clearance of cortisol in the immediate newborn period (Reynolds et al. 1962), treatment of infants with hydrocortisone just before or after delivery results in an extended period of elevated glucocorticoid concentrations. The efficacy of the larger doses of hydrocortisone for prevention of RDS has not been established. It is unlikely that they would be more effective than the standard treatment regimens since Liggins (1976) found similar clinical results with 24 mg of betamethasone vs. the 12 mg regimen. Furthermore, it is likely that high doses of hydrocortisone therapy increase the risk for potential adverse effects in the infant (discussed in Chap. 5).

6.4 Effect on Other Endogenous Hormones

Table 6.8 summarizes the effect of maternal corticosteroid thereapy on other endogenous hormones that have been examined. The summary is limited to studies employing doses and treatment regimens which are currently used or potentially could be used for routine prophylactic therapy. After treatment with 150 mg hydrocortisone 12 h prior to cesarean section, ACTH was similarly decreased in both maternal and umbilical arterial and venous plasma of term infants (Simmer et al. 1974). In the study by Huhtaniemi et al. (1982), mothers received 12, 8 and 4 mg dexamethasone for 3 consecutive days. The mean plasma ACTH in treated infants who delivered less than 24 h after the last dose of steroid was not different from the mean value in untreated infants. It is not reported whether cortisol values were suppressed in the treated infants.

Concentrations of dehydroepiandrosterone (DHEA) and DHEA sulphate are suppressed in both fetal and maternal circulation. The degree and time

Table 6.8. Effect of maternal glucocorticoid therapy on endogenous hormone concentrations. The data represent the range of maximal effects observed with maternal glucocorticoid treatment. In these studies women in the third trimester of pregnancy received dexamethasone (8-12 mg/day), betamethasone (12 mg daily) or hydrocortisone 150 mg over 12 h (Simmer 1974; Tulchinsky and Okada 1975) or 500 mg intramuscularly (Lefebvre et al. 1976)

Hormone	Change in concentration with therapy (% of untreated)			References
	Fetal plasma	Maternal plasma	Amniotic fluid	
Cortisol	23-42 (see Fig. 6.5)	15-30 (see Fig. 6.1)	22-40	Ballard et al. 1975a; Ballard et al. 1980; Collab. Group 1981; Genns[illegible] et al. 1976; Liggins & Howie 1972; Maltau et al. 1979; Ohrlander et a 1975; Osathanondh et al. 1977; Parker et al. 1982; Sybulski 1977; Kream et al. 1983
ACTH	39	40	-	Simmer et al. 1974
	100	-	-	Huhtaniemi et al. 1982
Dehydroepiandrosterone	28	21	-	Simmer et al. 1974
Dehydroepiandrosterone sulfate	13-35 (see Fig. 6.7)	28	-	Simmer et al. 1974; Ballard et al 1980; Parker et al. 1982
Esterone	25	38-49	100	Ohrlander et al. 1976; Simmer et al. 1974;
	-	100	-	Negulescu et al. 1977
17 β-estradiol	15	15-50	100	Negulescu et al. 1977; Ohrlander et al. 1976; Simmer et al. 1974; Kauppila et al. 1979
Estriol	22-27	22-54	30-58	Collab. Group 1981; Maltau et al. 1979; Negulescu et al. 1976; Kjar & Hess 1983; Kauppila et al. 1979; Simmer et al. 1974; Lefebv et al. 1976
Progesterone	-	100	100	Ohrlander et al. 1976; Tulchinsky &
	456	100	274	Okada 1975; Mahajan et al. 1983; Lefebvre et al. 1976
17 α-hydroxyprogesterone	51	-	-	Mahajan et al. 1983
17 α,20α-dihydroxyprogesterone	49	-	-	Mahajan et al. 1983
Testosterone	100 (male)	100	-	Huhtaniemi et al. 1982; Kauppila ε al. 1979
Total cholesterol	129-147	-	-	Anderson & Friis-Hansen 1977; Parker et al. 1982
Human chorionic somatomammotropin	-	100	-	Maltau et al. 1979; Ohrlander et al 1975
Growth hormone	47 (see Fig. 6.8)	-	-	Ballard et al. 1980
Prolactin	100	-	-	Ballard et al. 1980
T_4	100	100	100	Ballard et al. 1982a; Osathanondh al. 1978
T_3	100	-	-	Ballard et al. 1982a
	290	100	100	Osathanondh et al. 1978
rT_3	100	-	-	Ballard et al. 1982a
	180	100	100	Osathanondh et al. 1978

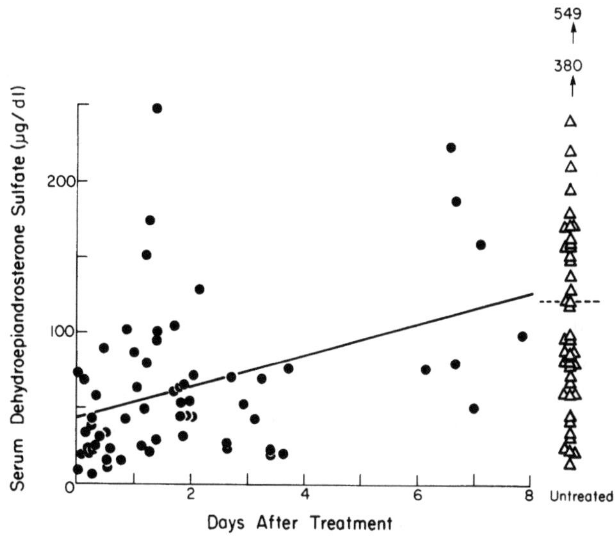

Fig. 6.7. DHEA sulfate concentrations in cord serum of premature infants delivering at various times after maternal treatment with 6 mg betamethasone. The mean ± SE value for the untreated population is 123.5 ± 14.3 µg/dl. Reproduced from Ballard et al. (1980), by permission

course of suppression for these steroids is similar to that observed for cortisol. Figure 6.7 shows the concentration of DHEA sulphate in cord serum of infants delivering at various times after exposure to maternal betamethasone therapy. By regression analysis, the steroid level was 43.3 µg/dl at the vertical intercept for treated infants vs. 123.5 ± 14.3 µg/dl in a population of untreated infants. DHEA sulphate concentrations in the treated infants returned to the untreated range by about 7½ days after the last dose of betamethasone.

Consistent with the role of DHEA as precursor for estrogens, most studies have found a suppression of estrone, 17β-estradiol, and estriol in both the fetal and maternal circulation. In addition, maternal urinary excretion of estriol and total estrogens is suppressed with glucocorticoid therapy (Ohrlander et al. 1975; Charles et al. 1971; Negulescu et al. 1977). In women who received 3 daily doses of 12 mg of betamethasone acetate and phosphate, excretion of estriol remained low for about 2 weeks following therapy (Ohrlander et al. 1975; Kjer and Hess 1983). It was noted that lower initial values of estriol excretion were associated with less of a decrease (expressed as mg/24 h) following betamethasone therapy. In other studies, using somewhat lower total doses of maternal glucocorticoid treatment, plasma and urinary estriol concentrations returned to the normal range in less than a week (Charles et al. 1971; Ylikorkala et al. 1978; Maltau et al. 1979; Negulescu et al. 1977; Kjer and Hess 1983). With repeated courses of betamethasone therapy, maternal estriol levels can remain low for prolonged periods (Elliman et al. 1981). In one case, a pregnant woman received 2 doses of 12 mg betamethasone (at 12-h intervals) on 5 separate occasions between weeks 27 and 31 of gestation. Plasma and amniotic fluid estriol concentrations were consistently low on repeated determinations during the next 6 weeks of gestation. On delivery at 39 weeks gestation, the cortisol concentration in cord blood was 2 μg/dl, increasing to the normal range by 2 h after birth. At 24 h of age, the cortisol response to administration of $ACTH_{1-24}$ was normal (A.W. Root, personal communication). This case illustrates that prolonged suppression of fetal adrenocortical function can occur with repeated courses of betamethasone therapy.

The suppression of maternal estrogen concentration with glucocorticoid treatment reflects decreased production of DHEA sulfate by the fetal adrenal rather than inhibition of placental enzymes catalyzing conversion of DHEA sulfate to estradiol. This is the conclusion of Kauppila et al. (1979), who administered DHEA sulfate to both untreated pregnant women and those treated with dexamethasone. The basal concentrations of estradiol were lower in the dexamethasone-treated group, but after injection of DHEA sulfate, estradiol increased to the same level in both groups of patients.

An increase in cord concentrations of cholesterol after corticosteroid therapy has been observed. Anderson and Friis-Hansen (1977) found an elevation of HDL-cholesterol but not other lipoprotein-cholesterol values, whereas Parker et al. (1982) report an increase in LBL-cholesterol (67 vs. 49 mg/dl). These workers speculate that inhibition of steroid secretion by the fetal adrenal after betamethasone therapy causes fetal plasma cholesterol levels to increase secondary to lower utilization by the adrenals. According to this mechanism, steroid therapy would increase fetal cholesterol concentration with a time course similar to that observed for suppression of cortisol and DHEA sulphate concentrations.

The proposed relationship between plasma cholesterol and DHEA sulfate is supported by the negative correlation for concentrations in cord plasma of normal infants, anencephalic newborns, and infants delivered of hypertensive mothers. Furthermore, there is a close inverse temporal relationship between concentrations of LDL-cholesterol and DHEA sulfate in cord plasma during the third trimester (Parker et al. 1980, 1983). These workers feel that the reduction of plasma LDL-cholesterol is probably not due to either maturation of the LDL-receptor system or diminished LDL-cholesterol production. A practical implication of this relationship between cholesterol and DHEA sulfate potentially exists with regard to screening of cord blood for familial hypercholesterolemia. In such a test, prenatal glucocorticoid therapy, as well as other in utero conditions which decrease steroidogenesis, would generate false positive results.

Maternal levels of progesterone are unaffected by corticosteroid therapy. This finding is consistent with other evidence that progesterone production by the human placenta is independent of both the fetal and maternal adrenal cortex. In one study, maternal concentrations of 17*a*-hydroxyprogesterone and 17*a*-, 20*a*-dihydroxyprogesterone decreased after treatment. During normal pregnancy in the human these steroids increase during the third trimester and with delivery (Tulchinsky and Simmer 1972; Mahajan et al. 1983). In the sheep, there is increased production of both steroids with either spontaneous labor or dexamethasone treatment (Anderson et al. 1975; Flint et al. 1975) due to induction of placental 17*a*-hydroxylase activity. Dexamethasone ap-

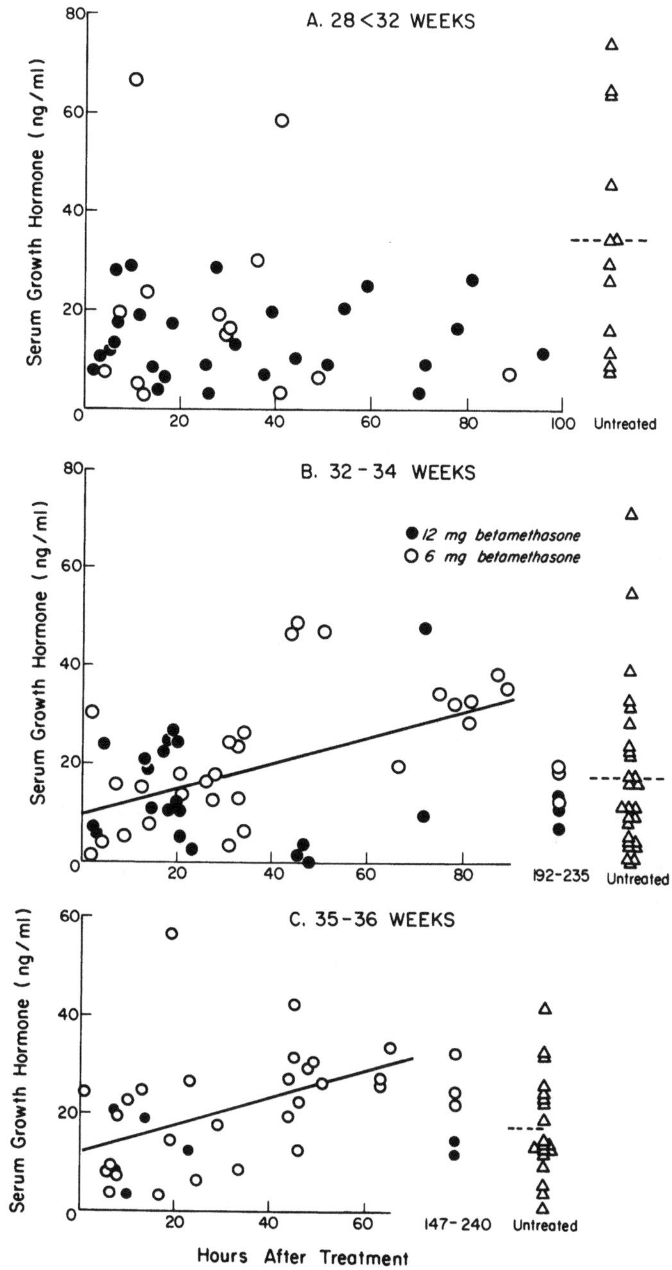

Fig. 6.8. Growth hormone concentrations in cord serum of infants delivering at various times after maternal treatment with betamethasone. Mean ± SE values for untreated populations are 34.9 ± 6.7, 17.9 ± 1.9, and 17.8 ± 2.4 ng/ml for parts A, B, and C, respectively. The P values for the slopes of the regression lines are <0.01. Reproduced from Ballard et al. (1980), by permission

parently does not stimulate this enzyme or 20α-hydroxysteroid dehydrogenase in the human, suggesting that the developmental increases in 17α-hydroxyprogesterone and 17α-, 20α-hydroxyprogesterone are not induced by endogenous corticosteroid.

An unexpected finding of steroid therapy was the suppression of fetal growth hormone concentrations. Figure 6.8 shows growth hormone values for infants of different gestational age groups. In treated infants of 28–30 weeks gestation the mean growth hormone concentration was 45 % of that in untreated infants. Less suppression of growth hormone was evident in the older groups of infants, and regression analysis suggested a prompt return to values equal to or greater than normal after the last dose of steroid. The transient decrease in growth hormone is unlikely to be physiologically important for the treated fetus, since growth hormone is apparently not essential for normal intrauterine growth (Liggins 1974; Lovinger et al. 1975).

As also indicated in Table 6.8, concentrations of T_4, T_3 and rT_3 in cord plasma of premature infants were not affected by exposure to prenatal betamethasone (Ballard et al. 1982a). In a study involving pregnant women at term, Osathanondh et al. (1978) found a 3- and 2-fold increase in T_3 and rT_3 concentrations, respectively, in umbilical plasma after maternal treatment with 8–16 mg dexamethasone given 3–48 h before cesarean section. T_4 concentrations in umbilical plasma, and concentrations of all three thyroid hormones in maternal plasma were not different for the control and dexamethasone-treated groups. The latter results are in contrast to the decrease in serum T_3 with dexamethasone treatment of non-pregnant adult subjects (Duick et al. 1974; Burr et al. 1976). Thus, glucocorticoids may have different effects on T_3 concentrations in the pregnant and non-pregnant state, and the effect in the fetus may be dependent on gestational age.

No effect of prenatal corticosteroid therapy has been noted on fetal concentrations of testosterone or prolactin. Also, therapy does not affect maternal concentrations of chorionic somatomammotropin.

6.5 Summary and Conclusions

Maternal treatment with corticosteroids causes a transient rise in fetal plasma glucocorticoid activity. To compare different regimens of corticosteroid therapy, steroid concentrations in the fetus can be expressed as cortisol equivalents, reflecting the intrinsic potency of the corticosteroids for receptor. The peak levels of unbound glucocorticoid activity (exogenous steroid plus endogenous cortisol) are similar after maternal treatment with 12 mg betamethasone acetate phosphate, 100 mg hydrocortisone sodium succinate, and 5 mg dexamethasone phosphate. Somewhat lower peak levels are obtained with 6 mg betamethasone alcohol, and much higher levels are achieved with the 125 mg dose of methylprednisolone succinate used in one study. The peak plasma levels in the fetus with the betamethasone and hydrocortisone regimens represent 3- to 5-fold increases over the untreated level of glucocorticoid activity. Based on the affinity of glucocorticoid binding to lung receptor, it is estimated that receptor occupancy approximately doubles after treatment.

The rise in unbound glucocorticoid activity with therapy is comparable to that occurring in untreated newborn infants who develop RDS, thereby representing a physiologic stress concentration of glucocorticoid. Higher doses of maternal hydrocortisone, as have been reported, expose the infant to pharmacologic concentrations of glucocortioid. Such regimens have not been shown to improve the efficacy of treatment and likely increase the risk for adverse effects.

There are substantial differences in the half-time for clearance of administered corticosteroids which result in different patterns of corticoid exposure. When dexamethasone phosphate or hydrocortisone sodium succinate is administered every 12 and 8 h, respectively, most of the administered steroid is cleared before the next injection. By contrast, about 24 h is required for clearance of betamethasone. Compared with the betamethasone regimen, therefore, the hydrocortisone and dexamethasone regimens produce greater fluctuations of serum levels and a shorter duration of elevated glucocorticoid concentration. The possible clinical effect of these differences will depend on the dissociation rate of glucocorticoid from receptor and the half-times of induced RNA's and proteins in fetal lung.

Maternal therapy with betamethasone (or hydrocortisone) suppresses endogenous cortisol in fetal and maternal circulation to 25 % or less of pretreatment levels. In the fetus, DHEA and DHEA sulphate are suppressed to a similar extent as cortisol, indicating that the fetal and definitive zones of the fetal adrenal are similarly affected. Secondary to this suppression, estrogen concentrations decrease transiently in both the fetal and maternal compartments. Fetal concentrations of cholesterol increase during steroid therapy, apparently due to decreased utilization by the fetal adrenal. Glucocorticoid therapy also suppresses plasma concentrations of growth hormone in the preterm fetus, but has no apparent effect on fetal prolactin or thyroid hormone levels. While these decreases in endogenous hormones are transient after the usual 2-day course of corticosteroid therapy, suppression can persist for more than a month following repeated courses of glucocorticoid treatment. One course of antenatal therapy does not interfere with the newborn infant's ability to produce cortisol in response to stress or ACTH administration.

References

Andersen CW, Cordero L (1980) Changes in amniotic fluid optical density at 450 mμ in Rh-sensitized patients after maternal hydrocortisone therapy. Am J Obstet Gynecol 137:820

Andersen GE, Friis-Hansen B (1977) Cord serum and lipoproteincholesterol values in normal and betamethasone-treated newborns of varying gestational age. Acta Paediatr Scand 66:355

Andersen GE, Friis-Hansen B (1978) Hypercholesterolemia in the newborn: Occurrence after antepartum treatment with betamethasone-phenobarbital-ritodrine for the prevention of the respiratory distress syndrome. Pediatrics 62:8

Anderson ABM, Flint APF, Turnbull AC (1975) Mechanism of action of glucocorticoids in induction of ovine parturition: Effect on placental steroid metabolism. J Endocrinol 66:61

Anderson ABM, Gennser G, Jeremy JY, Ohrlander S, Sayers L, Turnbull AC (1977) Placental transfer and metabolism of betamethasone in human pregnancy. Obstet Gynecol 49:471

Anderson GG, Rotchell Y, Kaiser DG (1981) Placental transfer of methylprednisolone following maternal interavenous administration. Am J Obstet Gynecol 140:699

Baden M, Bauer CR, Colle E, Klein G, Taeusch HW Jr, Stern L (1972) A controlled trial of hydrocortisone therapy in infants with respiratory distress syndrome. Pediatrics 50:526
Ballard PL, Granberg P, Ballard RA (1975a) Glucocorticoid levels in maternal and cord serum after prenatal betamethasone therapy to prevent respiratory distress syndrome. J Clin Invest 56:1548
Ballard PL, Carter JP, Graham BS, Baxter JD (1975b) A radioreceptor assay for evaluation of the plasma glucocorticoid activity of natural and synthetic steroids in man. J Clin Endocrinol Metab 41:290
Ballard PL (1979) Delivery and transport of glucocorticoids to target cells. In: Baxter JD, Rousseau GG (eds), Glucocorticoid Hormone Action, Springer, Berlin, Heidelberg, New York, pp 25–48
Ballard PL, Gluckman PD, Liggins GC, Kaplan SL, Grumbach MM (1980) Steroid and growth hormone levels in premature infants after prenatal betamethasone therapy to prevent respiratory distress syndrome. Pediatr Res 14:122
Ballard PL, Liggins GC (1982) Glucocorticoid activity in cord serum: Comparison of hydrocortisone and betamethasone regimens. J Pediatr 101:468
Ballard PL, Woeber KA, Klein AH (1982a) Thyroid hormone concentrations in cord serum after placental corticosteroid therapy. Pediatr Res 16:276A (abstract)
Ballard PL, Kitteman JA, Bland RD, Clyman RI, Gluckman PD, Platzker ACG, Kaplan SL, Grumbach MM (1982b) Ontogeny and regulation of corticosteroid binding globulin capacity in plasma of fetal and newborn lambs. Endocrinology 110:359.
Ballard PL, Ballard RA, Gonzales LK, Hümmelink R, Wilson CM, Gross I (1984) Corticosteroid binding by fetal rat and rabbit lung in organ culture. J Steroid Biochem 21:117
Beitins IZ, Bayard F, Ances IG, Kowarski A, Migeon CJ (1972) The transplacental passage of prednisone and prednisolone in pregnancy near term. J Pediatr 81:936
Blanford AT, Murphy BEP (1977) In vitro metabolism of prednisolone, dexamethasone, betamethasone, and cortisol by the human placenta. Am J Obstet Gynecol 127:264
Block MF, Kling R, Crosby WM (1977) Antenatal glucocorticoid therapy for the prevention of respiratory distress syndrome in the premature infant. Obstet Gynecol 50:186
Burr WA, Ramsden DB, Griffiths RS, Black EG, Hoffenberg H, Meinhold H, Wenzel KW (1976) Effect of a single dose of dexamethasone on serum concentrations of thyroid hormones. Lancet ii:58
Carson GD, Bolle JD, Challis JRG (1979) The availability of cortisone in amniotic fluid to the fetus and chorionic and amniotic membranes. Endocrinology 104:1053
Charles D, Pinkus JL, Fanous R, Chattoraj SC (1971) The effect of dexamethasone on the urinary excretion of steroids during pregnancy. J Obstet Gynecol Br Comm 78:241
Collaborative Group on Antenatal Steroid Therapy (1981) Effect of antenatal dexamethasone administration on the prevention of respiratory distress syndrome. Am J Obstet Gynecol 141:276
Duick DS, Warren DW, Nicoloff JT, Otis CL, Croxson MS (1974) Effect of single dose dexamethasone on the concentration of serum triiodothyronine in man. J Clin Endocrinol Metab 39:1151
Elliman D, Browning MCK, Forsyth CC (1981) Adrenal axis suppression due to maternal corticosteroid therapy. Pediatr Res 15:1187 (abstract)
Elsner CW, Buster JE, Preston DL, Killam AP (1979) Interrelationships of circulating maternal steroid concentrations in third trimester pregnancies. III. Effect of intravenous cortisol infusion on maternal concentrations of estriol, 16α-hydroxyprogesterone, 17α-hydroxyprogesterone, progesterone, 20α-dihydroprogesterone, Δ^5-pregnenolone, Δ^5-pregnenolone sulfate, dehydroepiandrosterone sulfate, and cortisol. J Clin Endocrinol Metab 49:30
Flint APF, Goodson JD,Turnbull AC (1975) Increased concentration of 17α-, 20α-hydroxypregn-4-en-3-one in maternal and foetal plasma near parturition in sheep. J Endocrinol 67:89
Gennser G, Ohrlander S, Eneroth P (1976) Cortisol in amniotic fluid and cord blood in relation to prenatal betamethasone load and delivery. Am J Obstet Gynecol 124:43
Gross I, Ballard PL, Ballard RA, Jones CT, Wilson CM (1983) Corticosteroid stimulation of phosphatidylcholine synthesis in cultured fetal rabbit lung: evidence for de novo protein synthesis mediated by glucocorticoid receptors. Endocrinology 112:829
Huhtaniemi I, Koivisto M, Pakarinen A, Tuimala R, Kauppila A (1982) Pituitary-adrenal and testicular function in preterm infants after prenatal dexamethasone treatment. Acta Paediatr Scand 71:425

Kauppila A, Koivisto M, Pukka M, Tuimala R (1978) Umbilical cord and neonatal cortisol levels: Effect of gestational and neonatal factors. Obstet Gynecol 52:666

Kauppila A, Tuimala R, Ylikorkala O, Reinila M, Ylostalo P (1979) Placental steroid synthesis from DHEAS during dexamethasone therapy. Obstet Gynecol 54:39

Kjer JJ, Hess J (1983) Serum estriol level during treatment with betamethasone in the last trimester of human pregnancy. Acta Obstet Gynecol Scand 62:307

Kream J, Mulay S, Fukushima K, Solomon S (1983) Determination of plasma dexamethasone in the mother and the newborn after administration of the hormone in a clinical trial. J Clin Endocrinol Metab 56:127

Lan NC, Baxter JD (1982) A radioreceptor assay for direct measurement of plasma free glucocorticoid activity. J Clin Endocrinol Metab 55:516

Lefebvre Y, Marier R, Amyot G, Bilodeau R, Hotte R, Raynault P, Durocher JG, Lanthier A (1976) Maternal, fetal, and intra-amniotic hormonal and biologic changes resulting from a single dose of hydrocortisone injected in the intra-amniotic compartment. Am J Obstet Gynecol 125:609

Levitz M, Jansen V, Dancis J (1978) The transfer and metabolism of corticosteroids in the perfused human placenta. Am J Obstet Gynecol 132:363

Liggins GC, Howie RN (1972) A controlled trial of antepartum glucocorticoid treatment for prevention of the respiratory distress syndrome in premature infants. Pediatrics 50:515

Liggins GC (1974) The influence of the fetal hypothalamus and pituitary on growth. In: Elliott K, Knight J (eds), Size at Birth, Elsevier-Excerpta Medica, North Holland, Amsterdam, pp 165–182

Liggins GC (1976) Prenatal glucocorticoid treatment: Prevention of Respiratory Distress Syndrome. In: Moore TD (ed), Proceedings of the 70th Ross Conference on Pediatric Research, Columbus, Ohio, Ross Laboratories

Lovinger RD, Kaplan SL, Grumbach MM (1975) Congenital hypopituitarism associated with neonatal hypoglycemia and microphallus: Four cases secondary to hypothalamic hormone deficiencies. J Pediatr 87:1171

Mahajan DK, Anderson G, Poole WK, Billiar RB, Little B (1983) Changes in the concentration of 17α, 20α-dihydroxypregn-4-en-3-one during pregnancy, labor and delivery and the effect of dexamethasone treatment during the third trimester of pregnancy. J Clin Endocrinol Metab 57:585

Maltau JM, Stokke KT, Moe N (1979) Effects of betamethasone on plasma levels of estriol, cortisol and HCS in late pregnancy. Acta Obstet Gynecol Scand 58:235

Meikle AW, Tyler FW (1977) Potency and duration of action of glucocorticoids. Effects of hydrocortisone, prednisone and dexamethasone on human pituitary-adrenal function. Am J Med 63:200

Migeon CJ, Bertrand J, Gemzell CA (1961) The transplacental passage of various steroid hormones in mid-pregnancy. Rec Prog Horm Res 17:207

Morrison JC, Whybrew WD, Bucovaz ET, Schneider JM (1978) Injection of corticosteroids into mother to prevent neonatal respiratory distress syndrome. Am J Obstet Gynecol 131:358

Negulescu RI, Strecker JR, Lauritzen C, Pal S (1977) The influence of betamethasone on the feto-placental unit. A preliminary report. J Perinat Med 5:120

Noguchi A, Reynolds JW (1978) Serum cortisol and dehydroepiandrosterone sulfate responses to adrenocorticotropin stimulation in premature infants. Pediatr Res 12:1057

Ohrlander SAV, Gennser GM, Grennert L (1975) Impact of betamethasone load given to pregnant women on endocrine balance of fetoplacental unit. Am J Obstet Gynecol 123:228

Ohrlander S, Gennser G, Batra S, Lebech P (1976) Effect of betamethasone administration of estrone, estradiol-17β, and progresterone in maternal plasma and amniotic fluid. Obstet Gynecol 49:148

Ohrlander S, Gennser G, Nilsson KO, Eneroth P (1977) ACTH test to neonates after administration of corticosteroids during gestation. Obstet Gynecol 49:691

Osathanondh R, Tulchinsky D, Kamali H, Fencl M deM, Taeusch HW Jr (1977) Dexamethasone levels in treated pregnant women and newborn infants. J Pediatr 90:617

Osathanondh R, Chopra I, Tulchinsky D (1978) Effects of dexamethasone on fetal and maternal thyroxine, triiodothyronine, reverse triiodothyronine, and thyrotropin levels. J Clin Endocrinol Metab 47:1236

Parker CR Jr, Simpson ER, Bilheimer DW, Leveno K, Carr BR, MacDonald PC (1980) Inverse relation between low-density lipoprotein-cholesterol and dehydroisoandrosterone sulfate in human fetal plasma. Science 208:512

Parker CR Jr, Herbert WNP, Morrison JC (1982) The effect of glucocorticoid therapy on fetal cholesterol (C) and adrenal steroids. Soc Gynecol Invest Meeting, page 129 (abstract)

Parker CR Jr,Carr BR, Simpson ER, MacDonald PC (1983) Decline in the concentration of low-density lipoprotein-cholesterol in human fetal plasma near term. Metabolism 32:919

Peets EA, Staub N, Synchowica C (1969) Plasma binding of betamethasone-^{3}H, dexamethasone-^{3}H and cortisol-^{14}C. A comparative study. Biochem Pharmacol 18:1655

Peterson MC, Nation RL, Ashley JJ, McBride WG (1980) The placental transfer of betamethasone. Eur J Clin Pharmacol 18:245

Reynolds JW, Colle E, Ulstrom RA (1962) Adrenocorticosteroid metabolism in newborn infants. V. Physiologic disposition of exogenous cortisol loads in the early neonatal period. J Clin Endocrinol Metab 22:245

Schatz M, Patterson R, Zeitz S, O'Rourke J, Melan H(1975) Corticosteroid therapy for the pregnant asthmatic patient. J Am Med Assoc 233:804

Schmidt PL, Sims ME, Strassner HT, Paul RH, Mueller E, McCart D (1984) Effect of antepartum glucocorticoid administration upon neonatal respiratory distress syndrome and perinatal infection. Am J Obstet Gynecol 148:178

Simmer HH, Tulchinsky D, Gold EM, Frankland M, Greipel M, Gold AS (1974) On the regulation of estrogen production by cortisol and ACTH in human pregnancy at term. Am J Obstet Gynecol 119:283

Sybulski S (1977 Effect of antepartum betamethasone treatment on cortisol levels in cord plasma, amniotic fluid, and the neonate. Am J Obstet Gynecol 127:871

Tait JF, Burstein S (1964) In vivo studies of steroid dynamics in man. In: Pincus G,Thimann KV (eds), The Hormones, Academic Press, New York, Vol 5, p 441

Tauesch HW Jr, Avery ME, Sugg J (1972) Premature delivery without accelerated lung development in fetal lambs treated with longacting methylprednisolone. Biol Neonate 20:85

Teramo K, Hallman M, Raivio KO (1980) Maternal glucocorticoid in unplanned premature labor. Controlled study on the effects of betamethasone phosphate on the phospholipids of the gastric aspirate and on the adrenal cortical function of the newborn infant. Pediatr Res 14:326

Tulchinsky D, Simmer HH (1972) Source of plasma 17α-hydroxyprogesterone in human pregnancy. J Clin Endocrinol Metab 35:799

Tulchinsky D, Okada DM (1975) Hormones in human pregnancy. IV. Plasma progesterone. Am J Obstet Gynecol 121:293

Warrell DW, Taylor R (1968) Otcome for the fetus of mothers receiving prednisolone during pregnancy. Lancet i:117.

Whitt GG, Buster JE, Killam AP, Scragg WH (1976) A comparison of two glucocorticoid regimens for acceleration of fetal lung maturation in premature labor. Am J Obstet Gynecol 124:479

Ylikorkala O, Dawood MY, Kauppila A, Tuimala R (1978) Effect of maternal dexamethasone therapy on the levels of oestrogens, progesterone and chorionic gonadotrophin in amniotic fluid and maternal serum. Br J Obstet Gynaecol 85:334

Zuspan FP, Cordero L, Semchyshyn S (1977) Effects of hydrocortisone on lecithin-spingomyelin ratio. Am J Obstet Gynecol 128:571

7 Thyroid Hormones: Effects and Binding

The effects of thyroid hormones on postnatal growth, differentiation, and metabolism are well known. It is also recognized that thyroid hormones and glucocorticoids have complementary, and sometimes synergistic, effects on specific enzymes in several organs. Given this background information, it is not surprising that thyroid hormones were evaluated for effects on lung maturation and function shortly after recognition of glucocorticoid action. In this chapter I review the action of thyroid hormones in fetal and postnatal lung, describe properties of pulmonary T_3 receptors and the correlations between binding and effect, and discuss preliminary information regarding clinical application.

7.1 Effects in Vivo

7.1.1 Fetal Treatment

In one of the first studies of thyroid hormone action in fetal lung, Wu et al. (1973) injected rabbit fetuses at 24 days gestation with 2 µg T_4. Control fetuses in the other uterine horn received saline. The fetuses were delivered by cesarean section 2 days later for analysis of lung histology and function. Fetuses treated with thyroxine had more air retention after passive deflation, a greater bubble stability ratio in lung wash fluid, and enhanced morphologic development by both light and electron microscopy. These findings provided the first evidence for a stimulatory effect of thyroid hormone in the fetal lung. Using a similar treatment protocol, Rooney et al. (1975) also found enhanced morphologic development.

In retrospect, it is evident that the technique of direct fetal injection in itself stimulates lung maturation, apparently by increasing endogenous corticoids (see Chap. 4). Thus, studies employing fetal injection assessed T_4 effects in the presence of elevated corticoids and possibly other stress-related hormones. In view of the synergistic interaction between corticosteroids and thyroid hormones on PC synthesis (Chap. 10), this experimental approach probably overestimates the effects of T_4 in the undisturbed fetus.

Hitchcock (1979) injected T_4 (67 µg) intra-amniotically in rats and subsequently carried out electron microscopy on fetal lung. To evaluate the influence of the surgical stress, some groups of animals received metopirone, the 11β-hydroxylase inhibitor, or underwent adrenalectomy. Accelerated lung development was observed in all groups receiving T_4. With the maneuvers to decrease endogenous corticosteroids, stimulatory effects of T_4 were still evident but less pronounced. The greatest effect was observed in animals receiving both intra-amnoitic T_4 and maternal treatment with hydrocortisone.

In a similar study with rats, Torday and Dow (1984) injected amniotic fluid with 0.1, 1 or 2 μg T_3 on day 17 and examined the pups on day 20. Compared with saline-injected littermates, T_3 produced a dose-dependent *decrease* in both lung weight and rate of choline incorporation into saturated PC. These findings contrast with the morphologic maturation noted after T_4 treatment (Hitchcock 1979).

Das et al. (1984) injected fetal rabbits on day 26 with approximately 20 μg T_3 or saline. This dose of hormone increased the levels of epinephrine, norepinephrine, β-adrenergic receptor, cAMP, and adenylate cyclase activity in lung tissue obtained 4 h later. The concentration of saturated PC in lavage fluid of treated fetuses was twice that of control littermates; this effect was completely blocked by simultaneous administration of propranolol. Except for the increase in adrenergic receptors, these results are consistent with a mechanism whereby high doses of T_3 increase endogenous catecholamines which cause secretion of surfactant. The relationship of this effect to changes in concentrations of endogenous thyroid hormones is uncertain.

There have been no in depth studies of thyroid hormone effects in fetal sheep. Such information would be useful for comparison with the data for glucocorticoid treatment in this species. However, preliminary reports do suggest that thyroid hormones are stimulatory to lung maturation in the sheep.

Nwosu et al. (1980), administered daily pulses of T_3 or T_4 to catheterized fetuses at 120–130 days gestation. In two fetuses receiving two courses of therapy, a substantial rise in the L/S ratio was detected. It is likely that daily intravenous pulses of thyroid hormone are not the optimal approach for treatment.

Lorijan et al. (1980) treated 13 chronically catheterized fetal lambs with T_3 by subcutaneous osmotic mini-pump. T_3 was released at a rate of 67 μg/h and increased serum T_3 concentrations from 20 ng/dl to about 200 ng/dl after 2 days of infusion. Serum concentrations of both T_4 and rT_3 decreased during infusion of T_3. Although this study was not specifically designed to evaluate lung maturation, several observations of interest were reported. In these animals of 125–135-days gestation, T_3 infusion increased cardiac output by 22 % compared with control fetuses. There was a similar rise in umbilical flow, coronary flow, and fetal oxygen consumption, and an apparently greater increase in pulmonary blood flow. On light microscopy, the lungs of five fetuses treated with T_3 were felt to show advanced maturation. During the treatment period there was no change in serum cortisol, epinephrine, norepinephrine or dopamine concentrations. This experimental approach has the advantages of exposing the fetuses to a continuous elevation of plasma T_3 without influencing cortisol levels. The increase in pulmonary blood flow may represent an effect of T_3 on either pulmonary vessels or the ductus arteriosus.

Korda et al. (1984) examined effects of intra-amniotic T_3 treatment of fetal lambs. At 130 days gestation saline or T_3 (50–1000 μg) was injected into the amniotic fluid; the fetuses were studied after cesarean delivery 48 h later. With the highest dose of T_3, lungs from 3 of 4 treated lambs demonstrated greater deflation stability than observed in control animals; phospholipid in a surfactant fraction of lung tissue was not significantly increased by T_3. Interpretation of these data is complicated by an increase in cord levels of cortisol

(3.2 vs. 1.6 µg/dl) in treated animals. Lung maturity may have been enhanced by T_3 alone, cortisol alone, or by a combined effect of the hormones.

Ikegami et al. (1983) examined lung phospholipids in fetal sheep thyroidectomized at 120 days with and without T_3 treatment for 8 days by mini-pump infusion. No effect of thyroidectomy or T_3 treatment on tissue phospholipid content was detected at this gestational age.

Additional experiments are required to define in vivo thyroid hormone effects on fetal lung. The chronic in utero fetal lamb model provides a suitable system to examine the flux of surfactant in tracheal fluid with particular regard to the time course of hormonal effect, reversibility, and the influence of gestational age. The ability to increase plasma T_3 concentrations without affecting plasma concentrations of either total cortisol (Lorijan et al. 1980; Ballard et al. 1982) or free cortisol (Ballard et al. 1982) provides an opportunity to test the effects of T_3 both alone and with administered glucocorticoid.

7.1.2 Maternal Treatment

Although iodothyronines do not readily cross the placenta in most species (Fisher et al. 1977), some passage occurs in the rat. Gross et al. (1984) injected pregnant rats with 0.7, 7, or 70 mg of T_3/kg daily on days 18 and 19 of gestation. On day 20, the concentration of T_3 in fetal plasma was 1.8, 33.5 and 188 ng/ml, respectively, compared with 1.2 ng/ml in control fetuses. The 7 mg regimen resulted in maximal (34 %) stimulation of choline incorporation into PC by fetal lung. The activity of cholinephosphate cytidylyltransferase (assayed in the absence of phosphatidylglycerol) was also increased (42 %) by T_3 treatment. Although high doses of T_3 were required in this study, the results indicate that maternally administered thyroid hormone stimulates PC synthesis in fetal lung. It is noteworthy that the T_3 effect occurred without a change in endogenous corticosterone concentrations.

An alternative approach to maternal therapy is the use of non-halogenated thyronine analogs. The synthetic compound 3,5-dimethyl-3′-isopropyl-L-thyronine (DIMIT) is one of the more potent analogs, exhibiting approximately 20 % the activity of T_4 in the tadpole (Frieden and Yoshizato 1974) and rat anti-goiter (Jorgensen et al. 1974) assays. The weak binding of DIMIT to plasma TBG facilitates placental passage. Administration of DIMIT to pregnant rats suppresses fetal thyrotropin levels, prevents propylthiouracil-induced fetal goiter, and increases the activity of thyroid hormone inducible enzymes in the fetal liver (Comite et al. 1978; Benson et al. 1978; Kriz et al. 1978). These effects in the fetus occur at doses which are not thyrotoxic to the mother; T_4 and T_3 also prevent fetal goiter, but only at doses which produce maternal hyperthyroidism. These early observations with DIMIT suggested unrestricted transfer across the rat placenta.

More recently, the distribution of DIMIT after maternal administration has been examined using the tritiated compound. In the rat, peak concentrations of radioactivity in fetal plasma were noted by 1 h after maternal administration (Ballard et al. 1980). As shown in Fig. 7.1, by 7 h after administration of ^{3}H-DIMIT similar concentrations of radioactivity were found in amniotic fluid, maternal plasma, and fetal plasma of both the rat and rabbit. Compar-

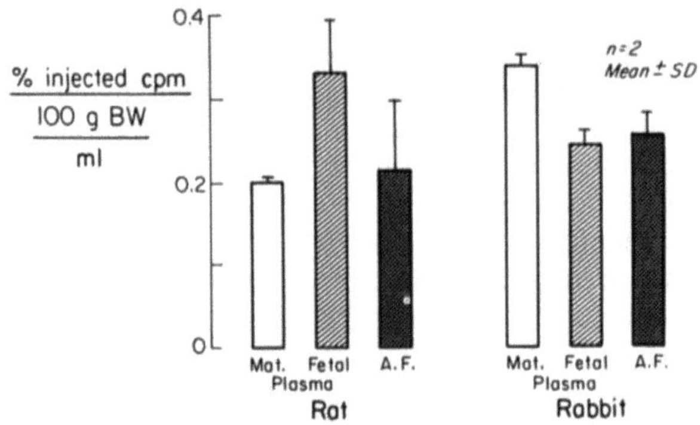

Fig. 7.1 Distribution of radioactivity after administration of [^{3}H]DIMIT to pregnant rats and rabbits. Rats (19 days gestation) and rabbits (25 days) received $\sim 1.5 \times 10^6$ cpm (6 µg) and $\sim 23 \times 10^6$ cpm (9 µg) of [^{3}H]DIMIT, respectively, and radioactivity was determined 7 h later. The proportion of radioactivity due to unmetabolized DIMIT (60–80 %) was similar in maternal and fetal compartments of both species. Data from Ballard et al. (1980)

able data were obtained in rats by radioimmunoassay (Chopra et al. 1984). There appeared to be preferential fetal localization of DIMIT in the rat, consistent with the greater biologic effects of DIMIT in rat fetuses than in their mothers. In the rabbit, maternal levels were slightly higher than in the fetus. The half-life for clearance of DIMIT from plasma of the adult rat is 6–7 h (Ballard et al. 1980; Chopra et al. 1984), which is slower than for T_3. A relatively slow clearance of DIMIT also occurs in adult humans (Tamagna et al. 1979).

Serum concentrations of DIMIT, T_4, and TSH have been determined in non-pregnant rats after treatment with various doses of DIMIT (Fig. 7.2). A statistically significant increase in DIMIT concentration occurred after a dose of 0.8 µg/100 g body weight once a day for 3 days (0.26 µg/dl vs. 0.12 in the control group). With a dose of 200 µg/100 g, the serum DIMIT concentration 15 h after the last dose was 44 µg/dl. There was a dose-dependent decrease in both serum T_4 and TSH concentrations with a half-maximal effect noted at about 3.5 µg DIMIT/100 g. Serum concentrations of DIMIT were also determined after rats were given 0.8 or 3.2 µg/100 g in once daily doses, or in divided doses at 8-h intervals. With both doses, equivalent serum concentrations were found for the single vs. divided therapy regimens (Chopra et al. 1984). DIMIT, like T_3, was more or less equally distributed among various tissues of the adult rat (lung was not examined), with tissue concentrations similar to that in serum. By comparison, tissue levels of T_4 were generally lower than the serum concentration, particularly in the case of skeletal muscle and brain (Chopra et al. 1984).

When ^{3}H-DIMIT was injected into pregnant sheep, a 4:1 maternal:fetal gradient of radioactivity was observed at 6 h, suggesting that transfer of DIMIT across the ovine placenta is restricted (Bachrach et al. 1982). Moreover, treatment of pregnant ewes with 1–2 mg DIMIT daily failed to prevent cretinism in their thyroidectomized fetuses.

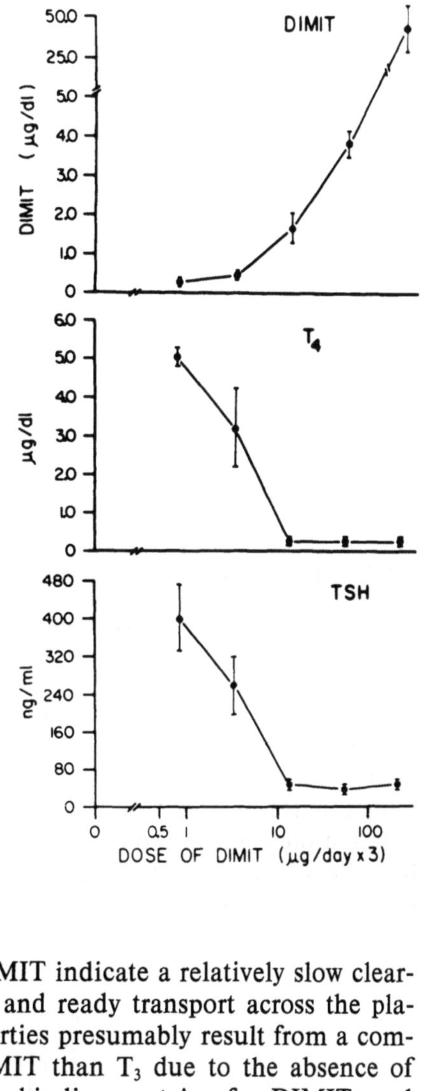

Fig. 7.2. Concentrations of DIMIT, T_4, and TSH in serum of rats given various doses of DIMIT. Data are mean ± SE (n = 4) and the dose of DIMIT is shown on a logarithmic scale as µg/100 g body weight given daily for 3 days. From Chopra et al. (1984), by permission

Thus, the pharmacokinetic data on DIMIT indicate a relatively slow clearance, free diffusion into various tissues, and ready transport across the placenta in at least two species. These properties presumably result from a combination of 1) slower metabolism of DIMIT than T_3 due to the absence of iodide groups, 2) a low affinity of serum binding proteins for DIMIT, and 3) binding of DIMIT by nuclear T_3 receptors. These characteristics support the potential usefulness of DIMIT and similar thyroid hormone analogs for treatment of the fetus through maternal administration.

Maternally administered DIMIT is thyromimetic in fetal lung. Ballard et al. (1980) injected pregnant rabbits with various doses of DIMIT for 1 or 2 days before the fetuses were studied on day 26 or 27 of gestation. Treatment did not affect fetal viability, birthweight or lung weight. In the fetal liver, DIMIT treatment increased the specific activity of NADPH cytochrome-C reductase by 64 % and reduced the glycogen content to 27 % of that in controls; these effects are similar to those described in fetal rats. In fetal lung, administration of DIMIT caused a dose-dependent increase in choline incorporation with a maximum response of 100 % at the highest dose. The activity of lung phosphatidic acid phosphatase (PAPase), a glucocorticoid inducible enzyme, also

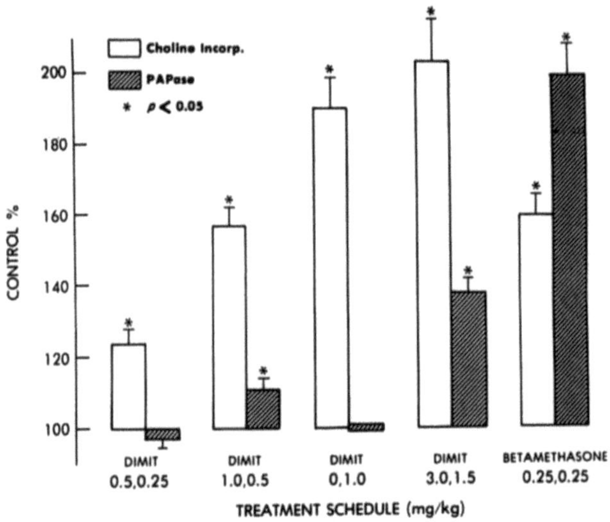

Fig. 7.3. Effect of DIMIT and betamethasone on choline incorporation and PAPase activity in lung of rabbit fetuses. Values are mean ± SE for determinations made on day 26 in lung tissue of fetuses exposed to daily maternal treatment as indicated. Data from Ballard et al. (1980)

increased, but the maximal response was less (38 %) and occurred only after 2 days of treatment with the higher doses of DIMIT (Fig. 7.3). By contrast, betamethasone treatment produced a doubling of PAPase activity in fetal lung homogenates. With two of the treatment regimens, the rate of choline incorporation increased without a detectable change in PAPase activity. It is likely that the stimulation of PAPase is secondary to the increase in endogenous corticoids (both total and free) which occurs with DIMIT treatment. In con-

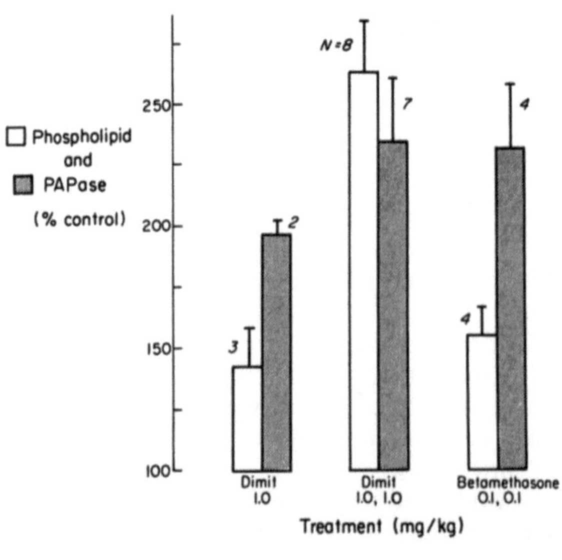

Fig. 7.4. Effect of DIMIT and betamethasone treatment on phospholipid content and PAPase activity in lung lavage of fetal rabbits. Lung lavage was performed in 27-day fetuses following maternal treatment as shown. Values are mean ± SE with the number of litters shown. Data from Ballard et al. (1980)

trast to the effect of betamethasone, stimulation of choline incorporation by DIMIT does not correlate closely with an increase in PAPase activity. These data suggest that glucocorticoids and thyroid hormones have different enzymatic sites of action in PC biosynthesis (discussed further in Chap. 10).

The effect of DIMIT treatment on phospholipid content and PAPase activity of lavage fluid is shown in Fig. 7.4. One dose of DIMIT 24 h before delivery increased phospholipid content by 36 %, and 2 days of treatment produced a 163 % increase over control levels. By comparison, betamethasone for 2 days increased phospholipids by about 50 %. PAPase activity in lavage fluid, presumably associated with lamellar bodies (Spitzer and Johnston 1978), is increased by both DIMIT and betamethasone. As shown in Fig. 7.5, DIMIT treatment was associated with an increased percentage of PC and saturated PC, and a decrease in sphingomyelin, in lavage fluid. Each of these changes with treatment is in the direction of enhanced maturity.

Neufeld and Melmed (1981) used DIMIT in pregnant alloxan-diabetic rabbits. Maternal DIMIT therapy reduced both maternal and fetal glucose levels and fetal insulin concentrations. DIMIT did not affect glucose or insulin levels in non-diabetic control animals and their fetuses. Alloxan diabetes was associated with decreased lung weight, protein/g lung, and total phospholipids/mg DNA. Exposure for 2 days to DIMIT increased each of these values toward control levels. Lungs of diabetic fetuses contained lower concentrations per mg DNA of sphingomyelin, phosphatidylserine, PC and saturated PC. DIMIT treatment increased the amounts of each of these phospholipids; however, the percentage composition of phospholipids was not altered by either diabetes or DIMIT. Similarly, DIMIT treatment did not alter the composition of tissue phospholipids in control, non-diabetic animals. Thus, alloxan diabetes in the rabbit was associated with smaller pulmonary cells con-

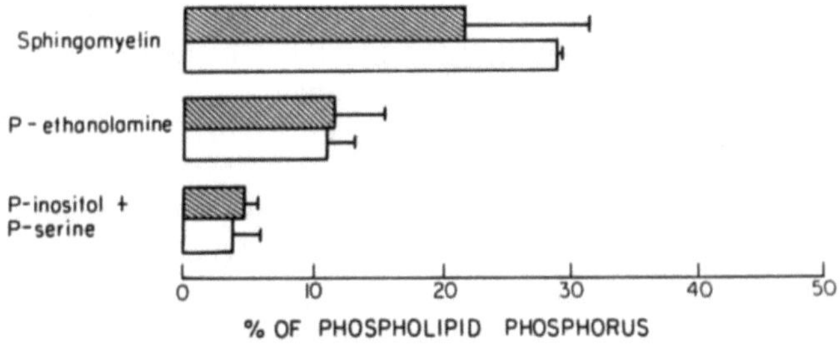

Fig. 7.5. Effect of DIMIT treatment on phospholipid composition of lavage fluid. Phospholipids were separated by two dimensional thin layer chromatography after extraction from lung lavage of control and DIMIT-treated (1 mg/kg, 2 doses) fetal rabbits. Data from Ballard et al. (1980)

taining less protein and phospholipid; DIMIT treatment for 2 days increased both of these parameters to levels similar to those in controls. Presumably this effect of DIMIT results from correction of fetal glucose and insulin concentrations. The relationship of these observations to surfactant production is uncertain, but it is conceivable that smaller type II cells in the diabetic animal contain less surfactant which is available for secretion. Information regarding lavage phospholipids in this experimental model would be of interest.

7.1.3 Postnatal Effects

In adult rat lung, Redding and Douglas (1972) observed effects of both T_4 treatment and thyroidectomy on the type II cell. Thyroidectomy of adult animals for 6 weeks reduced the diameter of type II cells by approximately one-third, and T_4 treatment (1 mg/kg) of intact animals for 6 days increased cell diameter compared with euthyroid controls. The number and size of lamellar bodies were proportionately changed in the two groups of animals. A striking finding of the study was that other cell types in the lung parenchyma were relatively unchanged, whereas T_4 appears to affect several cell types in the fetus. Hypothyroidism decreased, and T_4 treatment increased the quantity of surfactant isolated by lung lavage. Two other groups have found no effect of hypothyroidism in adult rats on lung tissue content of PC and saturated PC (Mason et al. 1972; Ruel et al. 1982a).

Das (1983) found that hypophysectomy of adult rats reduced the concentration of total phospholipids, PC and saturated PC in the lung. Treatment with T_3 (1 mg/kg) increased the phospholipid values to above normal levels within 3 days. Similar treatment of the intact animal increased these lipids by 33–51 %. The specific activities of palmitoyl-CoA synthetase, phospholipase A_2, and lyso PC acyltransferase enzymes were also low in hypophysectomized rats and restored by administration of T_3. The optimal response was observed 3–4 days after treatment and there was evidence that the increase reflected de novo synthesis. These findings suggest that T_3 stimulates production of many classes of phospholipids in lung, including dipalmitoyl PC through the deacylation-reacylation cycle. The possible relationship of these findings to the role of thyroid hormones in surfactant synthesis in fetal lung is only speculative.

The influence of thyroid hormones on the lung has also been studied in the suckling rat. Effects during this postnatal period may relate to the prenatal action of thyroid hormones in other species. Although surfactant synthesis and release increase prenatally in the rat, morphologic differentiation of the lung continues after birth and mature alveoli are not formed until the second week of postnatal life (Kauffman et al. 1974). Ruel et al. (1982a) found that hypothyroid rat pups had less tissue phospholipid per DNA and wet lung weight, without alteration of the PC and sphingomyelin percentages. Administration of T_4 to hypothyroid rats for 3 days increased both total phospholipid content and the percentage of PC. In apparent contrast with these data, Morishige et al. (1982) found that thyroidectomy increased and replacement T_3 therapy decreased the rate of choline incorporation into phospholipid. The T_3 effect was dose-dependent and required 48–72 h for maximal effect (approximately 45 % suppression). Lungs from hypothyroid pups incorporated less ^{3}H-thymidine into DNA than euthyroid controls, and exogenous T_3 markedly stimulated thymidine incorporation. This effect was observed during the period of alveolar type II cell proliferation (6–9 days), indicating a possible effect of endogenous T_3 in this process.

The studies in postnatal lung suggest that thyroid hormones are required for both cell division and growth. Possible effects of thyroid hormone on phospholipid synthesis are not yet defined, and none of the available data relate specifically to surfactant synthesis or content. The overall impression from the existing literature is that thyroid hormones stimulate growth of type II cells, including phospholipid synthesis, and thus indirectly influence surfactant levels.

7.1.4 Fetal Thyroidectomy

Observations on lung growth and maturity have been made in several studies in which thyroidectomy was performed on fetal lambs late in the second trimester and the fetuses assessed 3 to 6 weeks later. Hypothyroidism decreases body weight and lung weight proportionately (Erenberg et al. 1974; Bhakthavathsalan et al. 1981; Erenberg et al. 1979). The protein/DNA ratio in lung tissue is reduced, indicating a reduction in cell size compared with controls. Hypothyroid fetuses survive after birth, suggesting that adequate development of lung structure and surfactant can occur by term without the influence of endogenous fetal thyroid hormones (Hopkins and Thorburn 1972).

In *premature* fetuses, hypothyroidism apparently delays both morphologic maturation and surfactant appearance (Erenberg et al. 1979; Ayromlooi et al. 1983). As shown in Table 7.1, thyroidectomized fetuses delivered at 137–142 days gestation had substantially lower L/S ratios in tracheal fluid compared with euthyroid controls. The delay in L/S ratio and structural development (Ayromlooi et al. 1983) occurred even though thyroidectomized fetuses had normal levels of serum cortisol. Among euthyroid fetuses the L/S ratio correlated closely with serum cortisol concentration, whereas there was

Table 7.1. Effect of thyroidectomy of the fetal lamb on lung and body weights, hormone concentrations, and L/S ratio. Fetuses were thyroidectomized or underwent non-thyroid related surgery (euthyroid) at 95–99 days, and were delivered by cesarean section between 137 and 142 days. Data from Erenberg et al. (1979)

	Euthyroid (n = 5)	Thyroidectomized (n = 5)
Body weight (kg)	4.46	3.0[a]
Lung + heart weight (g)	200.0 ± 14.3	130.0 ± 22.5[a]
(% of body weight)	4.5	4.3
Serum T_4 (μg/dl)	14.2 ± 2.2	1[a]
Serum cortisol (μg/dl)	9.8 ± 2.1	9.8 ± 2.3
Tracheal fluid L/S	4.9 ± 1.4	1.0 ± 0.3[a]

[a] $p < 0.05$

no correlation among thyroidectomized fetuses. In the intact fetus near term there is a close correlation between cortisol levels and both maximal lung volume and tissue content of saturated PC (Kitterman et al. 1981). Thus, the data from thyroidectomy studies are consistent with both a primary and permissive role for thyroid hormones in lung development.

7.1.5 Ontogeny of Endogenous Thyroid Hormones

Serum concentrations of T_3 increase in fetal sheep during the third trimester when terminal lung differentiation is occurring (Fisher et al. 1977). The major increase in T_3 begins approximately one week prior to delivery (Klein et al. 1978; Nwosu et al. 1978). There is an associated decrease in serum concentrations of T_4 and rT_3, consistent with increased conversion of T_4 to T_3 by fetal tissues. This change in thyroid hormone concentration is temporally related to the pre-partum surge in fetal cortisol. Thomas et al. (1978) demonstrated that the increase in T_3 is precociously induced in fetal lambs by infusion of hydrocortisone at doses which produce serum concentrations of cortisol comparable to those at term. These findings are consistent with glucocorticoid induction of outer ring deiodination activity in fetal tissues. Thus, the effects of endogenous cortisol on lung differentiation near term occur in the presence of increasing concentrations of T_3.

There is less information regarding the pattern of endogenous thyroid hormones in other species. In the rat and rabbit, a major increase in T_3 and T_4 occurs after birth. Organically bound iodine is present in both the thyroid gland and extrathyroidal tissues of fetal rabbits and rats as early as 17 (55 % of gestation) and 19 days (90 % of gestation), respectively (Gorbman and Evans 1943; Waterman and Gorbman 1956). Both T_4 and T_3 plasma concentrations are low at birth in the rat (Dussault and Labrie 1975; Wrutniak and Cabello 1983); however, the latter workers report an exponential increase in T_4 during the last 5 days of gestation. Levels in the fetal rabbit also increase during the last week of gestation (U. Devaskar, personal communication). The data regarding occupancy of rabbit lung T_3 receptors by endogenous thyroid hormones, as discussed later in the chapter, provide additional evidence that thyroid hormones are present at biologically important levels before birth.

7.2 Uptake and Metabolism

The tissue/plasma ratio for T_3 and T_4 has been examined in adult and newborn rats (Hitchcock and Reichlin 1978; Hitchcock et al. 1980). Animals were injected with labeled hormones and then thyroid hormones were extracted from both plasma and tissues at various intervals. The lung/plasma ratio of T_3 in newborn rats was about 4, which is similar to the uptake by adult liver, kidney and lung. Tissue/plasma ratios for T_4 were low in all three tissues at every age examined. These findings are consistent with the presence of T_3 receptor in lung cells. The failure of rat lung and other tissues to concentrate T_4 contrasts with the binding of this hormone by isolated nuclei from lung. The lack of T_4 uptake, as compared with T_3 localization, may reflect the high affinity of TBG and the lower affinity of receptor for T_4 vs. T_3. Alternatively, lung cells may actively transport T_3 but not T_4 across the cell membrane.

Additional evidence for in vivo uptake of T_3 is provided by immunohistochemical studies (Wilson et al. 1979). L-2 cells, which originated from adult rat lung, were grown in the presence or absence of thyroid hormone, and reacted with anti-T_3 or anti-T_4 antibody. By immunofluorescence, T_3 was localized in both the cytoplasm and nucleus of cells grown with hormone, but not in those without hormone.

In liver and other tissues, T_4 may undergo deiodination of the outer ring to form T_3 or be deiodinated in the inner ring to form rT_3. These products may be further metabolized to 3,3'-T_2 and T_1. The relative amounts of outer vs. inner ring deiodination influences the level of thyromimetic activity resulting from T_4 uptake by a given tissue. The high concentrations of rT_3 in the fetus are well recognized, and it has been postulated that production of rT_3 instead of T_3 protects fetal tissues from the calorogenic effects of T_4 in utero (reviewed in Chopra 1981).

There is relatively little information on metabolism of thyroid hormones in lung. In a study with adult rats, there was no apparent generation of T_3 from T_4 by lung, whereas deiodination activity was detected in seven other tissues, with particularly high levels in liver and kidney (Chopra 1977). These data were obtained in tissue homogenates in the absence of added sulfhydryl compounds. The monodeiodination reaction is influenced by sulfhydryl compounds (Chopra 1978), and adult lung has relatively low levels of endogenous sulfhydryls (Granberg and Ballard 1977). Thus, it is not clear whether the absence of T_3 generation in adult lung represents low in vivo content of enzyme and/or low concentrations of tissue sulfhydryls which are rapidly oxidized in vitro.

Segall-Blank et al. (1983) investigated T_4 metabolism by fetal rat lung cells in culture. When cells were incubated with T_4 (6 nM), there was some generation of T_3, but the major metabolites of T_4 were rT_3 and its degradation products. The relatively small amount of T_3 which was generated appeared to localize in the nuclear fraction, consistent with binding to receptor.

Thus, the findings in both fetal and adult lung suggest that there is limited conversion of T_4 to T_3. This implies that direct effects of T_4 in lung of rats, at least, are mediated primarily through T_4 itself rather than through conversion to T_3. This interpretation is supported by two observations. First, exposure of cultured lung tissue to ^{125}I-T_4, with subsequent isolation of nuclei and extraction of thyroid hormones, reveals primarily T_4 present (L. Gonzales, personal communication). A second line of evidence is provided by dose-response studies for stimulation of PC synthesis in cultured lung. As discussed later in this chapter, there is a close correlation between the relative affinities of T_3 and T_4 for binding to receptor and their potencies in stimulating PC biosynthesis. If T_4 were acting in lung cells primarily through conversion to T_3, a relatively greater potency for T_4 would be expected.

7.3 Nuclear T_3 Receptor

Although the precise mechanism of thyroid hormone action in target tissues is not established, considerable data support the hypothesis that most effects of thyroid hormones in target tissues of the adult are mediated through interaction with specific receptors located in the cell nucleus. T_3 receptors are monomeric (MW ~50,000), non-histone, acidic proteins which are associated with chromatin. Binding of T_3 to receptor promotes de novo synthesis of specific mRNA's with subsequent de novo protein synthesis (reviewed recently by Baxter et al. 1979; Jump and Oppenheimer 1983; Oppenheimer and Samuels 1983). Recent studies from several laboratories have examined fetal and postnatal lung for the presence of nuclear T_3 receptors. These data, which are summarized in this section, establish that lung contains T_3 receptors and is a potential target tissue for thyroid hormones.

7.3.1 Species Distribution

Beginning with the initial report by Lindenberg et al. (1978), several studies have now established that T_3 receptors are present in rabbit, rat and fetal human lung (Table 7.2). Data have been obtained by dose response experiments with $[^{125}I]T_3$ for binding to isolated nuclei or solubilized nuclear receptor. The concentration of nuclear receptor ranges from about 900 to 2,500 sites/cell. This level is less than found in liver, kidney, and pituitary of adult rat (3900 to 5850 sites/cell) but is comparable to the concentration in other target tissues such as heart and brain (Oppenheimer et al. 1974). In the human fetus, lung contained the highest receptor concentration of four tissues examined (Bernal and Pekonen, 1984). Since the lung contains up to 40 different cell types, it is possible that certain cell types contain a higher concentration than others. Specific T_3 binding has been observed in nuclei of L-2 and A-549 cells

Table 7.2. Nuclear binding of T_3 in mammalian lung and pulmonary cell lines. Data were obtained by dose-response experiments with $[^{125}I]T_3$ and isolated nuclei, whole cells (L-2 and A-549 cells), or solubilized nuclear receptor (newborn rat). Values are the range in the studies referenced

Tissue	Sites/cell	K_D (pM)	References
Adult rat lung	900–1250	105–250	Morishige & Guernsey 1978
			Das & Ganguly 1981
			Ruel et al. 1982b
Newborn rat lung	1870	80	Ruel et al. 1982b
Adult rabbit lung	930–1410	70	Lindenberg et al. 1978
			Gonzales & Ballard 1982
			Das 1980
Fetal rabbit lung (28 days)	1500	110	Gonzales & Ballard 1982
	2580		Das 1980
Fetal human lung (16–19 weeks)	1520	40	Gonzales & Ballard 1981
	1980	60	Bernal & Pekonen 1984
L-2 cells	2280	280	Lindenberg et al. 1978
A-549 cells	1580	200	Lindenberg et al. 1978

(Table 7.2). These cell lines are felt to have originated from type II epithelial cells of adult rat and human lung, respectively. Thus, it is likely but not established that type II cells contain nuclear T_3 receptors.

T_3 binding to lung nuclei demonstrates high affinity in all species studied (Table 7.2). The K_D values of ~0.1 nM are comparable to those reported for other target tissues (Samuels and Tsai 1974). It is perhaps noteworthy that the K_D for binding in human lung (40–60 pM) is somewhat lower than values for both the rat and rabbit.

T_3 binding has also been described in nuclei and nuclear extracts of chick lung (Bellabarba et al. 1983). There is a marked decrease in binding capacity from day 12 in the embryo (2380 fmol/mg DNA) to 10 days post-hatching (190 fmol/mg DNA). The K_D (1.3 nM) did not change during development, and is considerably higher than observed in mammalian lung (Table 7.2).

7.3.2 Dose Response of Binding

An example of a dose response experiment with $[^{125}I]T_3$ and nuclei from fetal rabbit lung is shown in Fig. 7.6. Non-specific binding, as determined in the presence of excess non-labelled T_3, accounted for 5–31 % of $[^{125}I]T_3$ bound over the concentration range of 0.01–1.2 nM. Somewhat higher levels of background binding were observed in nuclei from *adult* lung (12–58 %) (Gonzales and Ballard 1982). Scatchard analyses of binding data from incubations of fetal nuclei at both 2 °C and 37 °C are linear, indicating the presence of a single class of high affinity binding sites. At the optimal incubation temperature for nuclei of adult lung (25 °C), the K_D determined by Scatchard analysis is similar to that for fetal lung.

The specificity of T_3 binding sites has been evaluated by competition studies with various thyroid hormone analogs. Figure 7.7 illustrates the displace-

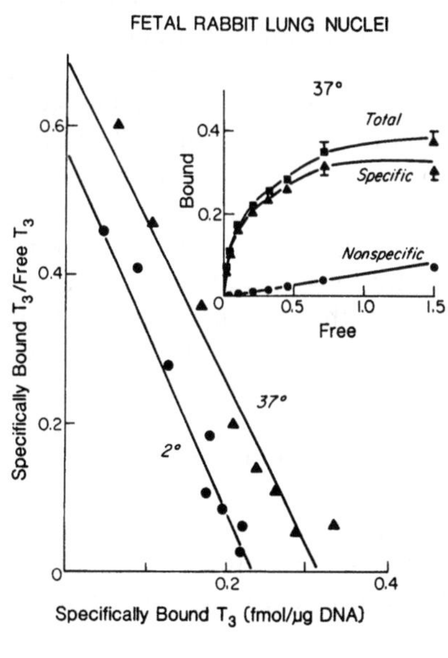

Fig. 7.6. Representative Scatchard plots for dose response studies of $[^{125}I]T_3$ binding to lung nuclei of fetal rabbit lung. Incubations were carried out for 90 min at 37 °C or for 4 h at 2 °C. The *inset* shows binding data plotted as a function of free T_3 concentration. The binding parameters in this experiment were K_D = 87 pM and capacity 0.322 fmol/µg DNA at 37 °C and K_D = 77 pM and capacity 0.235 fmol/µg DNA at 2 °C. Release of receptor was 7.1 % and 1.6 % at 37 and 2 °C, respectively. From Gonzales and Ballard (1982), by permission

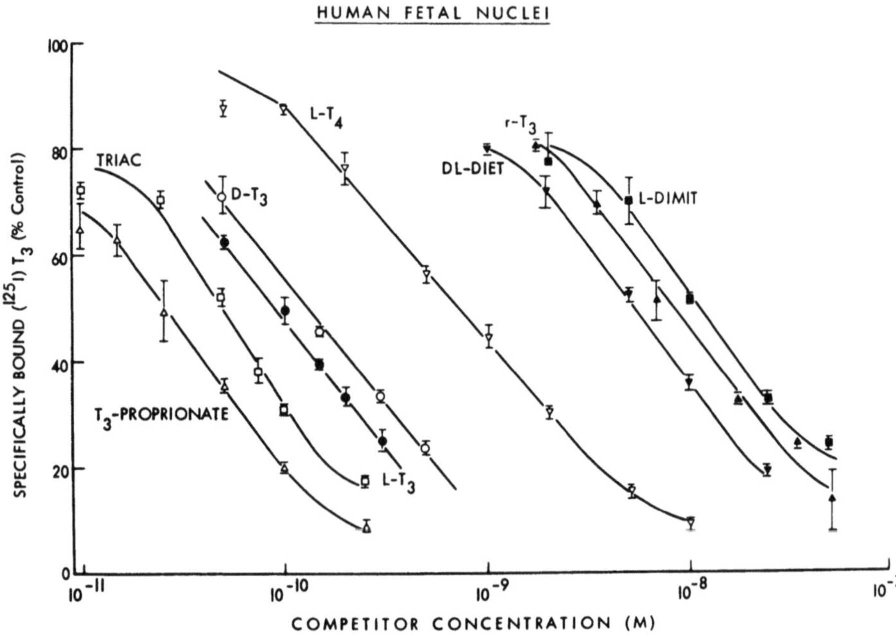

Fig. 7.7. Competition by various thyroid hormones for $[^{125}I]T_3$ binding in lung nuclei from human fetuses (17–19 wk). The assay systems contained nuclei (55–80 µg DNA), 45–112 pM $[^{125}I]T_3$, and various concentrations of unlabeled thyroid hormone. Abbreviations are shown in the legend of Table 7.3. From Gonzales and Ballard (1981), by permission

ment of $[^{125}I]T_3$ from binding sites of human lung nuclei by various concentrations of eight non-labelled thyroid hormone analogs. The dose response plots are parallel for all analogs and indicate that complete displacement occurs at high concentration in each case. The relative affinities of these and other analogs for binding to nuclear sites in lung of three species are presented in Table 7.3. Similar results have been obtained in all studies. Compared with L-T_3, T_3-proprionate and TRIAC have higher affinities. D-T_3 has 54–74 % the affinity of the L-isomer. The affinity of L-T_4 is 7–19 % of that for L-T_3, with somewhat higher values observed for fetal and newborn lung compared with adult tissue. It is of interest that both rT_3 and its metabolite, 3,3′-L-T_2, have 1 % or less the activity of L-T_3 for binding. rT_3 is present in relatively high concentrations in human cord blood compared to adult plasma, raising the possibility that this compound might be physiologically important during fetal life (Burman et al. 1976). This proposal is not supported by the finding of a low binding affinity in fetal lung similar to values obtained for adult rat liver (Papavasiliou et al. 1977; Koerner et al. 1975; Jorgensen et al. 1976) and cultured rat pituitary cells (Papavasiliou et al. 1977). The synthetic thyroid hormone analogs also have a relatively low affinity, with DIET being approximately 2–3 times more potent than DIMIT in each of three tissues. This difference in affinity may actually be underestimated, since L-DIMIT is compared with the mixed D,L-isomer of DIET. DIET is also more potent biologi-

Table 7.3. Relative affinities of thyroid hormone analogs for nuclear binding sites in lung. The data are from Gonzales and Ballard (1981) (human), Lindenberg et al. (1978) (fetal rabbit), Gonzales and Ballard (1982) (fetal and adult rabbit), Ruel et al. (1982b) (newborn rat); and Morishige and Guernsey (1978) (adult rat)

Compound	Relative affinity				
	Fetal human	Fetal rabbit	Adult rabbit	NB rat	Adult rat
L-T_3	100	100	100	100	100
T_3-proprionate	309	228	312		192
Triac	171	120	206	155	158
T_2-isopropyl		81			
D-T_3	62	74	56	68	54
Tetrac					10
L-T_4	15	11	8	19	7
D-T_4				9	4
3,5-L-T_2				0.7	0.1
3,3'-L-T_2		0.2			
rT_3	1.1	1.1	0.7	0.7	
L-DIMIT	0.7	0.7	0.8	2	
D,L-DIET	2.0	1.7	1.7		
Thyronine					< 0.01

L-T_3: 3,5,3'-triiodo-L-thyronine
T_3-proprionate: 3,5,3'-triiodothyroproprionic acid
Triac: 3,5,3'-triiodothyroacetic acid
T_2-isopropyl: 3,5,diiodo-3'-isopropyl-L-thyronine
D-T_3 : 3,5,3'-triiodo-D-thyronine
Tetrac: 3,5,3',5'-tetraiodothyroacetic acid
L-T_4: 3,5,3',5'-tetraiodo-L-thyronine
D-T_4: 3,5,3',5'-tetraiodo-D-thyronine
3,5-L-T_2: 3,5-diiodo-L-thyronine
3,3'-L-T_2: 3,3'-diiodo-L-thyronine
rT_3: 3,3',5'-triiodo-L-thyronine
L-DIMIT: 3,5-dimethyl-3'-isopropyl-L-thryonine
D,L-DIET: 3,5-diethyl-3'-isopropyl-D,L-thyronine

cally compared with DIMIT, as judged by choline incorporation into PC and glycogen depletion in fetal lung (Gonzales and Ballard 1981). The relative affinities of these analogs for binding sites in lung nuclei are comparable to results in other target tissues and in general reflect biologic potency (Oppenheimer et al. 1973; Papavasiliou et al. 1977; Koerner et al. 1975; Jorgensen et al. 1976). The data for fetal vs. adult rabbit and newborn vs. adult rat lung are in close agreement, consistent with the presence of identical binding sites in fetal and adult animals.

7.3.3 Kinetics of Binding

The time course of $[^{125}I]T_3$ binding to lung nuclei from fetal rabbits is shown in Fig. 7.8. Binding is temperature dependent, with equilibrium reached more quickly at 37 °C and 25 °C than at 2 °C. Non-specific binding is not temperature dependent. Similar kinetics of T_3 association with receptor occur in nuclei of rat lung (Das and Ganguly 1981). With nuclei from adult rabbit (Gon-

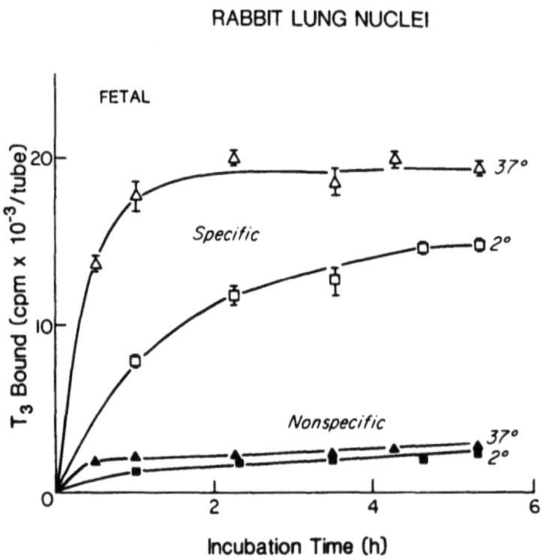

Fig. 7.8. Time course for $[^{125}I]T_3$ binding to lung nuclei from 28-day fetuses. Both specific and non-specific (in the presence of excess non-labeled T_3) binding are shown for two temperatures. From Gonzales and Ballard (1982), by permission

zales and Ballard 1982), and also from human lung (Gonzales and Ballard 1981), the time course of specific binding at 37 °C is biphasic, decreasing after about 60 min; this non-equilibrium situation is due to receptor instability.

The dissociation rate of $[^{125}I]T_3$-receptor complex is also temperature dependent as illustrated in Fig. 7.9. With nuclei isolated from fetal rabbit lung, the $t_{1/2}$ for dissociation at 37 °C, 30 °C, and 2 °C was 31 min, 2.5 h, and 24 h, respectively. The rate at 37 °C was the same whether dissociation was studied in the presence of excess non-labelled T_3 or after dilution, suggesting the ab-

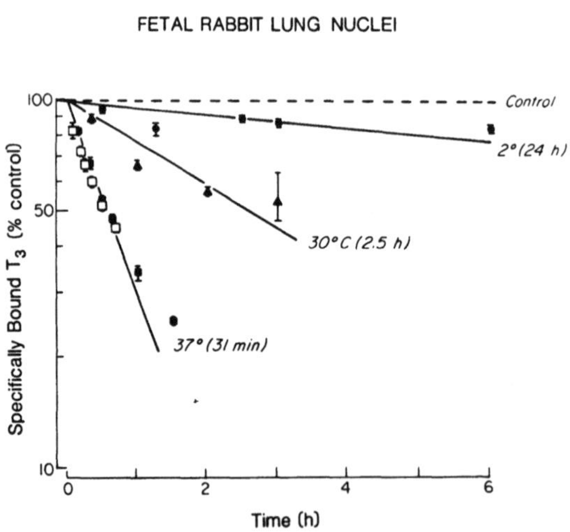

Fig. 7.9. Dissociation rate of T_3-receptor complex at various temperatures. Lung nuclei of 28-day fetal rabbits were incubated at 37 °C with 0.3 nM $[^{125}I]T_3$ and then either diluent (control) or excess unlabeled T_3 was added with incubation continued at the temperatures indicated. Alternatively, after equilibrium binding nuclei were washed and resuspended in fresh buffer to determine dissociation by dilution *(open squares)*. The half-times for dissociation are given in *parentheses*. From Gonzales and Ballard (1982), by permission

sence of cooperativity in the binding reaction. The slow dissociation at 2 °C indicates that only a small fraction of endogenously bound hormone dissociates from receptor during usual incubation periods (4h) at 2 °C, whereas nearly complete dissociation occurs in reactions carried out for 90 min at 37 °C. As discussed below, this temperature difference provides a means to assess receptor occupancy with endogenous thyroid hormone.

7.3.4 Release and Inactivation of Receptor

During incubation of isolated nuclei, receptor may be released into the incubation medium. In studies with liver nuclei, Bernal and DeGroot (1977) found substantial leakage of T_3 receptor. Release also occurs with lung nuclei, but at considerably lower levels. Receptor release is dependent on temperature and time, but independent of gestational age and the concentration of ligand. Under optimal binding conditions, release of receptor-T_3 complex from fetal and adult rabbit nuclei was 9.8 ± 0.4 and 10.3 ± 0.9 %, respectively. Unlike the situation in liver, the presence of 1 mM Ca^{+2} in the incubation medium did not prevent release of receptor from rabbit lung nuclei (Gonzales and Ballard 1982).

Inactivation of receptor also occurs during in vitro incubation of nuclei. Experimentally, this instability is a problem at elevated temperatures with nuclei of adult rabbit and fetal human lung, but not for fetal rabbit lung (Gonzales and Ballard 1981; Gonzales and Ballard 1982). The temperature-dependent decrease in binding with adult rabbit and human lung is primarily the result of inactivation or degradation of receptor sites rather than release into the incubation medium. With isolated nuclei from both species, receptor is stabilized by the presence of T_3. This effect is dependent on the concentration of T_3, with maximal protection provided by 1 nM T_3. The relevance of this finding to the situation in vivo is uncertain, but it represents a possible mechanism for regulation of receptor concentration.

7.3.5 Ontogeny

The developmental pattern of T_3 binding capacity in nuclei of rabbit lung is shown in Fig. 7.10. There is a 44 % increase between days 21 and 28 of gestation, with a subsequent decline in capacity by term. Capacity increases during the first three weeks of postnatal life, and is lower in the mature animal. A similar profile for binding capacity in lung was obtained by Das (1980). By contrast, T_3 binding capacity in liver shows only a slight gradual increase during development. In the rat, binding capacity decreases postnatally by about 60 % (Ruel et al. 1982b). Limited data with nuclei from human fetal lung indicate an increase in T_3 receptor concentration in the second trimester. Binding capacity was 0.227 and 0.282 fmol/µg DNA in two lungs of 12–13 weeks vs. a mean value of 0.42 ± 0.014 fmol/µg DNA in eight specimes of 16–19 weeks gestation (Gonzales and Ballard 1981).

The developmental data on binding capacity may indicate a change in number of receptors/cell. However, this interpretation is complicated by the heterogeneity of pulmonary cell types, possible developmental changes in the

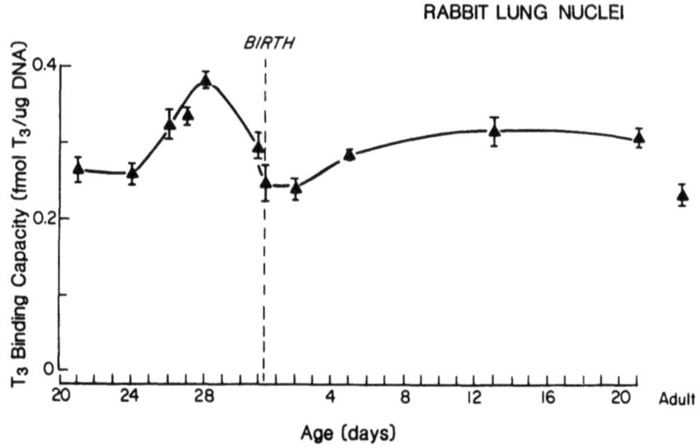

Fig. 7.10. T_3 binding capacity in rabbit lung during development. Dose response experiments were performed with isolated nuclei and the values are mean ± SE for 3–8 samples. From Gonzales and Ballard (1982), by permission

proportion of different cell types, and lack of information regarding distribution of T_3 receptors in pulmonary cells. It is unlikely that the increase in receptor concentration reflects a general increase in most nuclear proteins, or a decreasing average concentration of DNA/cell in late gestation (i. e., fewer cells in mitosis), since the protein/DNA ratio of nuclei does not change with age (Gonzales and Ballard 1982). It is also unlikely that the developmental changes in receptor concentration are an artifact of the in vitro assay. The binding reaction has been characterized for both fetal and adult tissue, and data were obtained under optimal conditions. Binding in fetal and adult nuclei are similar with regard to thyroid hormone binding specificity and affinity, reversibility and rates of dissociation, temperature dependence of dissociation, and receptor release under optimal reaction conditions. Furthermore, the recovery of tissue DNA in the isolated nuclei and the purity of the nuclei are similar at both ages (Gonzales and Ballard 1982). Although the physiologic relevance of the changes in receptor concentration are uncertain, the increase in fetal rabbit lung correlates temporally with both alveolarization and the increase in surfactant synthesis.

7.3.6 Hormonal Regulation

The possible factors influencing T_3 receptor concentration in fetal lung are unknown. It is of interest, however, that the prenatal increase in binding capacity occurs in parallel with increasing occupancy of lung receptor (Sect. 7.3.7). The relationship between thyroid hormones and receptor capacity has been examined in several studies (Table 7.4). Das and Ganguly (1981) found that T_3 binding capacity in adult lung is reduced in conditions which lower serum T_3 and T_4, with a close correlation between serum thyroid hormone concentration and binding capacity. These conditions did not influence purity and recovery of nuclei, receptor release, or either the kinetics or K_D of the binding

Table 7.4. Studies of thyroid hormone status on T_3 binding capacity in rat lung

Investigator	Age of animal	Method for hypothyroidism	Thyroid hormone		T_3 binding capacity	
			Method of treatment	Serum concentration (ng/dl)	System	Capacity (fmol/mg DNA)
Das & Ganguly 1981	Adult	None (control)	None	T_3 : 120	Isolated nuclei	321
		Streptozotocin diabetes	None	79[a]		224
		Hypophysectomy	None	60[a]		195
		Thyroidectomy	None	30[a]		102[a]
Ruel et al. 1982b	Adult	None (control)	None	T_4 : NR	Nuclear extract	296
		Propylthiouracil	None	ND		318
		None	40 µg T_4/100 g BW for 6 days	>13,000		430[a]
	Suckling (5 days)	None (control)	None	T_4 : NR	Nuclear extract	521
		Propylthiouracil	None	ND		554
		None	40 µg T_4/100 g BW for 5 days	>13,000		496
Bellabarba et al. 1984	Suckling (16–24 days)	None (control)	None	T_3 : NR	Isolated nuclei	303
		Radiotherapy	None	ND		606[a]
		Radiotherapy	5 µg T_3/100 g BW from day 8	"normal"		507[a]
Morishige et al. 1982	Suckling (9 days)	Propylthiouracil	None	100%	Isolated nuclei	100%
		Propylthiouracil	1 µg T_3 (one dose)	300%[a]		40%[a]

NR, not reported; ND, not detected

[a] $p < 0.05$ vs. control

[b] Note that the data of Morishige et al. are normalized

reaction. The effect of replacement T_3 therapy on receptor capacity, however, was not reported. Contrasting results have been obtained in the other studies. Ruel et al. (1982b) found that hyperthyroidism produced a 45 % increase in T_3 binding capacity of lung nuclear extract with no change in K_D. However, hypothyroidism induced with propylthiouracil treatment for six weeks did not alter T_3 binding capacity. In neonatal rats, neither hypo- nor hyperthyroidism influenced receptor capacity. According to Bellabarba et al. (1984), hypothyroidism was associated with increased T_3 binding capacity of nuclei; however, these levels were not affected by replacement T_3 treatment. Hypothyroidism also increased binding capacity in nuclei of liver and brain, but there was no change when binding was assayed in nuclear extracts. In a study by Morishige et al. (1982), however, T_3 treatment (1 μg) of hypothyroid pups reduced T_3 binding by lung nuclei.

In view of these conflicting results, the possible effect of T_3 on receptor concentration in lung remains uncertain. It is possible that differences in assay methodology or doses of thyroid hormone accounts for some of the different findings. Since there was no apparent influence of thyroid hormone levels on the K_D in each case, possible artifacts due to receptor occupancy are unlikely to have influenced the values for binding capacity. There is a similar lack of agreement for other tissues which have been examined; with elevated levels of thyroid hormone the binding capacity for T_3 was unchanged (Bernal et al. 1978), or increased (Hamada et al. 1979) in liver, and decreased in cultured pituitary cells (Samuels et al. 1977).

7.3.7 Occupancy by Endogenous Thyroid Hormones

The temperature dependence of T_3 dissociation from receptor has been used to assess occupancy of receptor by endogenous hormone. With this method, binding of $[^{125}I]T_3$ to isolated nuclei is determined at both 2 °C and 37 °C. At the lower temperature, binding approaches a plateau value by 5 h as free sites are occupied; during this period there is little dissociation of endogenous T_3 from receptor. At 37 °C, the level of binding at equilibrium reflects total binding capacity (free plus occupied sites). The difference in binding level at the two temperatures provides an estimate of occupancy.

Several observations support the validity of this assay. First, pre-incubation of nuclei at 37 °C increases $[^{125}I]T_3$ binding during subsequent incubation at 2 °C, consistent with dissociation of endogenous T_3 during pre-incubation. Second, when nuclei are shifted from 2 °C to 37 °C, there is a time-dependent increase in $[^{125}I]T_3$ binding. Third, when nuclei are exposed to increasing concentrations of non-labelled T_3, there is a progressive decline in subsequent $[^{125}I]T_3$ binding at 2 °C but not 37 °C. Fourth, occupancy of lung receptors as assessed by the 37°–2 °C difference assay increases following in vivo injection of newborn rabbits with T_3. Finally, occupancy as determined by this method has been compared with direct binding of $[^{125}I]T_3$ to isolated nuclei. As shown in Fig. 7.11, there is a close correlation between the two methods for occupancy up to approximately 60 % (Gonzales and Ballard 1982).

Using this method, occupancy was assessed in nuclei from fetal rabbit lungs

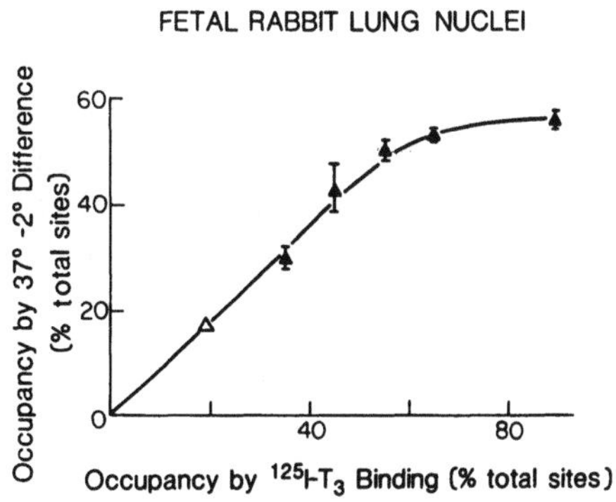

Fig. 7.11. Correlation of receptor occupancy as estimated directly ($[^{125}I]T_3$ binding) and by the temperature difference assay. Lung nuclei of 28-day rabbit fetuses were incubated at 2 °C for 4 h with various concentrations of unlabeled T_3 (0–0.4 nM) and then specific binding was determined by the two approaches. The *open triangle* is the occupancy determined in nuclei not exposed to added unlabeled T_3. From Gonzales and Ballard (1982), by permission

during the last 10 days of gestation. Occupancy increased from 11.3 % of total sites at 21 days to about 23 % at day 28–31 (Table 7.5). Using the data for receptor capacity (Fig. 7.10), the number of occupied receptor sites/cell was calculated to increase from 110 at 21 days to a maximum of 330 at 28 days. These values reflect average concentrations for all lung cells, and assume that there is no change in distribution of receptor among different cell types with advancing gestational age.

In the rat, occupancy of lung receptors was found to be 26 % in the newborn animal, and 48 % in the adult. During the second and third postnatal weeks, occupancy increased from 25 to 60 % during the same time that serum T_3 and T_4 concentrations increased (Ruel et al. 1982b). The estimate of occupancy in adult lung is similar to values previously reported for other tissues of the rat (35–50 %) (Coulombe et al. 1979; Oppenheimer et al. 1974; Bernal et al. 1978; Silva et al 1977).

Estimates of occupancy by the temperature difference method also have been made for human fetal lung. In lungs at 16–19 weeks gestation, a maximum of 30 % occupancy by endogenous thyroid hormone was found (Gonzales and Ballard 1981). The relative amount of endogenous T_3 vs. T_4 in lung nuclei of human and other species is not yet known. These observations in both fetal and adult lung suggest that occupancy of nuclear receptors correlates closely with serum concentrations of thyroid hormones. A linear rela-

Table 7.5. Occupancy of nuclear receptors in fetal rabbit lung by endogenous thyroid hormones. Occupancy was determined by incubation of isolated nuclei with $[^{125}I]T_3$ at 37 °C and 2 °C, and occupied sites/cell were calculated from data for receptor capacity (Fig. 7. 10). Data from Gonzales and Ballard (1982).

Gestational age (days)	n	Occupancy (% of total sites)	Occupied sites/cell
21	3	11.3 ± 4.7	110
25–26	8	14.5 ± 4.2	165
28	42	23.8 ± 1.4	330
31	10	23.0 ± 2.8	227

tionship between occupancy of receptor with T_3 and response has been demonstrated in hepatocytes (Mariash and Oppenheimer 1983) and pituitary cells (Samuels et al. 1976). The same relationship has recently been established for PC synthesis in cultured fetal lung (Sect. 7.4). Thus, it is reasonable to speculate that endogenous thyroid hormones exert increasing influence within the lung during both prenatal and postnatal life. This implies that endogenous thyroid hormones share with glucocorticoids, and possibly other hormones, the role of stimulating lung maturation prior to term.

7.4 Effects in Culture

In several investigations using cultured tissue, it has been established that the lung is a direct target tissue for thyroid hormones in vitro and also, therefore, in vivo. Organ culture of fetal lung has been particularly useful for studies of the mechanism of T_3 effects on PC synthesis.

7.4.1 Biochemical Responses

T_3 and/or T_4 has been shown to stimulate the rate of PC synthesis in organ cultures of fetal lung from the rat (Gross et al. 1980; Gross and Wilson 1982), rabbit (Ballard et al. 1984) and human (Gonzales and Ballard 1984). In addition, Longmuir et al. (1982) found that T_4 enhanced the rate of glycerol incorporation into phosphatidylglycerol by cultured rabbit lung. In an earlier study, T_4 at a high concentration (1 μM) increased choline incorporation by mixed monolayer cultures of rabbit lung (Smith and Torday 1974).

Table 7.6 compares the stimulation by T_3 and dexamethasone of precursor incorporation into PC of cultured rabbit lung. T_3 increases incorporation of choline, glucose and acetate by 25–50 % but only a small effect is observed with glycerol. Dexamethasone stimulates incorporation of choline, glycerol and acetate by 29–62 %, but has a minimal effect on glucose incorporation. T_3 stimulates choline incorporation in organ cultures of rat lung by 37 % after 2 days vs. 100 % increase with dexamethasone (Gross and Wilson 1982). In the case of choline, at least, the rate of incorporation into PC correlates

Table 7.6. Comparison of T_3 and dexamethasone effects on precursor incorporation into PC of rabbit lung. Explants of 23-day rabbit lung were cultured 3 days without hormones (control) or with T_3 (2 nM) or dexamethasone (10 nM), and then exposed to [^{3}H]precursor for 4 h. Data from Ballard et al. (1984)

Precursor	Control (nmol/4 h/mg DNA) mean ± SE	T_3 (% stimulation)	Dexamethasone (% stimulation)
Choline	13.17 ± 0.89	50.0 ± 5.8	62.1 ± 6.5
Glucose	6.14 ± 0.70	25.5 ± 9.7	8.3 ± 6.1
Glycerol	11.88 ± 1.06	8.1 ± 5.5	28.9 ± 4.4
Acetate	34.60 ± 4.64	28.9 ± 6.5	33.4 ± 10.9

closely with PC content (Ballard et al. 1984). In these studies employing organ culture, the tissue is washed and maintained in serum-free medium, indicating that thyroid hormone acts in the absence of added glucocorticoids or other hormones. By contrast, T_3 stimulates choline incorporation by mixed monolayer cultures of fetal rat lung only in the presence of cortisol (Smith and Sabry 1983).

T_4, like dexamethasone, stimulates the incorporation of choline into each of the choline-containing phospholipids of rat lung. Whereas dexamethasone causes a differential enhancement of label into saturated PC vs. unsaturated PC, an increase was not observed with T_4 or T_3 (Gross et al. 1980; Gross and Wilson 1982). In cultured *rabbit* lung, neither glucocorticoid nor thyroid hormone preferentially influences saturated vs. unsaturated PC (Gross et al. 1983; Ballard et al. 1984).

The distribution of radioactivity from [^{3}H]acetate among phospholipid fractions has been determined in both rat and rabbit lungs (Table 7.7). Whereas dexamethasone increases the percentage of radioactivity incorporated into PC in both species, thyroid hormone has no effect. T_3 does not alter the distribution of counts for any phospholipid in rabbit cultures, but changes were noted for several phospholipids with T_4 treatment in rat lung. The decrease for phosphatidylglycerol with T_4 was not seen in subsequent experiments using T_3 (Gross and Wilson 1982). Thus, in both species, thyroid hormones stimulate synthesis of all choline-containing phospholipids without a preferential effect on surfactant-associated phospholipids with regard to either choline or acetate incorporation.

T_4 decreases the glycogen content of cultured rat lung by about 40 %, which

Table 7.7. Comparison of thyroid hormone and glucocorticoid effects on distribution of radioactivity from [^{3}H]acetate into selected phospholipids. Explants of 18-day rat lung were cultured for 48 h and exposed to tracer amounts of [^{3}H]acetate (Gross et al. 1980). Rabbit lung was cultured 72 h and incubated with 1 mM [^{3}H]acetate (Ballard et al. 1984). Hormone concentrations were: T_3, 2 nM (rabbit); T_4, 10 μM (rat); and dexamethasone, 10 nM

Phospholipid	Distribution of radioactivity		
	Control	T_3/T_4 (% of total cpm)	Dexamethasone
Phosphatidylcholine			
rabbit	74.1 ± 0.05	75.5 ± 0.5	77.2 ± 0.5[a]
rat	74.1 ± 2.6	75.5 ± 2.9	78.4 ± 2.1[a]
Sphingomyelin			
rabbit	3.3 ± 0.07	3.4 ± 0.04	2.7 ± 0.0[a]
rat	3.2 ± 0.2	3.8 ± 0.3[a]	3.0 ± 0.3
Phosphatidylglycerol			
rabbit	2.0 ± 0.2	2.1 ± 0.02	1.5 ± 0.06
rat	4.2 ± 0.4	2.4 ± 0.2[a]	5.5 ± 0.5[a]
Phosphatidylethanolamine			
rabbit	9.0 ± 0.3	8.5 ± 0.2	8.3 ± 0.0
rat	12.8 ± 0.3	11.0 ± 0.7[a]	8.0 ± 0.5[a]

[a] $p < 0.05$ vs. control

is similar to the influence of dexamethasone. Exposure to T_4 did not affect the specific activity of various enzymes involved in phospholipid synthesis. These include phosphatidic acid phosphatase, choline phosphotransferase, choline kinase, 1-acylglycerolphosphate, acyltransferase, and lysolecithin acyltransferase. In addition, there was no effect of T_4 on activity of cholinephosphate cytidylyltransferase when assays were carried out in the presence of phospholipid cofactor (Gross et al. 1980). However, when this enzyme was assayed in the absence of added cofactor, T_3 treatment of cultures enhanced activity by 57 %, which is similar to the increase observed in vivo. Similar results also occur with corticosteroid exposure (Gross et al. 1984). These observations suggest that T_3 increases the activity of cholinephosphate cytidylyltransferase by increasing the amount of endogenous cofactor, rather than increasing the amount of enzyme protein.

7.4.2 Evidence for Receptor Mediation

The properties of thyroid hormone influence on choline incorporation have been examined for rabbit lung (Ballard et al. 1984). In these experiments, fetal lung was maintained in organ culture in serum-free medium and choline incorporation into PC and saturated PC was assayed after 24–72 h. The optimal response to T_3 (50 % increase compared with controls) occurred with 23-day lung. Stimulation with T_3 (and with dexamethasone) was greater for cultures maintained in oxygen vs. room air.

A representative time course of response to T_3 and dexamethasone is shown in Fig. 7.12. Fetal lung was cultured for 68 h and exposed to hormones for the last, 14, 28, and 46, or the entire 68 h. There is a lag period in the response (8–12 h) and stimulation by T_3 continues over the entire period, similar to the effect of dexamethasone.

The effect of removing T_3 during incubation is illustrated by the data in Table 7.8. Cultures were exposed to a low concentration of T_3 (0.2 nM) for 24 or 48 h, and then T_3 was washed out of some of the cultures. The results illus-

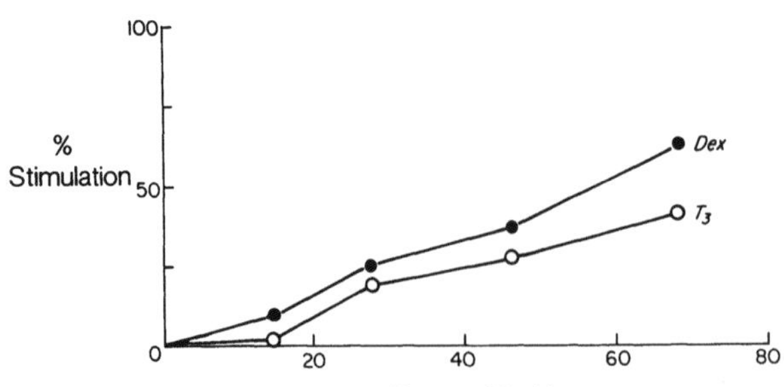

Fig. 7.12. Time course for stimulation of choline incorporation in cultured fetal rabbit lung by T_3 and dexamethasone. Lungs from 23-day rabbit fetuses were cultured for 68 h with T_3 (1 nM) or dexamethasone (10 nM) added for the last 14, 28, 46 or entire 68 h of culture. Values are mean ± SE for percent stimulation compared with control cultures. From Ballard et al. (1984)

Table 7.8. Effect of removing T_3 during culture. Lung from 23-day rabbit fetus was cultured with T_3 (0.2 nM) as shown. After 24 and 48 h, some cultures were switched to T_3-free medium (wash out). All media contained 10 nM dexamethasone. Data from Ballard et al. (1984).

Hormone exposure	Choline incorporation into PC	
	nmol/4 h/mg DNA mean ± SE	% stimulation
48 h incubation		
Control	10.5 ± 0.28	–
+ T_3 (48 h)	13.86 ± 0.54[a]	32
72 h incubation		
Control	21.75 ± 0.39	–
+ T_3 (72 h)	32.22 ± 0.63[a]	48.1
+ T_3 first 24 h only	22.85 ± 1.67[b]	5.1
+ T_3 first 48 h only	26.12 ± 1.72[b]	20.1

[a] $p < 0.05$ vs. control
[b] $p < 0.05$ vs. T_3 for 72 h

trate that the continued presence of T_3 is required for optimal stimulation, and that the hormonal effect is partially reversible within 24 h.

A dose-response experiment with T_3 is shown in Fig. 7.13. Stimulation occurs at concentrations as low as 0.01 nM T_3, and choline incorporation is half-maximally increased at a concentration of 0.12 ± 0.02 nM. For comparison, the K_D for T_3 binding to receptor in nuclei isolated from fetal rabbit lung is 0.11 ± 0.04 nM (Gonzales and Ballard 1982). There is a similar correlation be-

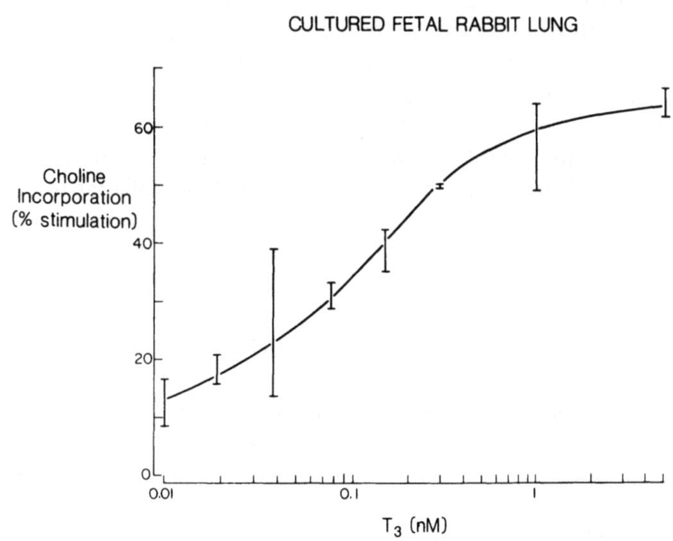

Fig. 7.13. Effect of T_3 dose on stimulation of choline incorporation by cultured lung of 23-day fetal rabbit. The range of duplicate determinations in a representative experiment are shown. Half-maximal stimulation occurs at about 0.09 nM. From Ballard et al. (1984), by permission

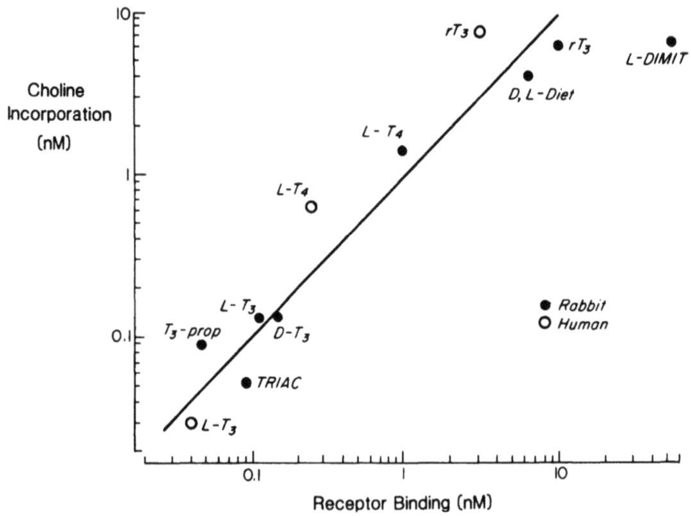

Fig. 7.14. Comparison of potency and binding affinity for various thyroid hormones. Dose-response experiments for stimulation of incorporation were performed for each hormone (Ballard et al. 1984; Gonzales and Ballard 1984) and mean values are plotted vs. the K_D for binding to receptor by isolated nuclei (Gonzales and Ballard 1981; Gonzales and Ballard 1982). The *solid symbols* are data for 23-day fetal rabbit lung in culture and the *open symbols* are results with human fetal lung in organ culture

tween T_3 affinity and potency in human fetal lung (Gonzales and Ballard 1984).

The effect of various thyroid hormone analogs was also studied. At optimal concentrations, each analog stimulated choline incorporation to a similar extent in both the absence and presence of dexamethasone. The data shown in Fig. 7.14 summarize dose-response experiments. Both T_3-proprionic acid and TRIAC are more potent than L-T_3, and these analogs have lower K_D values than T_3 for receptor binding. L- and D-T_3 are similar in both potency and receptor affinity. The potency of L-T_4 is 8.8 % of that for L-T_3. rT_3 and the synthetic analogs demonstrate potencies between 1 and 2 % of that for T_3. The values for the analogs are grouped around the line of identity, indicating a close correlation between potency and binding affinity.

To examine the requirement for RNA and protein synthesis, studies have been carried out with actinomycin D and cycloheximide, respectively. Representative data are shown in Table 7.9. Both inhibitors decrease the response to T_3 in a dose-dependent fashion. The response to T_3 was abolished by 0.2 μg/ml actinomycin D, while stimulation by dexamethasone was decreased but not eliminated. When cultures were first exposed to T_3 for 48 h, and then actinomycin D added for the last 24 h of culture, the same dose of actinomycin D was less effective. Cycloheximide at 0.04 μg/ml was similarly effective in blocking the response to T_3, whether present during the entire time of hormone exposure or when added only during the last 24 h of culture. The effect of dexamethasone was also less sensitive to this inhibitor (Ballard et al. 1984).

Table 7.9. Inhibition of T_3 stimulation of PC synthesis by cycloheximide and actinomycin D. Data from representative experiments of Ballard et al. (1984) with fetal rabbit lung are shown. Cycloheximide (0.04 μg/ml) was present for the last 24 h of a 72-h culture period. Actinomycin D (0.2 μg/ml) was added along with hormone during 48 h of culture.

Addition	Choline incorporation (nmol/4 h/mg DNA)	
	Control	Plus inhibitor
Experiment 1: Cycloheximide		
None	9.84	8.46
T_3	13.45	8.78
Dexamethasone	17.09	11.19
Experiment 2: Actinomycin D		
None	10.57	7.13
T_3	12.48	7.16
Dexamethasone	13.25	9.19

These findings lend strong support to the proposal that T_3 stimulation of PC synthesis is mediated through receptor involving de novo RNA and protein synthesis. The response to T_3 has a lag phase, consistent with new synthesis of macromolecules. Half-maximal stimulation of choline incorporation occurs at the same concentration of T_3 which produces half-maximal saturation of nuclear receptors. This finding indicates that there is a linear relationship between occupancy of receptor and response, similar to T_3 effects on enzyme induction in cultured hepatocytes (Mariash and Oppenheimer 1983) and growth hormone synthesis in GH_1 cells (Samuels et al. 1976). Furthermore, the potency of seven other thyroid hormones for stimulation of PC synthesis in cultured lung correlates closely with their affinity for receptor. Continued stimulation of choline incorporation depends on continued presence of the hormone in the culture medium, consistent with the reversibility of receptor binding. The effects with inhibitors suggest that there is sequential stimulation of RNA and protein synthesis on addition of T_3.

7.5 Human Studies

The involvement of endogenous thyroid hormones in human lung development is not fully defined. As discussed below, there are temporal associations between the ontogenesis of thyroid function and pulmonary maturation, and there is an indication that low serum levels of T_3 and T_4 are associated with RDS. Administration of thyroid hormones to accelerate lung development has been attempted, but the response to the treatment is not yet established. Nevertheless, available information regarding the human situation, in conjunction with the animal data, support the possibility that thyroid hormones influence the rate of pulmonary differentiation in the human fetus.

7.5.1 Development of Thyroid Function

The developmental pattern for hypothalamic-pituitary-thyroid function in the human has been recently reviewed (Fisher et al. 1977; Fisher and Klein 1981; Chopra 1981). Serum concentrations of TSH increase late in the first half of human gestation, and peak values are obtained between 20 and 24 weeks. Both total and free serum T_4 concentrations increase progressively from mid-gestation to term, with the major increase occurring between 20 and 30 weeks. Total T_4 is approximately 2, 9, and 11.5 μg/dl at 20, 30 and 40 weeks gestation, respectively. This increase appears to reflect increasing responsiveness of the thyroid to TSH during the second half of gestation.

T_3 is not detected (<15 ng/dl) in fetal serum until about 30 weeks of gestation. Subsequently, the concentration increases to a value of approximately 50 ng/dl at term. Serum concentrations of rT_3 decrease progressively during the last trimester to a value of about 150 ng/dl at term. These developmental patterns for thyroid hormones in the human are illustrated in Fig. 7.15. In amniotic fluid, T_4 and rT_3 levels are highest during the second trimester, whereas the concentration of T_3 increases throughout gestation (Klein et al. 1980). Occupancy of nuclear T_3 receptors in the fetal lung by endogenous hormone is detected by the beginning of the second trimester (Gonzales and Ballard 1981).

In the sheep, at least, the prenatal increase in serum T_3 reflects in part a maturational change in extrathyroidal conversion of T_4 to T_3 induced by cortisol. The increased conversion of T_4 to T_3 is presumably due to an increase in hepatic outer ring iodothyronine monodeiodinase activity. This could occur by increased synthesis of enzyme, or by increased concentrations of sulfhydryl cofactors such as glutathione which stimulate enzyme activity. This regulatory mechanism may not occur in the human, since betamethasone treatment of women in preterm labor did not affect either T_3 or rT_3 concentrations in fetal serum (discussed in Chap. 6).

After birth at term, there is a rapid surge in the serum concentration of T_3 and subsequent increases in both TSH and T_4. By 24–36 h of age, serum T_3 and free T_3 concentrations increase 3- to 6-fold. Based on studies in newborn sheep, it appears that the initial increase in T_3 is primarily due to enhanced peripheral conversion of T_4 to T_3. Although the stimulus for this change is not known, it seems likely to reflect activation of enzyme rather than de novo synthesis. Preterm infants have a similar pattern of increase in serum TSH and iodothyronine concentrations; however, the levels obtained are less than observed at term. The low levels of T_4 in the premature infant occur without elevated TSH, and thus apparently represent hypothyroidism of hypothalamic origin. The normal TSH responsiveness to TRH treatment supports this conclusion (Jacobson et al. 1976, 1977; Cuestas and Engel 1979; Hadeed et al. 1981; Chowdhry et al. 1984). Thus, normal thyroid function as judged by responsiveness to TRH, TSH, and to birth is established by the beginning of the third trimester; however, premature infants appear to have a maturational delay in hypothalamic-pituitary feedback control.

The documentation of thyroid hormone effects on lung maturation in animals has raised the possibility of prenatal treatment in the human for preven-

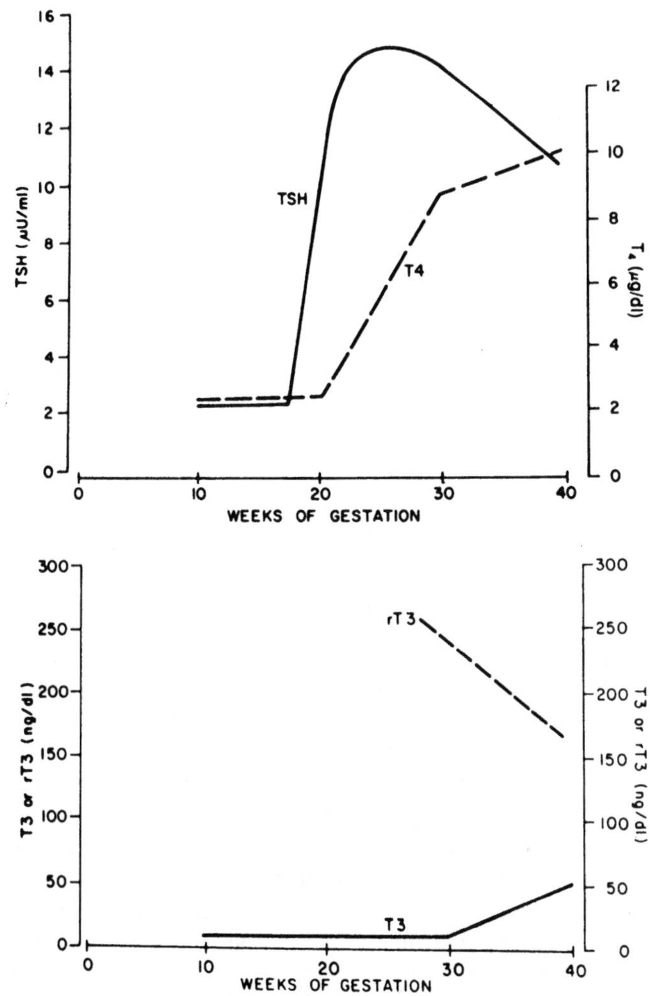

Fig. 7.15. Developmental patterns for TSH and thyroid hormones in serum of the human fetus. TSH values are maximal at 20–24 wk when T_4 begins a progressive increase. T_3 concentrations are normally unmeasurable (<15 ng/dl) before 30 wk and increase during the last trimester while serum rT_3 fall progressively. From Fisher and Klein (1981), by permission.

tion of RDS. However, the best approach for treating the fetus is not certain. There is little passage of either iodothyronines or TSH across the human placenta. Although earlier studies indicated that fetal concentrations of thyroid hormones are increased after maternal treatment (Raiti et al. 1967; Fisher et al. 1964), large doses of T_3 (300 μg/day) or T_4 (8,000 μg/day) were used. These doses produce transient hyperthyroidism in the mother, which could possibly have adverse effects during the stress of labor. Another approach to treatment is intra-amniotic administration of thyroid hormone (Mashiach et al. 1978; Sack et al. 1979; Schreyer et al. 1982). Although this approach avoids hyperthyroidemia of the mother, amniocentesis is required and absorption of thyroid hormone from amniotic fluid may be variable. This method obviously would not be suitable for women with ruptured membranes.

Synthetic thyroid hormone analogs such as DIMIT might be useful in prenatal treatment. These compounds freely transverse the placenta in several species, and have been shown to be thyromimetic in the human (Tamagna et al. 1979). DIMIT is under commercial development, but further human testing would be necessary before clinical trials for prevention of RDS could be initiated.

TRH could be useful in treating the fetus (Rooney et al. 1979; Ballard 1984). Treatment of pregnant women at term with 200–400 μg TRH increases T_3 in cord blood maximally about 3-fold, and levels remain elevated for at least 12 h (Roti et al. 1981). It is likely that a similar effect would occur in preterm fetuses, since TSH and T_4 increase in response to TRH administration in newborn preterm infants (Jacobsen et al. 1976, 1977; Cuestas and Engel 1979; Hadeed et al. 1981; Chowdhry et al. 1984). Studies in both sheep and monkeys also indicate that the preterm fetus is responsive to exogenous TRH in utero (Klein and Fisher 1980; Melmed et al. 1979; Azukizawa et al. 1976).

7.5.2 Thyroid Function and RDS

Several studies have addressed the question of whether RDS in premature infants is associated with decreased thyroid function. Thyroid hormones have been assayed in cord blood of infants with and without RDS. Interpretation of these data, summarized in Table 7.10, is complicated by deficiencies in sample size, selection of controls, or statistical analysis in the various studies. For example, infant groups were not matched for incidence of asphyxia (Redding and Pereira 1974), birthweight (Cuestas et al. 1976), or gestational age (Klein et al. 1979), and the sample size was small in two studies (Abbassi et al. 1977; Klein et al. 1979). The recent report by Klein et al. (1981) attempted to avoid these complications by using matched groups of infants and applying a global test to statistically evaluate differences in thyroid function. Their data for concentrations of T_4, T_3 and rT_3 produced a P value of 0.1–0.05 in testing for decreased thyroid function in infants with RDS. Despite the various deficiencies in the available data, it is noteworthy that mean values for both T_3 and T_4 were lower in infants with RDS in each report, and none of the studies found a difference in TSH concentration. Thus, there is an indication that premature infants who develop RDS have lower levels of circulating thyroid hormones than unaffected infants. Maturation of the hypothalamic-pituitary-thyroid axis, as well as peripheral metabolism of thyroid hormones, may be delayed in infants with retarded pulmonary development.

Thyroid hormones have also been assayed in the immediate newborn period after premature delivery. The postnatal rise in T_3 and T_4 is less marked in premature infants with RDS compared with well premature infants, and values remained lower in a study extended to 2 months of age (Klein et al. 1979; Cuestas and Engel 1979). The depressed thyroid function immediately after birth in infants with RDS may be secondary to the onset of RDS, intrapartum asphyxia, or reduced thyroid function preexisting in utero. Klein et al. (1979) speculate that metabolic effects of RDS are responsible for the fall in T_3 con-

Table 7.10. Thyroid function studies in cord blood of premature infants with and without RDS

Determination	Gestational age (weeks)	No RDS	RDS	P	References
T_4 (μg/dl)	30–33	8.5 ± 1.3	7.2 ± 1.4	< 0.05	Redding & Pereira 1974
	33–37	7.3 ± 0.3	6.3 ± 0.3	< 0.025	Cuestas et al. 1976
	24–35	7.8 ± 0.2	6.6 ± 0.6	NS	Abbassi et al. 1977
	[a]	11.0	9.9	NS	Klein et al. 1979
	31–34	10.6	10.2	[b]	Klein et al. 1981
	28–35	[c]	[c]		Hadeed et al. 1981
	26–36	7.1 ± 0.4	5.9 ± 0.4	< 0.05	Dhanireddy et al. 1983
	26–36	6.4	5.5	NS	Abbassi et al. 1984
Free T_4 index		2.54 ± 0.18	1.99 ± 0.31	< 0.01	Redding & Pereira 1974
	30–35	5.8	5.1	NS	Cuestas & Engel 1979
T_3 (ng/dl)		20.1 ± 2.4	13.4 ± 1.6	< 0.05	Cuestas et al. 1976
		36 ± 5	22 ± 2.6	< 0.025	Abbassi et al. 1977
		18	13	NS	Klein et al. 1979
		32.2	22.0	[b]	Klein et al. 1981
		40.3	16.8	0.008	Abbassi et al. 1984
TSH (μU/ml)		14.3 ± 1.6	18.1 ± 2.3	NS	Cuestas et al. 1976
		9.4 ± 2	7.2 ± 2	NS	Abbassi et al. 1977
		11.0	9.9	NS	Klein et al. 1979
		10.0	11.5	NS	Klein et al. 1981
		9.7	9.9	NS	Abbassi et al. 1984

[a] Mean gestational age was 33.2 ± 0.3 and 31.8 ± 0.5 weeks for no-RDS and RDS, respectively
[b] p = 0.1–0.05 for thyroid function by Hotelling T^2 test performed on 19 infants in each group who had assays for T_4, T_3, and rT_3
[c] Incidence of values < 6.5 μg/dl similar in two groups

centrations and increase in rT_3 level during the first 24 h of life. These effects are consistent with decreased peripheral conversion of T_4 to T_3, as well as decreased metabolism of rT_3.

Clinical observations support the involvement of thyroid hormones in lung maturation. Smith et al. (1975) reviewed the clinical course of infants who were subsequently found to have congenital hypothyroidism. Neonatal respiratory distress occurred in five of the 15 hypothyroid infants. This is an unexpectedly high incidence of RDS among infants of gestational age 36–44 weeks. Of interest, RDS occurred in at least three of four infants less than 39 weeks gestation, suggesting that thyroid status may be of particular importance with regard to lung maturity in the infant born somewhat prematurely. Many athyrotic infants are born after a prolonged gestation, perhaps explaining the general clinical impression that respiratory distress is not a clinical feature of hypothyroidism. There is also a case report of an infant delivered at 38 weeks gestation who developed RDS despite an L:S ratio of 3:1 and the presence of phosphatidylglycerol in amniotic fluid (Anderson et al. 1982). This infant was subsequently diagnosed as having congenital hypothyroidism.

7.5.3 Prenatal Treatment with Thyroid Hormone

To date there are only preliminary data available regarding the therapeutic application of thyroid hormones for prevention of RDS. Mashiach et al. (1978) have reported their experience with intra-amniotic administration of T_4 to eight women before delivery of their infants at 30–36 weeks gestation. Fetal lung maturity was evaluated by microviscosity determinations on amniotic fluid. Treatment with 200 µg of T_4 was associated in most cases with a fall in the microviscosity value, indicating enhanced lung maturity. None of the infants exposed to intra-amniotic T_4 developed RDS. Subsequent treatment of 16 premature infants produced similar results (Mashiach et al. 1979). In cord blood of premature infants delivering 4–24 h after intra-amniotic T_4 treatment (250 µg), serum T_4 was significantly elevated (17.0 vs. 11.6 µg/dl in untreated infants); the T_4 level was normal in infants delivering 3–7 d after therapy (Sack et al. 1979).

Schreyer et al. (1982) injected 40 µg of T_3 into the amniotic fluid of 15 women with severe hypertensive disease and anticipated preterm delivery. All of the infants delivered within 6 to 72 h after treatment at gestational ages between 28 and 34 weeks. Seven of the infants developed RDS and three died. T_3 concentrations were high in the amniotic fluid (275–600 ng/dl) of seven cases examined. However, the mean T_3 concentration in cord blood of treated infants (70.2 ng/dl) was not different from the value for an untreated group. There was also no difference in TSH values for treated and untreated infants. These results indicate that there was little fetal uptake of T_3 from the amniotic fluid in these pregnancies characterized by severe hypertension and fetal depression, and suggest that variable fetal absorption will be a complication of thyroid hormone therapy by intra-amniotic instillation.

Although additional controlled studies are needed to define the efficacy of thyroid hormones in preventing RDS, the preliminary data regarding in utero treatment support the potential usefulness of this therapy. In particular, combined glucocorticoid and thyroid hormone treatment may provide greater benefit than corticosteroid therapy alone as currently used. This possibility is discussed in Chap. 10.

7.6 Conclusions

Several studies over the past 10 years have established that lung maturation is influenced by thyroid hormones. Experimental approaches have involved direct in utero administration of T_4 and maternal treatment with T_3 or synthetic analog. A number of dose-dependent effects of treatment have been observed. These include enhanced morphologic development, increased rate of synthesis of PC and other phospholipids, enhanced surface activity and saturated PC content of lung lavage, and depletion of lung glycogen. Each of these changes is consistent with accelerated development. In adult animals, endogenous thyroid hormones appear to be necessary for normal division and growth of lung cells. The type II cell may be particularly sensitive to this hormonal influence. Thyroid hormones may influence pulmonary phospholipid synthesis in suckling animals, but their effect on phospholipids in the adult is not established.

At least three general properties of thyroid hormone action in fetal lung are known. First, studies with cultured tissue indicate that at least some effects of T_3 and T_4 result from direct action of hormone in lung cells. Thus, stimulation of PC synthesis in vivo is a direct effect of thyroid hormone in the lung and is not mediated through effects of T_3 in other tissues. It is likely, but not proven, that morphologic effects of thyroid hormone are also direct. Second, it is apparent that thyroid hormones have actions which are independent of glucocorticoids. In vivo, both T_3 and DIMIT stimulate PC synthesis under conditions in which there is no change in circulating corticosteroid levels. Furthermore, glucocorticoids need not be present to observe a response to T_3. In organ culture studies, fetal lung responds to T_3 after several days in culture and repeated changes of the culture medium which effectively removes endogenous corticosteroids. These data do not rule out the possibility that prior exposure of lung to corticosteroids in vivo influences later responsiveness to T_3. Third, data from three species indicate that thyroid hormones stimulate synthesis of all classes of phospholipids. By contrast, glucocorticoids have a preferential effect on saturated PC and phosphatidylglycerol, the major phospholipids of surfactant. Thus, T_3 appears to influence both membrane and surfactant phospholipids equally. In this regard, the stimulatory effect of thyroid hormone on surfactant may be viewed as indirect rather than specific.

The action of T_3 on PC synthesis is mediated through nuclear receptor. Thyroid hormone receptors have been identified and characterized in fetal and adult lung of several species. It is likely but not proven that they occur in type II cells as well as other pulmonary cell types. The T_3 binding sites in fetal lung have the properties expected of a receptor of physiologic importance. Binding of hormone occurs relatively rapidly at physiologic temperatures and is reversible. T_3 binds with high affinity, and the affinities of other thyroid hormones correlate with their biologic potencies. Receptor is present in lung early in gestation and there is a developmental increase in concentration in the two species examined thus far. The factors regulating this increase are not known. The response to T_3, in culture systems at least, is sensitive to inhibitors of RNA and protein synthesis. This implies that T_3 induces the synthesis of specific proteins such as occurs in other target tissues. The proteins induced in fetal lung have not been identified. Although the activity of cholinephosphate cytidylyltransferase increases, this results from increased amounts of cofactor rather than enzyme protein.

The following model may be proposed based on the data reviewed in this chapter. An early event in thyroid hormone action in fetal lung is the binding of hormone by nuclear receptor of type II cells. Both T_3 and T_4 interact with receptor, although in some species there may be conversion of T_4 to T_3 in the cytoplasm prior to binding. The interaction of thyroid hormone with receptor stimulates the synthesis of specific mRNAs. These molecules are translated with the resulting accumulation of specific proteins. The number and identity of induced proteins in lung cells is open to speculation, but presumably some are enzymes involved in phospholipid biosynthesis. Since thyroid hormones stimulate all classes of phospholipids, the induced enzymes probably catalyze reactions early in the biosynthetic pathway (e.g., fatty acid synthesis) rather than later events (e.g., enzymes involved in remodeling of PC to form saturated PC). Furthermore, thyroid hormones apparently influence different enzymes than those stimulated by glucocorticoids. The overall biochemical effect of thyroid hormone would be increased synthesis and accumulation of both surfactant and membrane phospholipids. The increased production rate would lead to accelerated accumulation of surfactant in alveoli.

Do endogenous thyroid hormones have a physiologic role in regulation of lung development? Several lines of evidence are consistent with this possibility. 1) Since T_3 effects in cultured lung are mediated by receptor, physiologic concentrations of hormone in vivo would be sufficient to exert effects. In human lung, for example, half-maximal stimulation of PC synthesis occurs with a T_3 concentration of 0.03 nM. At birth, circulating free T_3 reaches levels of 0.023 and 0.046 nM in preterm and term infants, respectively. 2) The thyroid begins to produce T_4 relatively early in gestation. Serum levels of T_4 increase early in gestation and T_3 rises later, providing increased exposure of lung cells to thyroid hormone. 3) Consistent with the above, occupancy of lung T_3 receptor by endogenous thyroid hormone increases during gestation in both the rabbit and human. 4) Thyroidectomy delays lung development in the fetal sheep without affecting levels of endogenous cortisol. 5) There is an apparent association between occurrence of RDS in premature infants and low levels of T_3 in cord blood. 6) Preliminary data from clinical trials indicate that T_4 therapy, producing elevations of plasma concentrations within the physiologic range, accelerates surfactant synthesis and reduces the incidence of RDS.

The possible impact of thyroid hormone therapy for prevention of RDS is only speculative at present. Controlled clinical trials are needed to establish the efficacy and determine the safety of such treatment. Possible therapeutic approaches include intraamniotic administration of T_3 or T_4, and maternal treatment with either a synthetic analog or TRH. It is possible that combined therapy with thyroid hormone and glucocorticoids will provide greater benefit than treatment with either hormone alone.

References

Abbassi V, Merchant K, Abramson D (1977) Postnatal triiodothyronine concentrations in healthy preterm infants and in infants with respiratory distress syndrome. Pediatr Res 11:802

Abbassi V, Adams J, Duvall D, Phillips E (1984) Prenatal thyroid function abnormalities in infants with idiopathic respiratory distress syndrome. Pediatr Res 18:926

Anderson CW, Conrad L, Cordero L (1982) Neonatal respiratory distress in the presence of amniotic fluid phosphatidylglycerol. Am J Obstet Gynecol 143:233

Ayromlooi J, Berg PD, Valderrama E, Tobias MD (1983) Midtrimester thyroidectomy in the ovine fetus. Pediatr Pharmacol 3:15

Azukizawa M, Murata Y, Ikenoue T, Martin CB Jr, Hershman JM (1976) Effect of thyrotropin-releasing hormone on secretion of thyrotropin, prolactin, thyroxine, and triiodothyronine in pregnant and fetal Rhesus monkeys. J Clin Endocrinol Metab 43:1020

Bachrach LK, Kudlow JE, Silverberg JDH, Kent G, Burrow GN (1982) Treatment of ovine cretinism in utero with 3,5-dimethyl-3′-isopropyl-L-thyronine. Endocrinology 111:132

Ballard PL, Benson BJ, Brehier A, Carter JP, Kriz BM, Jorgensen EC (1980) Transplacental stimulation of lung development in the fetal rabbit by 3,5-dimethyl-3′-isopropyl-L-thyronine. J Clin Invest 65:1407

Ballard PL, Kitterman JA, Bland RD, Clyman RI, Gluckman PD, Platzker ACG, Kaplan SL,

Grumbach MM (1982) Ontogeny and regulation of corticosteroid binding globulin capacity in plasma of fetal and newborn lambs. Endocrinology 110:359
Ballard PL (1984) Combined hormonal treatment and lung maturation. Seminars in Perinatology 8:283
Ballard PL, Hovey ML, Gonzales LK (1984) Thyroid hormone stimulation of phosphatidylcholine synthesis in cultured fetal rabbit lung. J Clin Invest 74:898
Baxter JD, Eberhardt NL, Apriletti JW, Johnson LK, Ivarie RD, Schachter BS, Morris JA, Seeburg PH, Goodman HM, Latham KR, Polansky JR, Martial JA (1979) Thyroid hormone receptors and responses. Rec Prog Horm Res 35:97
Bellabarba D, Bedard S, Fortier S, Lehous J-G (1983) 3,5,3'-triiodothyronine nuclear receptor in chick embryo. Properties and ontogeny of brain and lung receptors. Endocrinology 112:353
Bellabarba D, Fortier S, Belisle S, Lehous J-G (1984) Triiodothyronine nuclear receptors in liver, brain and lung of neonatal rats. Biol Neonate 45:41
Benson MC, Liu JP, Huang YP, Burger A, Rivlin RS (1978) Differential effects of triiodothyronine and 3,5-isopropyl-L-thyronine treatment of maternal rats upon hepatic L-triiodothyronine amino-transferase activity in fetal rats. Endocrinology 102:562
Bernal J, DeGroot LJ (1977) Thyroid hormone receptors: release of receptor to the medium during in vitro incubation of isolated rat liver nuclei. Endocrinology 100:648
Bernal J, Coleoni AH, DeGroot LJ (1978) Thyroid hormone receptors from liver nuclei: characteristics of receptor from normal, thyroidectomized, and triiodothyronine-treated rats: measurement of occupied and unoccupied receptors, and chromatin binding of receptors. Endocrinology 103:403
Bernal J, Pekonen F (1984) Ontogenesis of the nuclear 3,5,3'-triiodothyronine receptor in the human fetal brain. Endocrinology 127:278
Bhakthavathsalan A, Mann LI, Tang LC, Erickson ND, Delamater PV, Damm C (1981) The effects of fetal thyroidectomy during the second trimester in the ovine fetus. Am J Obstet Gynecol 141:436
Burman KD, Read J, Dimond RC, Strum D, Wright FD, Patow W, Earll JM, Wartofsky L (1976) Measurements of 3,3',5'-triiodothyronine (reverse T_3), 3,3'-L-diiodothyronine, T_3, and T_4 in human amniotic fluid and in cord and maternal serum. J Clin Endocrinol Metab 43:1351
Chopra IJ (1977) A study of extrathryoidal conversion of thyroxine (T_4) to 3,5,3'-triiodothyronine (T_3) in vitro. Endocrinology 101:453
Chopra IJ (1978) Sulfhydryl group and the monodeiodination of thyroxine and triiodothyronine. Endocrinology 199:904
Chopra IJ (1981) Triiodothyronines in health and disease. Monographs on Endocrinology, Vol. 18, Springer, Berlin, Heidelberg, New York
Chopra IJ, Huang T-S, Hurd RE, Solomon DH (1984) A radioimmunoassay of 3,5-dimethyl-3'-isopropyl-L-thyronine. Endocrinology 114:1295
Chowdhry P, Scanlon JW, Auerbach R, Abbassi V (1984) Results of controlled double-blind study of thyroid replacement in very low-birth-weight premature infants with hypothyroxinemia. Pediatrics 73:301
Comite F, Burrow GN, Jorgensen EC (1978) Thryoid hormone analogs and fetal goiter. Endocrinology 102:1670
Coulombe P, Ruel J, Dussault JH (1979) Analysis of nuclear 3,5,3'-triiodothyronine-binding capacity and tissue response in the liver of the neonatal rat. Endocrinology 105:952
Cuestas RA, Lindall A, Engel RR (1976) Low thyroid hormones and respiratory-distress syndrome of the newborn. Studies on cord blood. N Engl J Med 295:297
Cuestas RA, Engel RR (1979) Thyroid function in preterm infants with respiratory distress syndrome. J Pediatr 94:643
Das DK (1980) Fatty acid synthesis in fetal lung. Biochem Biophys Res Commun 92:867
Das DK, Ganguly M (1981) Diabetes, hypophysectomy, or thyroidectomy reduces nuclear L-triiodothyronine-binding capacity of rat lung. Endocrinology 109:296
Das DK (1983) Hormonal control of pulmonary surfactant synthesis. Arch Biochem Biophys 224:1
Das DK, Ayromlooi J, Bandyopadhyay D, Bandyopadhyay S, Neogi A, Steinberg H (1984) Potentiation of surfactant release in fetal lung by thyroid hormone action. J Appl Physiol: Respir Environ Exercise Physiol 56:1621
Dhanireddy R, Smith YF, Hamosh M, Mullon DK, Scanlon JW, Hamosh P (1983) Respiratory

distress syndrome in the newborn: Relationship to serum prolactin, thyroxine, and sex. Biol Neonate 43:9

Dussault JH, Labrie F (1975) Development of the hypothalamic-pituitary-thyroid axis in the rat. Endocrinology 97:1321

Erenberg A, Omori K, Menkes JH, Oh W, Fisher DA (1974) Growth and development of the thyroidectomized ovine fetus. Pediatr Res 8:783

Erenberg A, Rhodes ML, Weinstein MM, Kennedy RL (1979) The effect of fetal thyroidectomy on ovine fetal lung maturation. Pediatr Res 13:230

Fisher DA, Lehman H, Lackey C (1964) Placental transport of thyroxine. J Clin Endocrinol Metab 24:393

Fisher DA, Dussault JH, Sack J, Chopra IJ (1977) Ontogenesis of hypothalamic-pituitary-thyroid function and metabolism in man, sheep, and rat. Rec Prog Horm Res 33:59

Fisher DA, Klein AH (1981) Thyroid development and disorders of thyroid function in the newborn. N Engl J Med 304:702

Frieden E, Yoshizato K (1974) Thyromimetic activity of methyl thyronines in bullfrog tadpole. Endocrinology 95:188

Gonzales LW, Ballard PL (1981) Identification and characterization of nuclear 3,5,3′-triiodothyronine-binding sites in fetal human lung. J Clin Endocrinol Metab 53:21

Gonzales LW, Ballard PL (1982) Nuclear 3,5,3′-triiodothyronine receptors in rabbit lung: Characterization and developmental changes. Endocrinology 111:542

Gonzales LK, Ballard PL (1984) Glucocorticoid and thyroid hormone stimulation of phosphatidylcholine synthesis in cultured human fetal lung. Pediatr Res 18:310A (abstract)

Gorbman A, Evans HM (1943) Beginning of function in the thyroid of the fetal rat. Endocrinology 32:113

Granberg JP, Ballard PL (1977) The role of sulfhydryl groups in the binding of glucocorticoids by cytoplasmic receptors of lung and other mammalian tissues. Endocrinology 100:1160

Gross I, Wilson CM, Ingleson LD, Brehier A, Rooney SA (1980) Fetal lung in organ culture. III. Comparison of dexamethasone, thyroxine, and methylxanthines. J Appl Physiol: Respirat Environ Exercise Physiol 48:872

Gross I, Wilson CM (1982) Fetal lung in organ culture. IV. Super-additive hormone interaction. J Appl Physiol: Respirat Environ Exercise Physiol 52:1420

Gross I, Ballard PL, Ballard RA, Jones CT, Wilson CM (1983) Corticosteroid stimulation of phosphatidylcholine synthesis in cultured fetal rabbit lung: evidence for de novo protein synthesis mediated by glucocorticoid receptors. Endocrinology 112:829

Gross I, Dynia DW, Wilson CM, Ingleson LD, Gewolb IH, Rooney SA (1984) Glucocorticoid-thyroid hormone interactions in fetal rat lung. Pediatr Res 18:191

Hadeed AJ, Asay LD, Klein AH, Fisher DA (1981) Significance of transient postnatal hypothyroxinemia in premature infants with and without respiratory distress syndrome. Pediatrics 68:494

Hamada S, Nakamura H, Nanno M, Imura H (1979) Triiodothyronine-induced increase in rat liver nuclear thyroid-hormone receptors associated with increased mitochondrial α-glycerophosphate dehydrogenase activity. Biochem J 182:371

Hitchcock KR, Reichlin S (1978) Thyroid hormones in the adult rat lung. Am Rev Resp Dis 117:807

Hitchcock KR (1979) Hormones and the lung. I. Thyroid hormones and glucocorticoids in lung development. Anat Rec 194:15

Hitchcock KR, Harney J, Reichlin S (1980) Hormones and the lung. III. Thyroid hormone uptake kinetics of perinatal rat lung. Endocrinology 107:294

Hopkins PS, Thorburn GD (1972) The effects of foetal thyroidectomy on the development of the ovine foetus. J Endocrinol 54:55

Ikegami M, Klein AH, Padbury JF, Jobe AH (1983) Does lung surfactant respond to thyroid hormones in fetal sheep? Pediatr Res 17:134A (abstract)

Jacobsen BB, Andersen H, Dige-Petersen H, Hummer L (1976) Thyrotropin response to thyroxine-releasing hormone in fullterm, euthyroid and hypothyroid newborns. Acta Paediatr Scand 65:433

Jacobsen BB, Andersen H, Dige-Petersen H, Hummer L (1977) Pituitary-thyroid responsiveness to thyrotropin-releasing hormone in preterm and small-for-gestational age newborns. Acta Paediatr Scand 66:541

Jorgensen EC, Murray WJ, Block P Jr (1974) Thyroxine analogs. XXII. Thyromimetic activity of halogen-free derivatives of 3,5-dimethyl-L-thyronine. J Med Chem 17:434

Jorgensen EC, Bolger MB, Dietrich SW (1976) Thyroid hormone analogs: correlations between structure, nuclear binding, and hormonal activity. Proceedings of the Fifth International Congress of Endocrinology, Vol 1, Excerpta Medica International Congress, p. 117

Jump DB, Oppenheimer JH (1983) Association of thyroid hormone receptors with chromatin. Molec Cell Biochem 55:159

Kauffman SL, Burri PH, Weibel ER (1974) The postnatal growth of the rat lung. II. Autoradiography. Anat Rec 180:63

Kitterman JA, Liggins GC, Campos GA, Clements JA, Forster CS, Lee CH, Creasy RK (1981) Prepartum maturation of the lung in fetal sheep: relation to cortisol. J Appl Physiol: Respirat Environ Exercise Physiol 51:384

Klein AH, Oddie TH, Fisher DA (1978) Effect of parturition on serum iodothyronine concentrations in fetal sheep. Endocrinology 103:1453

Klein AH, Foley B, Kenny FM, Fisher DA (1979) Thyroid hormone and thyrotropin responses to parturition in premature infants with and without the respiratory distress syndrome. Pediatrics 63:380

Klein AH, Murphy BEP, Artal R, Oddie TH, Fisher DA (1980) Amniotic fluid thyroid hormone concentrations during human gestation. Am J Obstet Gynecol 136:626

Klein AH, Fisher DA (1980) Thyrotropin-releasing hormone-stimulated pituitary and thyroid gland responsiveness and 3,5,3′-triiodothyronine suppression in fetal and neonatal lambs. Endocrinology 106:697

Klein AH, Foley B, Foley TP, MacDonald HM, Fisher DA (1981) Thyroid function studies in cord blood from premature infants with and without RDS. J Pediatr 98:818

Koerner D, Schwartz HL, Surks MI, Oppenheimer JH, Jorgensen EC (1975) Binding of selected iodothyronine analogs to receptor sites of isolated rat hepatic nuclei. J Biol Chem 250:6417

Korda AR, Fleming SF, Senior C, Duck-Chong CG, Henderson-Smart DJ, Ramsey G, Shutt DA, Russell P, Shearman RP (1984) The effect of intra-amniotic injection of triiodothyronine on pulmonary maturity in lambs at 130 days gestation. Pediatr Res 18:932

Kriz BM, Jones AL, Jorgensen EC (1978) Effects of a thyroid hormone analog on fetal rat hepatocyte ultrastructure and microsomal function. Endocrinology 102:712

Lindenberg JA, Brehier A, Ballard PL (1978) Triiodothyronine nuclear binding in fetal and adult rabbit lung and cultured lung cells. Endocrinology 103:1725

Longmuir KJ, Bleasdale JE, Quirk JG, Johnston JM (1982) Regulation of lamellar body acidic glycerophospholipid biosynthesis in fetal rabbit lung in organ culture. Biochem Biophys Acta 712:356

Lorijan RHW, Nelson JC, Longo LD (1980) Induced fetal hyperthyroidism: cardiac output and oxygen consumption. Am J Physiol 239:H302

Mariash CN, Oppenheimer JH (1983) Interrelationship of triiodothyronine concentration, metabolism, protein binding, and nuclear occupancy in the induction of malic enzyme by cultured adult rat hepatocytes. Endocrinology 112:80

Mashiach S, Barkai G, Sack J, Stern E, Goldman B, Brish M, Serr DM (1978) Enhancement of fetal lung maturity by intra-amniotic administration of thyroid hormone. Am J Obstet Gynecol 130:289

Mashiach S, Barkai G, Sack J, Stern E, Brish M, Goldman B, Serr DM (1979) The effect of intra-amniotic thyroxine administration on fetal lung maturity in man. J Perinat Med 7:161

Mason RJ, Manganiello V, Vaughan M (1972) Effect of thyroxine on the disaturated lecithin content of lung. Am Rev Respir Dis 106:767

Melmed S, Harada A, Murata Y, Socol M, Reed A, Carlson HE, Azukizawa M, Martin C, Jorgensen E, Hershman JM (1979) Fetal response to thyrotropin-releasing hormone after thyroid hormone administration to the rhesus monkey: Lack of pituitary suppression. Endocrinology 105:334

Morishige WK, Guernsey DL (1978) Triiodothyronine receptors in rat lung. Endocrinology 102:1628

Morishige WK, Joun NS, Guernsey DL (1982) Thyroidal influence on postnatal lung development in the rat. Endocrinology 110:444

Neufeld N, Melmed S (1981) 3,5-dimethyl-3′-isopropyl-L-thyronine therapy in diabetic pregnancy. J Clin Invest 68:1605

Nwosu UC, Kaplan MM, Utiger RD, Delivoria-Papadopulos M (1978) Surge of fetal plasma triiodothyronine before birth in sheep. Am J Obstet Gynecol 132:489
Nwosu UC, Anday EK, Bolognese RJ, Bongiovanni AM, Delivoria-Papadopulos M (1980) Effect of in utero intravenous administration of thyroxine and other hormones on the lung fluid lecithin/spingomyelin ratio in the fetal lamb. Am J Obstet Gynecol 138:459
Oppenheimer JH, Samuels HH (eds) Molecular Basis of Thyroid Hormone Action, Academic Press, New York, 1983
Oppenheimer JH, Schwartz HL, Dillman W, Surks MI (1973) Effect of thyroid hormone analogs on the displacement of ^{125}I-L-triiodothyronine from hepatic and heart nuclei in vivo: possible relationship to hormonal activity. Biochem Biophys Res Commun 55:544
Oppenheimer JH, Schwartz HL, Surks MI (1974) Tissue differences in the concentration of triiodothyronine nuclear binding sites in the rat: liver, kidney, pituitary, heart, brain, spleen and testis. Endocrinology 95:897
Papavasiliou SS, Martial JA, Latham KR, Baxter JD (1977) Thyroid hormone-like actions of 3,3′,5′-L-triiiodothyronine and 3,3′-diiodothyronine. J Clin Invest 60:1230
Raiti S, Holzman GB, Scott RL, Moser RM (1967) Evidence for the placental transfer of tri-iodothryonine in human beings. N Engl J Med 277:156
Redding RA, Douglas WHJ (1972) Thyroid hormone influence upon lung surfactant metabolism. Science 175:994
Redding RA, Pereira C (1974) Thyroid function in respiratory distress syndrome (RDS) of the newborn. Pediatrics 54:423
Rooney SA, Gross I, Gassenheimer LN, Motoyama EK (1975) Stimulation of glycerolphosphate phosphatidyltransferase activity in fetal rabbit lung by cortisol administration. Biochim Biophys Acta 398:433
Rooney SA, Marino PA, Gobran LI, Gross I, Warshaw JB (1979) Thyrotropin-releasing hormone increases the amount of surfactant in lung lavage from fetal rabbits. Pediatr Res 13:623
Roti E, Gnudi A, Braverman LE, Robuschi G, Emanuele R, Bandini P, Benassi L, Pagliani A, Emerson CH (1981) Human cord blood concentrations of thyrotropin, thyroglobulin, and iodoothyronines after maternal administration of thyrotropin-releasing hormone. J Clin Endocrinol Metab 53:813
Ruel J, Coulombe P, Dussault JH (1982a) Thyroid hormones, malnutrition, and biochemical composition of developing rat lung. Am J Physiol (Endocrinol Metab):E378
Ruel J, Coulombe P, Dussault JH (1982b) Characterization of nuclear 3,5,3′-triiodothyronine receptors in the developing rat lung: Effects of hypo- and hyperthyroidism. Pediatr Res 16:238
Sack J, Mashiach S, Barkai G, Lunenfeld B, Brish M, Goldman B, Serr DM (1979) Intra-amniotic thyroxine absorption of the premature human fetus. Acta Endocrinol 90:361
Samuels HH, Tsai JS (1974) Thyroid hormone action. Demonstration of similar receptors in isolated nuclei of rat liver and cultured GH_1 cells. J Clin Invest 53:656
Samuels HH, Stanley F, Shapiro LE (1976) Dose-dependent depletion of nuclear receptors by L-triiodothyronine: evidence for a role in induction of growth hormone synthesis in cultured GH_1 cells. Proc Natl Acad Sci USA 11:3877
Samuels HH, Stanley F, Shapiro LE (1977) Modulation of thyroid hormone nuclear receptor levels by 3,5,3′-triiodo-L-thyronine in GH_1 cells: evidence for two functional components of nuclear-bound receptor and relationship to the induction of growth hormone synthesis. J Biol Chem 252:6052
Schreyer P, Caspi E, Letko Y, Ron-El R, Pinto N, Zeidman JL (1982) Intraamniotic triiodothyronine instillation for prevention of respiratory distress syndrome in pregnancies complicated by hypertension. J Perinat Med 10:27
Segall-Blank M, Douglas WHJ, Sanders RL, Hitchcock KR (1983) Thyroxine metabolism in cultured cells derived from fetal rat lung. Pediatr Res 17:596
Silva ES, Astier H, Thakare U, Schwartz H, Oppenheimer J (1977) Partial purification of the triiodothyronine receptor from rat liver nuclei. J Biol Chem 252:6799
Smith BT, Torday JS (1974) Factors affecting lecithin synthesis by fetal lung cells in culture. Pediatr Res 8:848
Smith BT, Sabry K (1983) Glucocorticoid-thyroid synergism in lung maturation: A mechanism involving epithelial-mesenchymal interaction. Proc Natl Acad Sci USA 80:1951
Smith DW, Klein AM, Henderson JR, Myrianthopoulos NC (1975) Congenital hypothyroidism – signs and symptoms in the newborn period. J Pediatr 87:958

Spitzer HL, Johnston JM (1978) Characterization of phosphatidate phosphohydrolase activity associated with isolated lamellar bodies. Biochem Biophys Acta 531:275

Tamagna EI, Hershman JM, Jorgensen EC (1979) Thyrotropin suppression by 3,5-dimethyl-3′-isopropyl-L-thyronine in man. J Clin Endocrinol Metab 48:196

Thomas AL, Krane EJ, Nathanielsz PW (1978) Changes in the fetal thyroid axis after induction of premature parturition by low dose continuous intravascular cortisol infusion to the fetal sheep at 130 days of gestation. Endocrinology 103:17

Torday JS, Dow KE (1984) Synergistic effect of triiodothyronine and dexamethasone on male and female fetal rat lung surfactant synthesis. Dev Pharmacol Ther 7:133

Waterman AJ, Gorbman A (1956) Development of the thyroid gland of the rabbit. J Exp Zoolog 132:509

Wilson M, Hitchcock KR, Douglas WHJ, DeLellis RA (1979) Hormones and the lung II. Immunohistochemical localization of thyroid hormone binding in type II pulmonary epithelial cells clonally-derived from adult rat lung. Anat Rec 195:611

Wrutniak C, Cabello G (1983) Changes in the concentration of thyroxine in the plasma of rat fetuses during late gestation: influence of ligation of the maternal uterine vein and artery. J Endocrinol 99:233

Wu B, Kikkawa Y, Orzalesi MM, Motoyama EK, Kaibara M, Zigas CJ, Cook CD (1973) The effect of thyroxine on the maturation of fetal rabbit lung. Biol Neonate 22:161

8 Beta-Adrenergic Agonists

Treatment of the fetus with adrenergic agonists causes both release of surfactant and fluid reabsorption by the lung. These effects have been investigated in both whole animal preparations and in culture systems. It is likely that endogenous catecholamines also stimulate these processes and thus have an important role in establishing normal lung function at birth. In the first half of this chapter I review the data supporting this hypothesis. Section 8.2 deals with β-adrenergic receptors in lung. In recent years there has been considerable interest and progress in defining the distribution, properties and regulation of these receptors.

8.1 Effects

Initial interest in the effects of catecholamines on surfactant release in fetal and newborn lung stemmed from observations in three areas. First, there was evidence that the birth process in experimental animals is associated with release of surfactant into the alveolar spaces (Kikkawa et al. 1968; Taeusch et al. 1974). Increased concentrations of circulating catecholamines are known to occur with birth. Second, there were reports that autonomic agents cause the release of surfactant in adult animals (Goldenberg 1969; Olsen 1972). Third, a report appeared in the literature in 1973 describing an unexpectedly low inci-

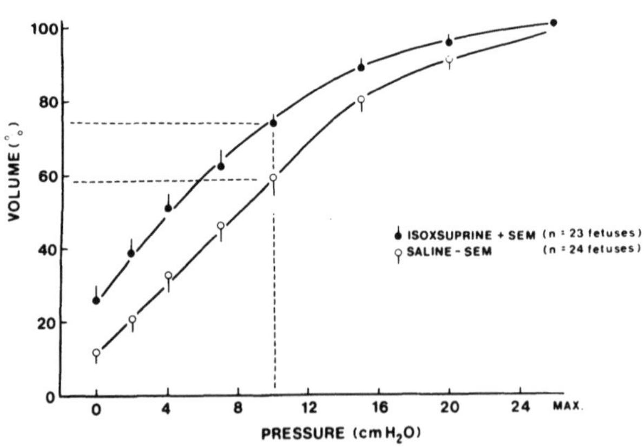

Fig. 8.1. Deflation pressure-volume curves for isoxsuprine vs. saline treated fetal rabbits. Fetuses at 28 days gestation were injected in utero with 0.5 mg isoxsuprine or saline and delivered 3 h later. After breathing air for 30 min, pressure-volume studies were performed. Data from Wyszogrodski et al. (1974), by permission

dence of RDS in infants whose mothers were treated with isoxsuprine (Kero et al. 1973). These findings set the background for experiments examining the effects of catecholamines on surfactant content and lung function in the newborn animal. At about the same time, it was noted that the incidence of respiratory distress and death from hyaline membrane disease was greatest among infants born by cesarean section before the onset of labor (Fedrick and Butler 1972; Usher et al. 1971). This observation suggested that both surfactant secretion and lung fluid reabsorption were influenced by labor. Subsequent experiments have confirmed the influence of catecholamines on both of these processes at birth. The following discussion also includes information on effects of both cAMP derivatives and the methylxanthines (e.g., aminophyllin). This topic is included because of the involvement of cAMP in mediation of adrenergic effects in fetal lung and also to allow comparisons between effects of catecholamines and cAMP.

8.1.1 Surfactant Release

8.1.1.1 In Vivo Studies

Wyszogrodski et al. (1974) performed the first study directly testing the hypothesis that catecholamines would stimulate release of pulmonary surfactant. They treated rabbit fetuses in utero with isoxsuprine (0.5 mg) or saline, and then delivered the fetuses 3 h later. On pressure-volume studies, fetuses at 28 days gestation treated with isoxsuprine demonstrated significantly greater stability on deflation (Fig. 8.1). Treatment had no effect in fetuses of 27 and

Table 8.1. Effects of catecholamines on surfactant in the fetal rabbit

Observation	Drug	(route)[a]	Investigator
Increased deflation stability	Isoxsuprine	(f)	Wyszogrodski et al. 1974
			Corbet et al. 1977
	Terbutaline	(f)	Bergman et al 1980
			Ekelund et al. 1981
			Ekelund et al. 1983
	Isoxsuprine	(m)	Kanjanapone et al. 1980
Decreased surface tension of lung lavage	Isoxsuprine	(f)	Enhorning et al. 1979
	Isoxsuprine	(m)	Enhorning et al. 1979
	Terbutaline	(f)	Bergman et al. 1980
			Ekelund et al. 1981
Increased L/S ratio or phospholipid in lung lavage	Isoxsuprine	(m)	Hayden et al. 1977
			Kanjanapone et al. 1980
	Isoxsuprine	(f)	Enhorning et al. 1977
	Terbutaline	(f)	Bergman 1981
			Ekelund et al. 1981
			Ekelund et al. 1983
Increased alveolar sudanophilic material	Isoxsuprine	(m)	Enhorning et al. 1979
	Terbutaline	(f)	Bergman 1981
Decreased lamellar bodies in type II cells	Isoxsuprine	(f)	Enhorning et al. 1977
Increased lung PC content	Isoxsuprine	(m)	Hayden et al. 1977
			Kanjanapone et al. 1980

[a] f, fetal; m, maternal

26 days gestation. This age effect is not surprising since there are relatively few lamellar bodies present in type II cells before 28 days, and the concentration of adrenergic receptor is relatively low.

The effect of beta-mimetics on surfactant content in potential airspaces of fetal lung has been confirmed and further characterized by several investigators. Methods used in the study of surfactant secretion, and effects of β-adrenergic agonists, have been recently reviewed by Hollingsworth and Gilfillan (1984). The data of Table 8.1 summarize observations in fetal rabbits exposed to either isoxsuprine or terbutaline. Increased amounts of surfactant in alveoli after exposure to catecholamine is indicated by increased stability of lungs in pressure-volume studies, lower surface tension of lung lavage as assessed by the pulsating bubble technique, and a higher L/S ratio in lung lavage. The increased amount of sudanophilic material in alveolar spaces indicates more lipid-containing material. One study found a lower number of mature lamellar bodies in type II cells of treated lungs, consistent with a rapid release of surfactant from these cells.

The influence of epinephrine on surfactant efflux in the lamb was studied by Lawson et al. (1978). Infusion of epinephrine at 3.3 μg/min for 6 h to fetal lambs was associated with increased surfactant concentration in tracheal fluid. This response was reversible and increased with gestational age. The studies in fetal rabbits were carried out at about 28 days gestation. The effect of age on responsiveness to catecholamines has not been systematically examined, except for the observations of Wyszogrodski et al. (1974) with younger fetuses.

For in utero treatment, isoxsuprine has been used at a dose of 0.5 mg and terbutaline at 0.1 mg. Maternal treatment with isoxsuprine has consisted of intravenous infusion at a rate of 2.5 mg/kg/h (Enhorning et al. 1979) or intramuscular treatment (3.3 mg/kg) at 8-h intervals (Hayden et al. 1977; Kanjanapone et al. 1980). The intravenous regimen likely results in considerably higher circulating concentrations of drug than with intramuscular administration and was associated with increased maternal heart and respiratory rate, and a decrease in blood pressure and pH. Possible maternal effects after fetal treatment have not been reported. Dose response studies for in vivo treatment have not been described.

The action of beta-mimetics on surfactant release in vivo is quite rapid. After fetal injection, the effects noted in Table 8.1 occur within $2^1/_2$–$4^1/_2$ h. This response time is consistent with accelerated release of preformed surfactant rather than increased synthesis with secondary secretion into alveoli. Glucocorticoid treatment also increases the surfactant content in alveolar spaces, but this effect requires a longer period of time and results from an increased rate of synthesis. For example, aminophyllin but not dexamethasone increases alveolar surfactant 2 h after treatment (Corbet et al. 1978), and corticosteroid does not stimulate secretion by isolated Type II cells (Dobbs, personal communication).

A detailed study of the time course of action of terbutaline on release of surfactant in the fetal rabbit has been performed recently (Ekelund et al. 1983). Fetuses at 27.75 days gestation were injected with 0.1 mg terbutaline or saline, and the lungs were studied at times thereafter. The time course of ef-

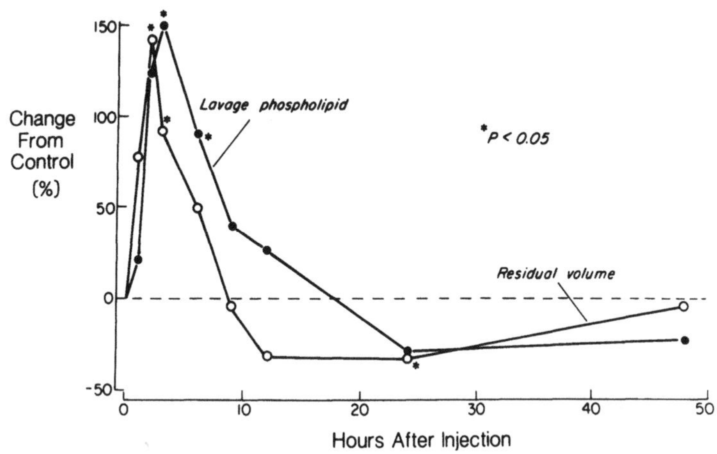

Fig. 8.2. Time course of terbutaline effect on lavage phospholipid and residual volume in fetal rabbit lung. Fetuses of 28 days gestation received 0.1 mg terbutaline or saline (control) in utero and were studied at various times thereafter by lavage (total phospholipid phosphorus) and pressure-volume measurements (residual volume at 0 cm H_2O pressure). Data from Ekelund et al. (1983)

fects on residual volume (ml/g dry lung at a deflation pressure of 10 cm H_2O) and phospholipid content of lavage fluid (μg/g dry lung) are summarized in Fig. 8.2. A statistically significant stimulation of both parameters was observed by 2 h. Analysis of complete pressure-volume curves indicated increased deflation stability after 1 h exposure to terbutaline. The effect of terbutaline is lost by approximately 12 h, and there is a deficit in residual volume of treated pups at 24 h. This delayed response was confirmed in full pressure-volume curves and in separate experiments with continuous maternal infusion of terbutaline. This study confirms the rapidity of catecholamine action after in vivo treatment. In addition, the data at 24 h suggest that there is a rebound phenomenon of surfactant deficiency in alveolar spaces. This may reflect continued release of lamellar bodies with resulting depletion of intracellular stores, and/or down regulation of beta-adrenergic receptors producing a relative insensitivity to endogenous catecholamines. It is not known whether this delayed effect occurs at all gestational ages and in other species. Nevertheless, these findings may have clinical implications for the newborn infant exposed to beta-mimetic treatment for tocolysis of premature labor. Whereas the infant might benefit from a short exposure to beta-agonists by enhanced release of surfactant, prolonged treatment might reduce the amount of surfactant available for stabilizing the lungs at birth.

Beta-mimetics appear to stimulate the *synthesis* of PC as well as secretion. Kanjanapone et al. (1980) report a ~ 50 % increase in both choline incorporation into PC and saturated PC content in lungs of fetal rabbits exposed to maternal isoxsuprine treatment for 24 h. Using a similar experimental protocol, Hayden et al. (1977) reported a 25 % increase in fetal lung PC content with isoxsuprine treatment. In both cases the data were calculated per g lung wet weight, which may complicate interpretation because of the effects of catecholamine on lung fluid. To date, there is no information regarding possible effects of *short-term* beta-mimetic treatment on the rate of PC synthesis in vivo. Nevertheless, it would appear that any effect of catecholamine on phospholipid synthesis is not involved in its action on surfactant release.

Several of the studies with beta-mimetics were performed with fetuses that were not allowed to breathe (Corbet et al. 1977; Enhorning et al. 1977; Enhorning et al. 1979; Bergman et al. 1980). Thus, release of surfactant by exogenous catecholamine occurs in utero prior to air inflation. This is noteworthy in view of the observations that ventilation increases the content of alveolar surfactant in both newborn and adult animals (Gluck et al. 1967; Kikkawa et al. 1968; Taeusch et al. 1974; Hildebran et al. 1975; Faridy 1976; Oyarzun and Clements 1977; Oyarzun and Clements 1978; McDonald et al. 1984). Liquid inflation of the lung in rabbit pups killed after 30 min air breathing, as used in lavage studies, also causes release of phospholipid. This response is decreased at low temperature and, in premature pups, by high concentrations of propranolol (1 mM) in the lavage fluid (Corbet et al. 1984), suggesting mediation in part by endogenous catecholamines. It has been proposed that endogenous beta-adrenergic agonists are also in part responsible for the normal release of surfactant after birth (Taeusch et al. 1974); evidence relating to this hypothesis is discussed below in Sect. 8.1.3.

The specificity of the catecholamine effect in vivo has received only limited investigation. Using pressure-volume measurements, Corbet et al. (1977) found improved deflation stability in fetal rabbits receiving pilocarpine and isoxsuprine, but not after treatment with muscarine or phenylephrine. The effect of isoxsuprine was blocked by simultaneous treatment with propranolol, but not by phenoxybenzamine, consistent with β vs. α stimulation. The response to pilocarpine, principally a cholinergic drug, originally suggested an influence of parasympathetic stimulation in surfactant release (Corbet et al. 1976). However, a subsequent study demonstrated that the effect of pilocarpine on lung stability was blocked by propranolol as well as by atropine and phenoxybenzamine, suggesting an indirect effect through stimulation of the sympathetic nervous system. Bergman et al. (1980) compared the effects of prenalterol and terbutaline, which are principally β_1- and β_2-adrenergic agonists, respectively. Rabbit fetuses were given 0.1 mg of drug or saline and studied 3 h later. Terbutaline treatment increased the maximal lung volume and air retention on deflation, whereas no effect was noted with prenalterol. However, both agents reduced the volume of pulmonary fluid recovered from the airways. These several observations support the proposal that surfactant release in the fetal rabbit is mediated through the β_2-receptor.

Adrenergic agonists also affect surfactant secretion in the adult animal. Oyarzun and Clements (1978) determined phospholipid concentration in lavage fluid of anesthetized adult rabbits breathing spontaneously. Continuous infusion of terbutaline (0.15 mg/kg/min) for 2 h significantly increased phospholipid content, and the effect was blocked by propranolol. An increase in lavage phospholipid also occurs with hyperventilation in this experimental model. This effect was prevented by both propranolol and sotalol, consistent with mediation by endogenous beta-agonists.

Effects of aminophyllin on secretion of surfactant have been described.

Treatment of fetal rabbits in utero with 5 mg of aminophyllin 2.5 h before cesarean section increased the deflation stability and the phospholipid content of lung lavage (Corbet et al. 1978). However, in similar experiments, using 10 mg aminophyllin intramuscularly to rabbit fetuses, Ekelund et al. (1981) found increased mortality and no effect on lung compliance or phospholipids of lavage fluid. In experiments where pregnant rabbits received a long course of aminophyllin treatment, the phospholipid content of alveolar wash was enhanced in fetuses at 29 and 30 days gestation (Karotkin et al. 1976). Although this treatment did not increase lavage phospholipid content of 28-day pups, more treated fetuses were alive 60 min after birth and these animals had more lavage PC than controls (Barrett et al. 1978). There is relatively little information on effects of in vivo treatment with cAMP. Hallman (1977) reported that dibutyryl cAMP given at the birth of premature rabbit pups enhanced the content of phospholipids and proteins in alveolar wash one h later. There is also preliminary morphologic evidence for a prompt effect of in vivo dibutyryl cAMP on secretion of lamellar bodies from adult type II cells (Stahlman et al. 1974). These observations support the proposal that cAMP, whether of endogenous or exogenous origin, is a stimulus to surfactant secretion. There seems to be little doubt that catecholamines stimulate secretion in lung as in other tissues through activation of adenylate cyclase. However, a possible role for other hormones acting through this second messenger cannot yet be ruled out.

In vivo treatment with aminophyllin also influences phospholipid synthesis in the lung. Prolonged maternal treatment stimulates the rate of glucose, choline, and palmitate incorporation into saturated PC, increases pulmonary tissue content of saturated PC as well as other lipids, and decreases glycogen content (Barrett et al. 1976; Sevanian et al. 1979). However, the magnitude of these effects (5–20 %) is considerably less than observed after in vivo treatment with glucocorticoids or thyroid hormones. Also, both cAMP analogs and phosphodiesterase inhibitors appear to stimulate the synthesis of most classes of phospholipids both in vitro and in vivo (discussed in 8.1.1.2.). These properties suggest that cAMP stimulation of phospholipid synthesis in vivo is not preferentially directed toward the surfactant system (Gross 1977).

Thus, it is apparent that both β-adrenergic agonists and cAMP increase the alveolar content of surfactant in fetal and adult animals. The rapidity of the response is consistent with stimulated secretion of preformed lamellar bodies from type II cells. These in vivo observations are supported and expanded by more recent studies with cultured lung tissue.

8.1.1.2 Cultured Lung

Secretion of surfactant has been studied in vitro using both isolated type II cells and tissue slices. In the first reported study of this type, Dobbs and Mason (1979) used type II cells isolated from adult rat lung by treatment with elastase. The cells were placed in primary culture and intracellular phospholipids were labeled by incubation with ^{14}C-choline. After changing the culture medium, aliquots of the medium were removed at various times for lipid extraction and isolation of saturated PC. Figure 8.3 shows the time course for appearance of radioactive saturated PC in the culture medium. The basal rate

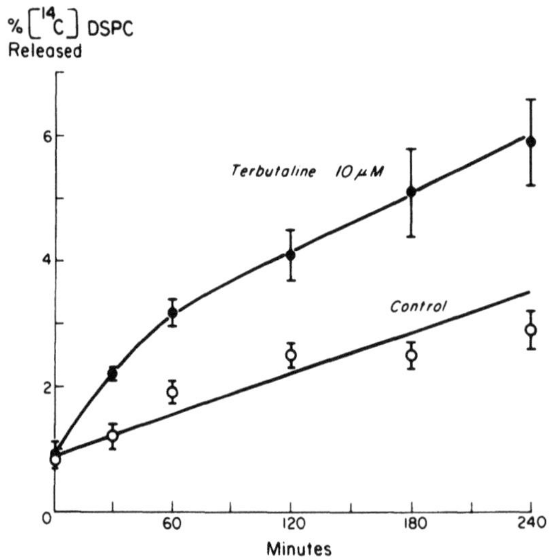

Fig. 8.3. Time course for release of labeled saturated PC from type II cells in culture. Cells were isolated from lungs of adult rats and exposed to [^{14}C] methyl choline to label phospholipids. After washing, the cells were exposed to terbutaline or diluent and saturated PC in the culture medium was determined at the intervals shown. Data from Dobbs and Mason (1979), by permission

of release in control cultures was ~0.6 % per h of total cellular saturated content. Within 30 min of exposure to terbutaline, release is stimulated. The material appearing in the culture medium under both basal and stimulated conditions is similar to surfactant obtained by lavage on the basis of phospholipid composition, apoprotein content, surface activity, and morphologic appearance (Dobbs et al. 1982).

The data in Fig. 8.4 compare dose-response characteristics for terbutaline and phenylephrine which are predominantly β- and α-adrenergic agonists, respectively. Terbutaline produced half-maximal stimulation at 0.8 μM, which is comparable to the potency described in other cellular systems. Phenylephrine was less potent than terbutaline. Stimulation by both agents was blocked by propranolol, indicating action through β-adrenergic receptors. By contrast, phentolamine and atropine did not prevent stimulation by terbutaline. The

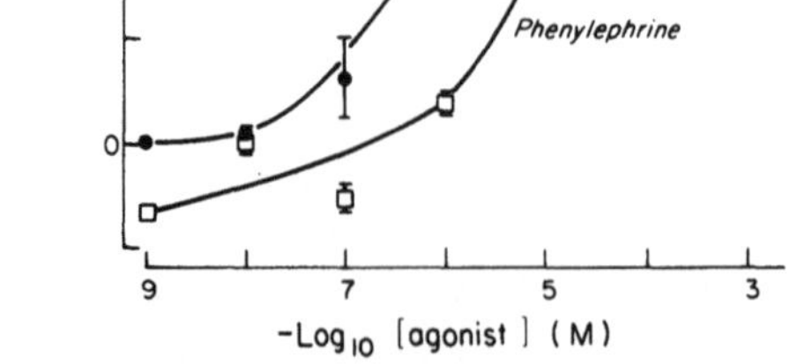

Fig. 8.4. Dose-response curves for DL-terbutaline and phenylephrine in stimulating secretion of saturated PC from isolated type II cells. The experimental approach is outlined in the legend of Fig. 8.3. Half-maximal effect occurred at 0.8 μM and 13 μM for terbutaline and phenylephrine, respectively. Data from Dobbs and Mason (1979), by permission

(−)-isomer of isoproterenol was approximately 50 times more potent than the (+)-isomer, indicating stereoselectivity. The effect of catecholamines in these cells did not involve cellular toxicity as monitored by release of cytoplasmic lactic dehydrogenase. Furthermore, as expected, there was no stimulation of saturated PC release by terbutaline in cultures of lung fibroblasts. Similar results with β-adrenergic agonists have been obtained in two other studies with isolated type II cells (Brown and Longmore 1981; Mettler et al. 1981).

Release of radioactive saturated PC from type II cells is also stimulated by 8-bromo-cAMP, N^6O^2-dibutyryl cAMP, and isobutomethylxanthine, but not by the bromo analog of cGMP (Dobbs and Mason 1979; Brown and Longmore 1981; Mettler et al. 1981). The magnitude of the stimulation seen with cAMP and phosphodiesterase inhibitor is similar to that achieved with β-agonist. An increase in cAMP levels in type II cells exposed to β-agonists has been demonstrated (Brown and Longmore 1981; Mettler et al. 1981; Mescher et al. 1983). Cyclic AMP levels are maximal (4.8-fold increase) approximately 2 min after addition of isoproterenol (Fig. 8.5). The kinetics and magnitude of this response are comparable to results in other tissues and in lung fragments (Moore 1977; Stoner et al. 1974; Palmer 1972).

The effect of terbutaline on PC *synthesis* in isolated type II cells was examined by Mettler et al. (1981). The rate of choline incorporation into phospholipid (predominantly PC) increased maximally about 40 % on exposure to terbutaline. No stimulation was observed after 1 h incubation, and the response appeared to plateau by 4 h. The half-maximal effect occurred at approximately 2 μM, similar to the dose-response relationship observed for secretion of saturated PC. Exposure of cells to 8-bromo cAMP (0.1 mM) also stimulated choline incorporation (29 %), whereas bromo-cGMP was ineffective at the same concentration. In A-549 cells derived from adult human lung, exposure to various cAMP analogs for 48 h increased both choline incorporation into PC and the content of saturated PC per cell. This effect was specific for analogs of cAMP and showed dose dependency with maximal stimulation occurring at about 10 μM (Niles and Makarski 1979). These observations in adult lung cells agree with data for cultured fetal lung, where exposure to

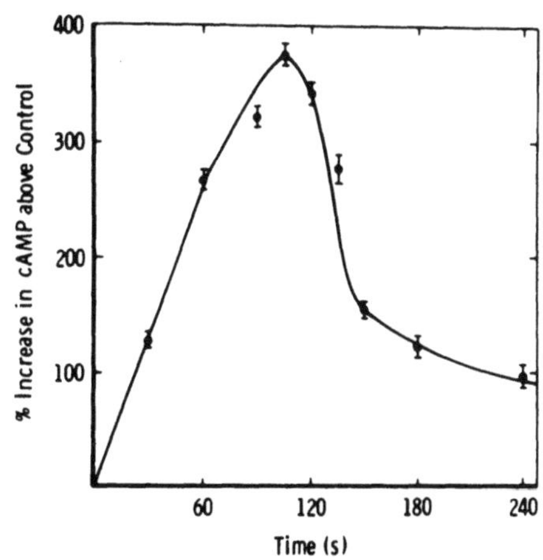

Fig. 8.5. Time course for cAMP concentration in type II cells exposed to isoproterenol. Cells were isolated from lungs of adult rats, placed in culture, and exposed to an optimal concentration (10 μM) of (-)-isoproterenol. cAMP was determined by RIA; the basal concentration was 0.9 pmol/10^5 cells. Data from Brown and Longmore (1981), by permission

either aminophyllin or cAMP enhances phospholipid synthesis and decreases glycogen content (Gross and Rooney 1977; Maniscalco et al. 1979; Gross et al. 1980; Aeberhard et al. 1984). The response in fetal lung appears to involve several classes of phospholipids (Gross 1977; Aeberhard et al. 1984).

To date, surfactant release in fetal and newborn lungs has been studied only using a lung slice model (Marino and Rooney 1980, 1981). In this approach, rabbits are delivered by cesarean section and injected with [^{3}H]choline to label pulmonary phospholipids. After 4 h, the lungs are perfused, sliced, and incubated in a culture system. Following several changes of the culture medium, the lipids which are released have a composition similar to that of lung lavage. Secretion of labeled PC was linear with time and did not occur in the cold. In the initial study with fetal rabbits at term, there was no stimulation of PC release by either isoxsuprine or terbutaline. Subsequently, however, the study was repeated using fetuses of 30 days gestation not exposed to labor. Under these conditions, terbutaline at 0.1 mM produced a 33 % stimulation in release. Possibly, the failure to see adrenergic effects at 31 days is due to maximal stimulation by endogenous catecholines. This interpretation is supported by the observations that the rate of PC secretion increases with gestational age, is further enhanced by labor, and is decreased by propranolol in fetuses delivered by oxytocin-induced labor. Thus, the available data suggest that the adrenergic response is similar in fetal and adult lung.

Table 8.2 summarizes the response of cultured type II cells (adult lung) and lung slices (fetal) to various agents. Secretion of PC is stimulated by various

Table 8. 2. Release of PC from lung cells in culture. Results are from studies with isolated type II cells from adult rat lung (Dobbs and Mason 1979; Brown and Longmore 1981; Mettler et al. 1981; Rice et al. 1984; Gilfillan and Rooney 1985), and/or from slices of lung from newborn rabbit lung as noted (Marino and Rooney 1980; Marino and Rooney 1981)

Stimulate	Decrease[a]	No effect
Epinephrine	Colchicine	Propanolol
Isoproterenol	Cytochalasin B	Pilocarpine
Terbutaline[b]	Indomethacin	Carbamylcholine
Phenylephrine	Flufenamic acid	Methacholine
	Propanolol	Acetylcholine
		Dibutyryl–cGMP
Isobutylmethylxanthine		Dibromo–cGMP
Dibutyryl–cAMP		
Dibromo–cAMP		
Tetradecanoyl phorbol acetate		
Calcium ionophore[b] (A23187)		
PGE_2[a]		
Arachadonic acid		
Cytochalasins A, B, C, D		

[a] Data from newborn lung slices only
[b] Data from both newborn lung and isolated type II cells

β-adrenergic agonists, by phosphodiesterase inhibitor, and by analogs of cAMP. The effect of phenylepherine, primarily an α-agonist, appears to be through the β-receptor, as judged by the high dose required and inhibition by propranolol. Lung cells also respond to tetradecanoyl phorbol acetate, a secretagogue of unknown mechanism in other tissues. In fetal lung, at least, secretion is stimulated by the calcium ionophor A23187 and by PGE_2, and decreased with inhibitors of prostaglandin synthesis and agents which disrupt microtubules and microfilaments; these effects have not been fully characterized. By contrast, no effect has been observed with analogs of cGMP, nor with cholinergic agents. Acetylcholine did increase cGMP and this effect was inhibited by atropine, suggesting that cholinergic receptors were present and functional. Although pilocarpine increased surfactant release in vivo, this is thought to be secondary to stimulation of catecholamine release. However, Brown and Longmore (1981) observed a stimulatory effect of pilocarpine in the isolated perfused lung. Unlike the observation in vivo, the β-adrenergic antagonist alprenolol did not block the effect of pilocarpine in the perfused lung whereas atropine was inhibitory as expected. It must also be noted that negative effects in isolated type II cells could result from alterations during cell preparation. Isolation by enzymatic treatment could alter membrane receptors, and there is disruption of cell polarity and cell-cell interaction which could be involved in hormonal responsiveness.

In summary, the evidence from both in vivo and culture experiments indicates that exogenous adrenergic agonists both stimulate surfactant release and enhance the rate of phospholipid synthesis in type II cells. Secretion is stimulated before enhanced synthesis can be detected, indicating that release is not secondary to accumulation of surfactant within type II cells. It is possible that secretion is a stimulus for surfactant synthesis. Both effects are mediated through adenylate cyclase and can be mimicked by treatment with analogs of cAMP. The dose-response characteristics, stereoselectivity, and inhibition by propranolol indicate that the responses are mediated through β-adrenergic receptor. The studies with isolated type II cells establish that catecholamines are acting directly on these cells to influence surfactant secretion. The next two sections discuss the other observed effect of adrenergic agonists (reabsorption of pulmonary fluid) and the separate question of whether endogenous catecholamines regulate surfactant release and fluid dynamics during normal development and birth.

8.1.2 Fluid Reabsorption

8.1.2.1 Fluid Dynamics

During fetal life the lung is a secretory organ. The fluid produced by the respiratory epithelium is characterized by a high concentration of chloride, low protein content, and a developmental increase in potassium concentration. Lung fluid is not a simple dialysate of plasma, but rather a specialized secretion which is transported into alveolar spaces by an active chloride ion pump. In the fetal lamb, lung liquid is formed at a rate of 2–5 ml/h/kg, and occupies a volume approximately equal to the functional residual capacity. The rate of fluid production is constant through the last 20 % of gestation in the lamb until several days prior to spontaneous delivery. At this time, the production rate decreases and reabsorption begins. Removal of fluid from the lung at birth happens over a period of several hours and occurs primarily through the vascular rather than the lymphatic system (Faure-Fremiet and Dragoiu 1923; Avery 1961; Aherne and Dawkins 1964; Humphreys et al. 1967; Adamson et al. 1969; Olver and Strang 1974; Mescher et al. 1975; Kitterman et al. 1979; Bland et al. 1980, 1982).

The physiologic mechanisms regulating lung fluid secretion and reabsorption are not fully understood. In preparation for birth and breathing, fluid production needs to be "switched off" and reabsorption initiated. Presumably, reabsorption continues through adult life to maintain relatively fluid-free airways. There is now convincing evidence that administration of catecholamines to the fetus near term will alter lung fluid dynamics, mimicking the changes which normally occur just prior to birth. The following section summarizes data obtained in the fetal rabbit and lamb treated with β-adrenergic agonists.

8.1.2.2 Treatment with Catecholamines in Vivo

The first demonstration of adrenergic influence on fetal lung fluid was made in fetal rabbits (Enhorning et al. 1977). Isoxsuprine (0.5 mg) was administered to rabbit fetuses on day 28 of gestation and the animals were studied 4 h later. Fetal lung fluid was collected through a tracheal catheter and lung weight was recorded. The data presented in Table 8.3 indicate that significantly less fluid was recovered from isoxsuprine-treated fetuses, and that these fetuses had a lower lung weight/body weight ratio than control animals. These results are consistent with dehydration of the fetal lung within 4 h after exposure to isoxsuprine. Comparable results were obtained in a subsequent study using maternal treatment with isoxsuprine for 4 h (Enhorning et al. 1979). Bergman et al. (1980) treated rabbit fetuses with terbutaline and delivered the animals 3 h later. Compared with control littermates, there was a 65 % reduction in the quantity of lung fluid which could be obtained through a tracheal catheter evacuated with a negative pressure of 5 cm H_2O. Some animals were also observed for up to 2 h after birth and wet lung weight/body weight ratios were determined. As shown in Fig. 8.6, control pups had about a 25 % decrease in this ratio over the first 60 min after birth. Pups treated with terbutaline in utero had values at birth equivalent to the steady state value reached later by con-

Table 8.3. Effects of Isoxsuprine treatment on lung fluid of the fetal rabbit (Enhorning et al. 1977). Mean ± SE values for 73 isoxsuprine-treated (0.5 mg) and 64 saline-treated fetuses who received injections in utero 4 h prior to delivery at 28 days gestation

Measurement	Isoxsuprine-treated	Saline-treated	p
Body weight (g)	32.8 ± 0.5	31.9 ± 0.6	NS
Lung fluid recovered (mg)	63 ± 7	161 ± 7	0.001
Lung weight (mg) (less lung fluid)	811 ± 20	910 ± 23	0.001
Lung weight/body weight ($\times 10^4$)	264 ± 6	331 ± 5	0.001

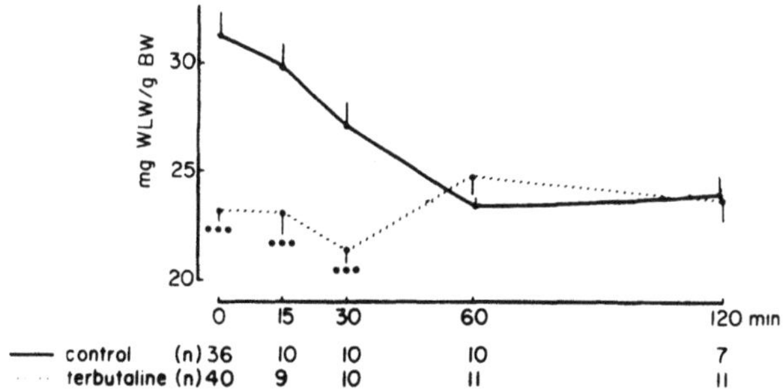

Fig. 8.6. Effect of terbutaline on lung fluid content of fetal rabbits after birth. Fetuses of 28 days gestation received 0.1 mg terbutaline or saline (control) in utero 3 h before delivery. At various times after birth the fluid content was estimated by determination of wet lung weight (WLW) per g body weight (BW). Values are mean ± SE; ***, $p < 0.001$. Data from Bergman et al. (1980), by permission

trol animals, indicating precocious clearance of lung fluid. By contrast, Kanjanapone et al. (1980) detected no effect of maternal isoxsuprine treatment for 24 h on the wet lung weight/body weight ratio of fetal rabbits. However, these studies were performed at 26 days gestation rather than 28 days and maternal treatment was used. Either or both of these differences in experimental protocol may have contributed to the difference in results.

The most complete description of in vivo catecholamine effects on lung fluid come from the studies by Walters and Olver (1978), and Brown et al. (1983). In these experiments, fetal sheep at 120–148 days gestation were used for in utero measurements of lung fluid secretion and reabsorption. Radiolabeled albumin was introduced into the fetal lung via a tracheal catheter, and aliquots of fluid were subsequently removed to determine rates of production and/or reabsorption. The effects of intravenous infusion of catecholamines in

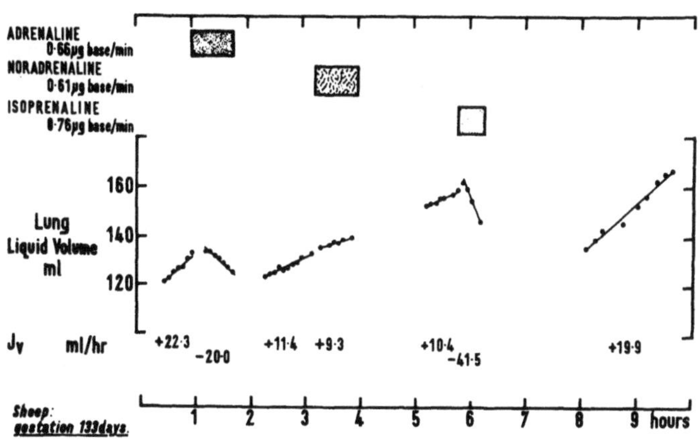

Fig. 8.7. Effect of catecholamines on fluid flux in a fetal lamb. Changes in lung fluid volume were obtained with and without intravenous infusion of catecholamines. Positive J_V values indicate fluid secretion and negative values reflect absorption. Data from Walters and Olver (1978), by permission

this experimental preparation are illustrated in Fig. 8.7. Infusion of epinephrine or isoproterenol produced a prompt and reversible resorption of lung fluid. At 120–130 days, the usual response was slower fluid secretion, whereas after 130 days absorption occurred (Table 8.4). Administration of norepinephrine at a similar concentration had little effect on the rate of fluid production. In fetuses that received a (relatively large) loading dose of propranolol (4 mg), the effect of isoproterenol and epinephrine was blocked. Propranolol alone did not affect flux of lung fluid. Comparable results of epinephrine infusions (3.3 μg/min) on fluid flow of fetal lambs were reported by Lawson et al. (1978).

A particularly interesting finding of Brown et al. (1983) was the influence of gestational age; responsiveness to epinephrine (0.5 μg/min) increased exponentially between 122 days gestation and term (Table 8.4). Based on dose-response studies, this change is due, at least in part, to a developmental increase in the sensitivity of fluid secretion/absorption to catecholamines. The data in Table 8.4 show a 10-fold increase in sensitivity during the last week of gestation. The apparent discrepancy between the timing for enhanced responsiveness to epinephrine infusion at 0.5 μg/min (prior to 140 days) and increased sensitivity to epinephrine (primarily occurring after 140 days – Table 8.4, last column) may relate to the occurrence of preterm labor (with accelerated maturation) among lambs of the first group. A similar change in responsiveness to isoproterenol was noted in fetuses who delivered prematurely at 132–137 days. The increase in catecholamine sensitivity before both preterm and term delivery is strikingly similar to the pattern for plasma concentrations of fetal cortisol. A causal relationship between cortisol and sensitivity to catecholamine is suggested by the finding that glucocorticoids induce β-adrenergic receptors (discussed in Sect. 8.2.3).

Although the site of action of catecholamines has not been determined by

Table 8.4. Effect of epinephrine infusion on secretion and absorption of lung fluid in the fetal lamb. Secretion rate of lung fluid was determined in fetuses before (control) and after infusion of epinephrine; the response increases with gestational age. In separate experiments, the response to various doses of infused epinephrine (0.1-1.0 μg/min) was used to calculate the sensitivity to epinephrine (last column). Data from Brown et al. (1983)

Gestational age		n	Secretion rate (ml/h)			Plasma epinephrine concetration to induce zero flow (ng/ml)
Range	Mean		Control	Epinephrine infusion (0.5 μg/min)	Change	
120-124	122.8 ± 0.5	9	11.7 ± 1.0	6.5 ± 0.6	5.2 ± 0.9	-
125-129	127.1 ± 0.4	12	13.2 ± 1.3	4.5 ± 1.0	8.6 ± 1.1	-
130-134	131.5 ± 0.4	10	17.3 ± 2.0	−1.3 ± 2.4	18.6 ± 1.6	
132-134	133.5 ± 0.2	11	-	-	-	0.43
135-139	136.2 ± 0.5	11	17.0 ± 1.5	−9.2 ± 3.3	26.2 ± 3.3	
135-137	135.9 ± 0.3	11	-	-	-	0.49
138-140	138.8 ± 0.3	10	-	-	-	0.28
≧ 140	141.8 ± 0.8	4	10.3 ± 2.8	−17.9 ± 4.8	28.2 ± 5.3	
	145.5 ± 0.9	4	-	-	-	0.029

these in vivo experiments, there is a strong suggestion that the β-agonists are acting at the level of the respiratory epithelium. Changes in pulmonary blood flow with catecholamine treatment could influence fluid flux, but other observations do not support this possible mechanism of action (Walters and Olver 1978). Catecholamines may affect the chloride pump mechanism responsible for lung fluid production. Action at this site might decrease fluid production and also allow reabsorption to occur by passive diffusion down the protein osmotic pressure gradient (Olver and Strang 1974). Alternatively, catecholamines may stimulate active reabsorption by the respiratory epithelium. This hypothesis is supported by the description of lumenal to basal transport of electrolytes and fluid by isolated type II cells (following section) and by additional data from the fetal lamb. In these studies, the electrical potential difference across the pulmonary epithelium (lung lumen vs. blood) became more negative with epinephrine infusion. Furthermore, amiloride, which blocks sodium on the apical aspect of cells and thereby inhibits sodium pump activity on the basolateral aspect, blocked the effect of epinephrine on fluid reabsorption in lungs of fetal lambs (Olver et al. 1981).

8.1.2.3 Studies in Isolated Cells

Recent investigations with alveolar type II cells indicate the presence of an active ion transport mechanism which drives fluid from the apical side of cells to their basal side. A visually striking demonstration of this process is the formation of domes by primary cultures of type II cells (Mason et al. 1982; Goodman et al. 1982). In these experiments, type II cells isolated from adult rat lung are grown in culture on dishes coated with extracellular matrix. After the cells flatten and become confluent (with formation of tight junctions), raised areas of approximately 1 mm diameter appear over the culture surface. Formation of such domes is generally thought to result from active fluid transport and accumulation of fluid beneath the layer of cells. For example, epithelial cells that transport fluid in vivo (e.g., kidney, mammary gland, colon, trachea, and choroid plexus) form domes in monolayer culture (Lever 1979; Handler et al. 1980). Other data with the cultured type II cells support this interpretation. There is a transepithelial potential difference with the apical surface negative with respect to the basolateral surface. Furthermore, amiloride abolished the potential difference when it was added to the apical side, but not when it was added to the basal side (Mason et al. 1982). The potential difference across the cells was increased by addition of terbutaline (10 µM). Extrapolation of these results to the situation in vivo is complicated by the dedifferentiation (loss of lamellar bodies and decreased content of saturated PC and phosphatidylglycerol) of type II cells during culture; this process may reflect formation of type I cells such as occurs in vivo after lung injury.

Studies with isolated type II cells (adult rat) in suspension confirm the presence of an active Na^+-K^+ pump which contributes to the electronegativity of the membrane potential (Jones et al. 1982; Castranova et al. 1983). Recently, ion transport has been examined in type II cells isolated from fetal and adult rabbits (Bland and Boyd 1984a,b,c) and adult rat (Gallo et al. 1984). Active uptake of rubidium was demonstrated, indicating extrusion of $3\,Na^+$ in exchange for $2\,K^+$. Cation exchange appeared to be activated by labor, and the rate of rubidium uptake by rabbit cells increased over time postnatally. The possible effects of adrenergic agonists in fetal cells remain to be examined. In type II cells of adult rat, the electrical potential across the plasma membrane, as estimated by Rb^+ distribution, is -63 mV which is similar to values in other secretory cells. Preliminary data indicate that there is a rapid and dose-dependent hyperpolarization induced by adrenergic agonists (Finkelstein et al. 1984). This suggests a possible biochemical association between transmembrane flux of ions, water, and surfactant.

Thus, several types of studies with isolated cells support the concept that there is reabsorption of fluid by alveolar epithelial cells. Type II cells may be a major site in the lung for active fluid transport, although the possible involvement of type I cells, which comprise a large proportion of alveolar surface area, has not been determined. It is likely that the effects of adrenergic agonists on fluid transport are mediated, at least in part, through stimulation of sodium transport by type II cells.

8.1.3 Physiologic Relevance

The effects of administered catecholamines on surfactant release and fluid absorption suggest that endogenous epinephrine and norepinephrine influence these processes during normal development. Although the precise role and involvement of endogenous catecholamines in preparing the lung for birth is not yet certain, several lines of evidence support this possibility.

8.1.3.1 Experimental Approaches

In the studies of Walters and Olver (1978) and Brown et al. (1983), epinephrine was infused at rates of 0.1–3.0 μg/min. These rates are within the range for endogenous epinephrine secretion from adrenals of fetal lambs exposed to asphyxia or splanchnic nerve stimulation, and are similar to the basal secretion rate of the newborn lamb (Comline and Silver 1961; Comline et al. 1965; Comline and Silver 1966). In addition, plasma concentrations of infused epinephrine are comparable to those found for endogenous epinephrine during spontaneous labor and delivery. In the latter situation, a highly significant negative correlation was found between fluid flux and the log of plasma epinephrine ($r = 0.81$, $p < 0.001$). Both the slope of the response curve and the concentration of endogenous epinephrine inducing zero fluid flow (~0.11 ng/ml) agree closely with results in animals receiving epinephrine infusion (Table 8.4). These findings indicate that fluid transport is sensitive to catecholamines at physiologic (stress) concentrations and are consistent with a causal relationship. Information on the effect of adrenergic blockade during spontaneous labor in this preparation would be of considerable interest.

In the fetal rabbit, the adrenal content of catecholamines increases severalfold during late gestation. The concentration of phenylethanolamine N-methyltransferase (PNMT), the final enzyme in epinephrine biosynthesis, also rises and is a likely explanation for increasing epinephrine content. The content of norepinephrine in fetal lung also increases markedly during late fetal and early postnatal life in the rat and rabbit, and PNMT activity has been identified in ovine fetal lung. This enzyme has different chromatographic and pharmacologic properties from the adrenal enzyme, but specific activity increases several-fold during the third trimester; possible responsiveness to glucocorticoids has not been examined (Padbury et al. 1981; Tordet et al. 1981; Padbury et al. 1983a; Padbury et al. 1983b). Thus, the fetal lung is exposed to increasing production of catecholamines by both the adrenal medulla and pulmonary sympathetic ganglia.

Two different experimental approaches have been utilized to evaluate the role of endogenous catecholamines in lung differentiation. Padbury et al. (1984) administered SKF-29661, an inhibitor of adrenal PNMT, to pregnant rabbits during the last trimester. At a dose of 50–100 mg/kg/day, the fetal adrenal content of epinephrine and PC in lung lavage were reduced by 57 % and 40 %, respectively, compared to controls. There was a positive correlation between epinephrine content and alveolar PC (r = 0.45). These results suggest that epinephrine of adrenal origin contributes to the regulation of surfactant release during fetal life.

An alternative approach to blocking endogenous adrenergic influence is treatment of fetal rabbits with the irreversible β-adrenergic antagonist (bromacyl-(1,8)diamino-β-menthone alprenolol) (BRALP). This compound binds covalently to β-adrenergic receptors with a relatively high affinity, thus blocking interaction with adrenergic agonists. MacDonald et al. (1985) injected fetuses at 28-days gestation and studied the pups 2-3 days later. At the doses of antagonist used ($\geqq$ 30 mg/kg), binding sites on fetal lung membranes were reduced by >50 % with only a small change in K_D (attributed to residual BRALP). Receptor blockade decreased (~30 %) the phospholipid content in lung lavage of 30 day fetuses delivered by cesarean section and prevented the increase associated with labor (vaginal delivery) (Fig. 8.8). Both control and treated pups showed the expected increase in lavage phospholipid after air

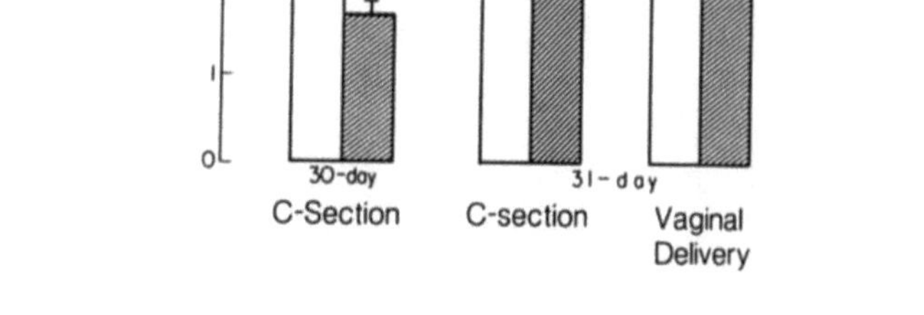

Fig. 8.8. Effect of treatment with irreversible β-adrenergic antagonist on the phospholipid content of lung lavage. Rabbit fetuses received an intraperitoneal injection of the β-antagonist BRALP (30 mg/kg) *(hatched bar)* or diluent *(open bar)* on day 28 of gestation. After delivery on day 30 or 31, tracheal lavage was performed with cold saline and the phospholipid content was determined. The concentration of available β-adrenergic receptor in treated lungs was <50 % of that in control animals. Mean ± SE values; * = $P < 0.05$. Data from MacDonald et al. (1985)

breathing consistent with results after propranolol treatment (Corbet 1981). Treatment did not affect fetal weight, lung weight or lung PC synthesis and content, indicating a specific effect of receptor blockade on surfactant release vs. synthesis. Surprisingly, treatment did not alter the amount of fetal lung fluid at birth or the postnatal rate of clearance.

8.1.3.2 Labor and Birth

Early studies on lung fluid concluded that clearance of fluid begins at birth (Aherne and Dawkins 1964; Adams et al. 1971). Subsequent work has established that this process starts before delivery and is apparently associated with the initiation of labor. In fetal sheep, the rate of fluid flow from the trachea decreases during the 2–3 days before delivery (Mescher et al. 1975; Kitterman et al. 1979). Lung lymph collected from fetal lambs becomes more dilute during labor, consistent with some reabsorption of fluid through lymphatics (Bland et al. 1982). In their study with fetal lambs during labor and delivery, Brown et al. (1983) found that reabsorption of lung fluid began in the hour before delivery; absorption continued after birth at an even greater rate. This change in fluid flux correlated closely with the concentration of epinephrine in fetal plasma. Other investigators have confirmed the responsiveness of the fetal adrenal medulla to stress (Comline et al. 1965) and a prepartum increase of catecholamines in the fetal lamb, although the exact timing of this rise is disputed (Jones 1980; Eliot et al. 1981; Brown et al. 1983).

In the rabbit, birth and air breathing are associated with increasing concentrations of alveolar surfactant and dehydration of the lungs (Gluck et al. 1967; Taeusch et al. 1974; Bland et al. 1980; Bergman et al. 1980). It is now evident, however, that these processes are initiated prior to birth. Rabbit pups delivered at term by cesarean section after oxytocin-induced labor versus delivery

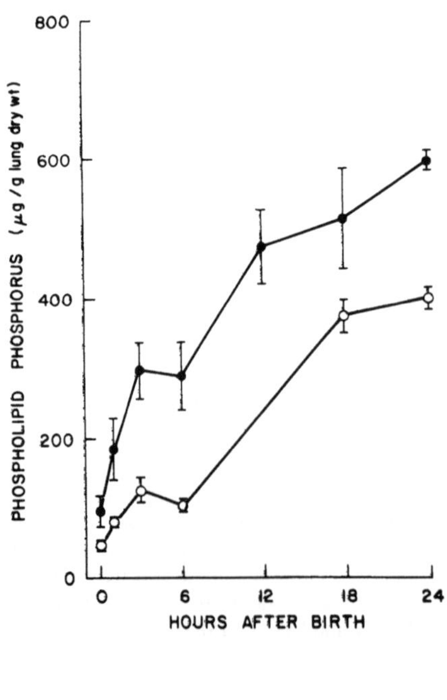

Fig. 8.9. Effect of labor on phospholipid content in lung lavage of newborn rabbits. Animals were delivered by cesarean section before *(open circles)* or after onset of oxytocin-induced labor *(closed circles)*. Mean ± SE values for 4–6 pups assessed at various times after birth. Data from Rooney et al. (1977), by permission

before labor, had substantially greater phospholipid content of lung lavage (Fig. 8.9). In these experiments, delivery took place within 15 min after administration of oxytocin, indicating a rapid effect of labor and/or oxytocin. Although plasma catecholamines were not determined, it is likely that they would be elevated under these circumstances. Bland et al. (1979) carried out similar experiments in rabbits to examine lung water content. Rabbit pups delivered after oxytocin-induced labor, whether by cesarean or vaginal delivery, had less extravascular lung water content (per g dry lung tissue) than animals which never experienced labor. The prepartum water loss associated with labor represented 38 % of the total fluid loss occurring during the first day of life in pups delivered without labor (Bland et al. 1980). The plasma protein concentration was increased in pups exposed to labor, and a similar increase occurs with spontaneous labor in fetal sheep (Ballard et al. 1982). Although the possible role of catecholamines in this hemoconcentration is only speculative, the increase in oncotic pressure may contribute to the process of fluid clearance from airways before birth.

8.1.3.3 Clinical Observations

A relationship between labor, endogenous catecholamines, and lung maturity apparently extends to the human infant. As reviewed recently by Olver (1981), there is general agreement that the incidence of RDS is greater among infants delivered by cesarean section, particularly before onset of labor, than those delivered vaginally. Cesarean section delivery is also associated with lower lung volumes than occurs with vaginal delivery. Thus, delivery without benefit of labor is apparently associated with greater lung immaturity with regard to both surfactant concentration and volume of lung fluid, increasing the risk for both RDS and transient tachypnea of the newborn.

At birth, plasma concentrations of norepinephrine greatly exceed those for epinephrine; levels of both hormones are greater in the umbilical artery than vein, indicating production by the fetus. There is a wide range in catecholamine concentrations observed at birth; most values are many-fold higher than in the adult and day-old infant. Catecholamine levels in fetal scalp blood samples increase during the second stage of labor and are elevated further at both preterm and term delivery by fetal distress producing acidosis; this response to intrapartum asphyxia increases with gestational age (Lagercrantz and Bistoletti 1977; Nylund et al. 1979; Eliot et al. 1980; Lagercrantz et al. 1981; Artal et al. 1982; Padbury et al. 1982; Bistoletti et al. 1983; Newnham et al. 1984). Cord arterial concentrations of epinephrine are similar in infants from vaginal and cesarean section deliveries when the mothers have labored (Eliot et al. 1980). However, in some studies, elective cesarean section without labor has been associated with lower levels of catecholamines in cord blood at birth (Irestedt et al. 1982; Falconer and Lake 1982). Intermittent fetal hypoxemia, occurring with fetal distress or normally with active labor, may be a stimulus to catecholamine release from sympathetic nerves and the adrenal medulla.

Catecholamines and their metabolites can be detected in amniotic fluid during human pregnancy, and concentrations increase with gestational age (Woodman et al. 1978; Artal et al. 1979; Lagercrantz et al. 1980; Artal et al. 1982; Divers et al. 1982). Levels of amniotic fluid free metanephrine, the

0-methylated metabolite of catecholamine, were higher in patients near term who were in labor compared to those without labor (Artal et al. 1979). The ratio of 4-hydroxy-3-methyoxyphenyl glycol (HMPG) to 4-hydroxy-3-methoxymandelic acid (VMA), which possibly reflects fetal:maternal catecholamine metabolism, was higher in amniotic fluid of 7 growth retarded infants (Lagercrantz et al. 1980). At 37 weeks gestation in diabetic pregnancies, both the L/S ratio and occurrence of phosphatidylglycerol in amniotic fluid were greater in patients with a normal amniotic fluid metanephrine concentration compared with patients having a low concentration. These results were interpreted as evidence for delayed sympatho-adrenal maturation in the diabetic pregnancy (Artal et al. 1982). Divers et al. (1982) determined amniotic fluid concentrations of epinephrine, norepinephrine, and 3,4-dihydroxyphenoglycerol, a norepinephrine metabolite. Patients with phosphatidylglycerol present in amniotic fluid had higher concentrations of each compound than a group of patients without phosphatidylglycerol of similar gestational age.

These several observations indicate a relationship between concentrations of amniotic fluid catecholamine and lung maturation in both normal and abnormal pregnancies. Since amniotic fluid catecholamines are felt to be primarily of fetal origin (Zuspan 1974), a role for the fetal adrenosympathetic system is suggested. It is perhaps not surprising that catecholamine levels were higher in complicated pregnancies. Such pregnancies undoubtedly represent a chronically stressful condition for the fetus which would stimulate both the adrenal cortex and medulla.

Several reports have appeared regarding the possible effect of β-sympathomimetic treatment, given to inhibit premature labor, on lung maturity. A low incidence of RDS is described for premature infants exposed to maternal treatment with isoxsuprine, ritodrine and terbutaline (Table 8.5). The possible significance of these reports is difficult to determine. None of the studies involved randomized, double-blind treatment of patients with tocolytics and with one exception the control population is either absent or poorly defined. The duration of treatment before delivery, likely an important factor, has not been controlled or analyzed. These reports have also not involved large numbers of infants at high risk for RDS (i.e., less than 30 weeks gestation). Despite these shortcomings, there is the suggestion of less RDS with prenatal exposure to a β-mimetic drug.

One study reports a decreased incidence of RDS and improved 7-day survival rate in premature infants whose mothers received aminophyllin (250 mg every 12 h) prior to delivery (Hadjigeorgiou et al. 1979). However, there are apparent discrepancies among data reported in the paper for the gestational age of treated and untreated groups, and the remarkable similarities of some of the mean values has been pointed out (Mortimer 1981). Further studies, prospective in design and suitably controlled, are required to establish and define possible benefits of both β-mimetics and aminophyllin for premature infants.

Other effects of β-mimetic therapy have been noted in mothers and infants. Wallace and Herrick (1981) reported no consistent rise in the amniotic fluid L/S ratio of 8 patients treated with terbutaline for 2–7 days. With longer treatment using fenoterol (greater than 7 days I. V. or greater than 14 days oral)

Table 8.5. Literature reports regarding maternal β-mimetic treatment and RDS in premature infants

Authors	Type of study	Drug	Dose and duration of treatment	Number of infants (treated/untreated)	Gestational age range	Incidence (%) of RDS (treated/untreated)
Kero et al. 1973	Retrospective	Isoxsuprine	Not stated	26/0	28–36	0/–
	Prospective without controls	Isoxsuprine	80 mg IV daily for 1–2 days	12/0	28–32	0/–
Boog et al. 1975	Retrospective; concurrent controls	Ritodrine	Not stated	20/18	25–36	25/67
Hastwell 1977	Retrospective	Salbutamol	8 mg q 6 h for >2 days	77/0	Not stated	3/–
Bergmann & Hedner 1978	Prospective; concurrent controls	Terbutaline	5–10 mg/day for <1 to >32 days	24/17	30–36	4/29
Brazy & Pupkin 1979	Retrospective; concurrent controls	Isoxsuprine	0.5 mg/min IV within 48 h of delivery	43/107	26–35	26/20
Curet et al. 1984	Control population (without premature rupture of membranes) of corticosteroid trial	Isoxsuprine	Not stated	61/35	30–34	9.8/28.6

substantially lower levels of amniotic fluid PC were found compared with untreated women (Dudenhausen et al. 1978). This finding, if confirmed, indicates a potentially adverse effect of prolonged adrenergic therapy on fetal surfactant production which is perhaps analagous to the observation in fetal rabbits (Ekelund et al. 1983). During 4 days of ritodrine therapy for premature labor, maternal levels of plasma ACTH decreased transiently but there was no change in concentrations of cortisol and prolactin. At term, a 30 min infusion of isoxsuprine (150 μg/min) or fenoterol (3 μg/min) did not affect either maternal or cord levels of ACTH, cortisol, or prolactin (Kauppila et al. 1981). Congestive heart failure with pulmonary edema has occurred in women receiving high doses of intravenous β-mimetic drug (Robertson et al. 1981). Finally, the outcome of premature infants exposed to maternal isoxsuprine within 48 h of delivery was reported by Brazy and Pupkin (1979). Compared with an untreated group of infants of the same gestational age range (26–31 wk), there was no difference in incidence of RDS (55 % vs. 50 %), but treatment was associated with an increased incidence of ileus and hypotension. At two years of age, treated and untreated groups had similar scores on mental and psychomotor testing (Brazy et al. 1983).

8.2 Receptor

Catecholamines, of both endogenous and synthetic origin, exert their physiologic and pharmacologic effects through interaction with receptors on plasma membranes of responsive cells. Earlier pharmacological studies, examining the potency and inhibitory activity of agonists and antagonists, indicated the existence of various types of adrenergic receptors. These subtypes have been designated α_1, α_2, β_1, and β_2 receptors. Since 1974, an enormous volume of information about these receptors has been generated by ligand-binding studies. A variety of radiolabeled agonists and antagonists has been developed, and binding properties of receptors have been characterized in intact cells, isolated membranes, and soluble preparations. More recently, research has been di-

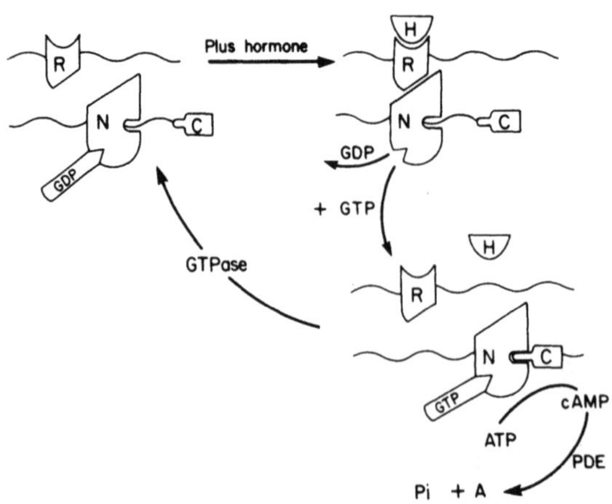

Fig. 8.10. Model of the β-adrenergic receptor-adenylate cyclase complex. The scheme is discussed in the text. Abbreviations: *R*, receptor; *H*, hormone (β-agonist); *N*, N-protein (regulatory protein); *C*, catalytic component of adenylate cyclase; *PDE*, phosphodiesterase. From Roberts (1981), by permission

rected toward studies of receptor-effector coupling, regulation of receptor number, and purification of receptor.

Of the many types of hormone receptors which are membrane-bound, few have received more attention than the β-adrenergic receptor. These receptors are widely distributed among tissues and species, mediate a diverse number of physiologic responses, and are involved in the therapy of certain human illnesses. The β-adrenergic receptor has been purified from several sources in recent years; a single subunit peptide of approximately 58,000–62,000 molecular weight has both the binding site and the capacity to couple in vitro with adenylate cyclase (Cerione et al. 1983).

Considerable effort has been directed toward understanding how the β-adrenergic receptor interacts with the adenylate cyclase system. The current model for this process is depicted in Fig. 8.10. In addition to receptor, the components of the hormone-responsive system include the catalytic moiety of adenylate cyclase, the nucleotide regulatory protein (N) and guanyl-nucleotides. Receptor resides in the outer plasma membrane and N-protein is localized to the inner region where it has access to the catalytic unit of adenylate cyclase. The N-protein is capable of activating the catalytic subunit only when complexed with GTP. In the absence of hormone, N-protein is inactive and occupied by GDP. Interaction of hormone with receptor increases the affinity of receptor for N-protein and binding occurs. This interaction reduces the affinity of N-protein for GDP, and it is replaced by GTP which is present in high concentrations intracellularly. This change in guanyl-nucleotide produces two results: 1) the affinity of N-protein for catalytic subunit is increased, the enzyme is activated, and production of cAMP from ATP occurs; 2) the affinity of hormone for receptor and receptor for N-protein decreases and there is dissociation of the complex. The activation of the catalytic subunits is reversed by the action of GTPase which hydrolyzes GTP to GDP, and cAMP is inactivated by the action of phosphodiesterase. Cholera toxin, which prevents hydrolysis of GTP, produces both irreversible activation of adenylate cyclase and prolonged stimulation, (e.g., intestinal secretion). Recent reviews of β-adrenergic receptors and coupling to adenylate cyclase include articles by Roberts (1981), Motulsky and Insel (1982), and Lefkowitz et al. (1983).

The effect of adrenergic stimulation on airway smooth muscle is well known, and β-adrenergic receptors have been described in adult lung tissue. More recently, information about adrenergic effects on surfactant and fluid flux in fetal lung has stimulated studies of adrenergic binding in fetal and neonatal tissue. The following discussion reviews the binding properties, ontogeny, and regulation of β-adrenergic receptors in perinatal lung tissue.

8.2.1 Binding Properties

Pulmonary β-adrenergic receptors have been investigated using either [^{3}H]dihydroalprenolol (DHA) or ^{125}[I]iodohydroxybenzylpindolol (HYP), potent β-antagonists, as ligand. Binding reactions are usually carried out with a lung particulate preparation (washed membrane fraction) prepared by homogenization and centrifugation. Assays are performed at either 30 or 37 °C followed by a rapid filtration through glass fiber filters to separate free and bound hormone. Nonspecific binding is assessed by addition of an access of nonlabeled β-agonist or by computer-assisted curve fitting of data for total binding. Adrenergic binding has been studied in fetal and neonatal lung of the rabbit (Cheng et al. 1980; Giannopoulos 1980; Whitsett et al. 1981a; Padbury et al. 1981; Giannopoulos and Sommers-Smith 1982), rat (Whitsett et al. 1980; Whitsett et al. 1981b; Whitsett et al. 1982a; Whitsett et al. 1982b), and human (Roberts et al. 1985).

Binding of radioligands to lung particulate preparations is rapid, saturable, of high affinity, and reversible. The K_D for DHA binding is 0.8–2.5 nM in rabbit tissue and 0.4–0.9 in rat. A value of 0.2–0.4 nM is reported for HYP binding in rabbit tissue. These values are consistent with results in other target tissues, including the adult lung. The binding of both agonists and antagonists exhibits the expected stereoselectivity, and Scatchard analysis of dose-response data indicates a single class of high affinity binding sites. The relative ability of adrenergic agonists to compete for binding sites in fetal lung is: $(-)$ isoproterenol $>$ $(-)$ epinephrine $\sim$ $(-)$ norepinephrine in rabbit lung and isoproterenol $>$ epinephrine $>$ norepinephrine in rat tissue. These results are consistent with primarily β_1-adrenergic binding in the rabbit and predominantly β_2-binding in rat lung. Equivalent results are reported in adult rabbit and rat lung where the relative distribution of β_1 and β_2 receptor subtypes is approximately 4:1 and 1:4, respectively (Lefkowitz et al. 1983).

Beta-adrenergic receptors have also been identified in membrane preparations from fetal human lung (Roberts et al. 1985). In tissue at 16–20 weeks gestation, the K_D for DHA binding was approximately 0.4 nM and the receptor concentration about 35 fmol/mg protein. Similar to adult lung, the predominant subtype in the fetus is β_2.

8.2.2 Cellular Distribution

The studies described above assayed binding in membrane fractions prepared from whole lung tissue. The question of whether receptors are present on alveolar type II cells has been investigated by two different experimental approaches. Barnes et al. (1982) developed an experimental system to localize binding sites by radioautography in frozen sections of tissue. In this procedure, frozen sections of tissue are mounted on glass slides, warmed and reacted with radio-labeled ligand, washed to remove unbound radioactivity, and subsequently analyzed by radioautography. Adjacent sections of tissue were used for assessment of nonspecific binding and light microscopy. The validity of this approach was established by experiments measuring binding parameters by direct isotopic counting rather than radioautography.

Figure 8.11 shows representative sections of lung from both fetal and adult rabbit which were incubated with [^{3}H]DHA. The distribution of silver grains clearly outlines alveoli, and the density appears greater than over bronchioles. Labeling is considerably greater in adult than fetal tissue, consistent with binding data using membrane preparations. In each specimen binding of labeled ligand was eliminated by the presence of propranolol. After exposure to betamethasone in vivo for 24 h, more labeling is observed. By grain count, there was a significant increase in density over alveoli with corticosteroid ther-

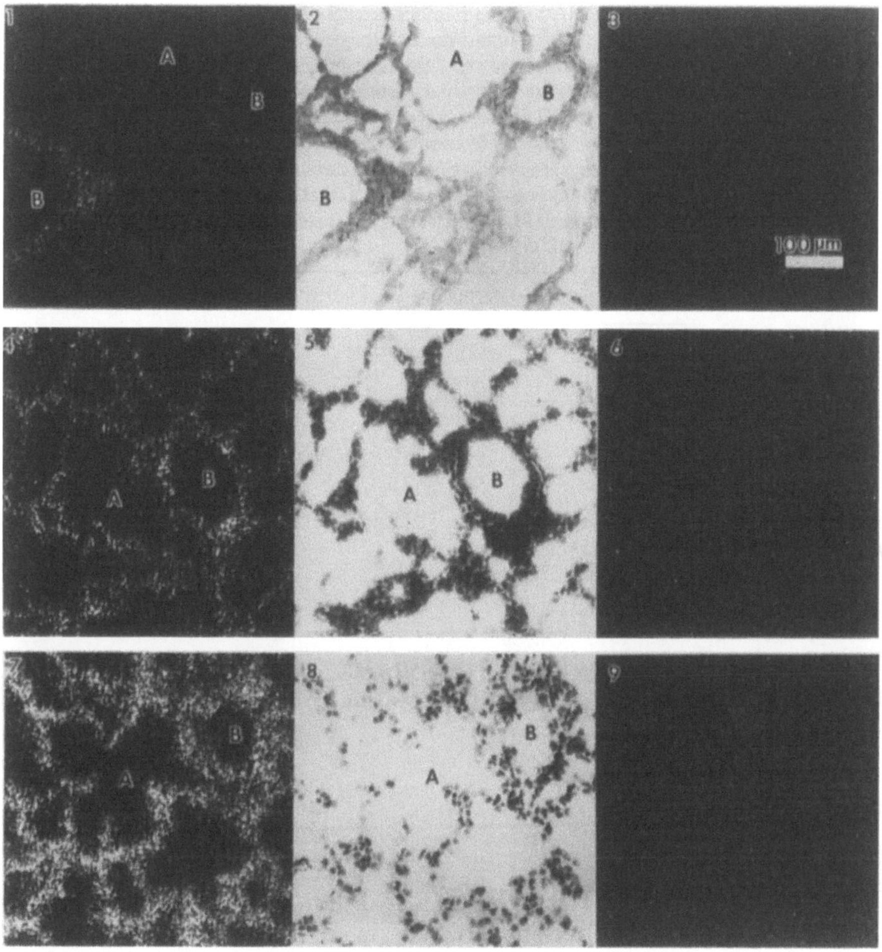

Fig. 8.11. Radioautography of [^{3}H]DHA binding in rabbit lung. Frozen sections of fetal and adult tissue were incubated with [^{3}H]DHA in the presence *(right)* and absence *(left)* of propranolol and exposed to photographic emulsion for 3 months. Adjacent sections of lung were stained with hemotoxylin-eosin *(middle)* and are shown for comparison. *1–3* Day 26, control; *4–6* day 26, treated; *7–9* adult, control. Treated fetuses were exposed to maternal betamethasone (0.15 mg/kg) 24 h prior to the binding studies on day 26 of gestation. *A*, alveoli; *B*, bronchiole. From Barnes et al. (1984), by permission

apy, but no change for bronchioles or myocardium (Table 8.6). The uniformly high concentration of DHA binding along the alveolus probably indicates the presence of β-adrenergic receptor on both type I and type II cells. Demonstration of β-adrenergic binding in alveolar epithelial cells of adult lung by radioautography has been recently confirmed (Smith and Sidhu 1984; Gatto et al. 1984; Conner and Reid 1984).

An alternative approach has been the study of isolated type II cells. Preliminary studies have identified specific adrenergic binding in populations of type II cells prepared from adult rat (Roberts et al. 1985) and from both fetal and adult rabbit (Sommers-Smith and Giannopoulos 1983). Further data are

Table 8.6. Grain counts of [^{3}H]DHA binding in autoradiographs of fetal and adult rabbit lung. Specific grain counts were determined by counting total silver grains/1000 μm^2 tissue area and subtracting non-specific counts in the same area of adjacent sections which were exposed to propranolol. Data shown are mean ± SD of three areas from three separate slides in two animals. By two-way analysis of variance counts were significantly higher over airways than over alveoli in both fetal and adult tissue ($p < 0.001$), counts in adult lung were greater than in fetal, and betamethasone treatment (0.15 mg/kg, 24 h) significantly increased counts over alveoli. Data from Barnes et al. (1984)

	Specific grain counts/1000 μm^2		P
	Control	Corticosteroid treated	
26–day fetal			
Alveoli	18.5 ± 3.8	39.2 ± 8.5	<0.001
Airways	43.4 ± 7.2	54.2 ± 6.8	NS
Heart	61.2 ± 10.5	56.7 ± 10.3	NS
Adult			
Alveoli	162.7 ± 27.5		
Airways	228.7 ± 23.5		

needed to establish the relative concentration of binding sites in these cells versus other cell types of the lung.

8.2.3 Concentration

8.2.3.1 Ontogeny

The concentration of β-adrenergic receptor in lung tissue has been examined during development of the rabbit (Cheng et al. 1980; Giannopoulos 1980; Whitsett et al. 1981a; Padbury et al 1981) and rat (Whitsett et al 1981b; Whitsett et al. 1982a; Whitsett et al. 1982b; Whitsett et al. 1983; Maniscalco and Shapiro 1983). In both species there is a progressive increase in receptor during both fetal and postnatal life. Figure 8.12 presents representative data for these two species. Compared with the third trimester fetus, the lung of adult animals contains 5- to 10-fold greater concentration of receptor expressed as specifically bound ligand per mg protein in a washed membrane preparation. A developmental increase in receptor was also demonstrated when binding to membranes was expressed per lung or per mg of lung (Whitsett et al. 1982b; Maniscalco and Shapiro 1983). However, in one study (Whitsett et al. 1982a), receptor concentration appeared to decrease during postnatal development of the rat when binding was carried out in crude homogenate and expressed per g of lung or protein. These results raise the possibility, albeit unlikely, that the developmental increase observed in membrane preparations represents increased recovery of membranes which are relatively enriched in receptor compared with other proteins. This interpretation would imply a developmental change in receptor location or grouping on cellular membranes rather than an increase in total number of binding sites per cell.

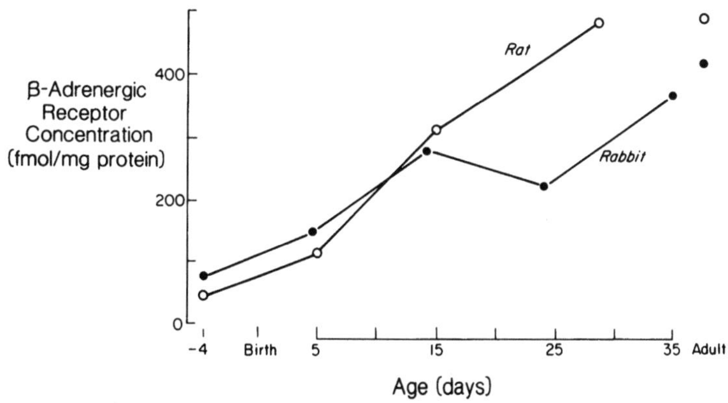

Fig. 8.12. Ontogeny of β-adrenergic receptor in rat and rabbit. Maximal binding capacity for [^{3}H] DHA was determined in washed membrane preparations from lung of fetal and postnatal animals. Data from Whitsett et al. (1980, 1981a, 1982a, b)

The striking increase in receptor concentration of fetal lung during late gestation is apparently tissue specific. Compared with a nearly 4-fold increase in binding sites of lung, receptor concentration doubled in the heart and did not change in the brain (Maniscalco and Shapiro 1983).

The developmental pattern for α-adrenergic and β-adrenergic receptors has been compared in rat lung (Whitsett et al. 1982b). The concentration of α-adrenergic receptors, as measured by binding of [^{3}H]-prazosin, doubled between day 18 in the fetus and postnatal day 15 when the adult level was achieved. This ontogenic pattern is quite different from that observed for β-adrenergic binding (Fig. 8.12). It is proposed that the increase in α-adrenergic binding reflects increased postsynaptic receptors during the perinatal period when sympathetic innervation is occurring.

8.2.3.2 Hormonal Influence

The possibility that glucocorticoids influence β-adrenergic receptors of fetal lung was investigated by Cheng et al. (1980). They injected pregnant rabbits with betamethasone on day 25 of pregnancy. After 24 h, the fetuses were obtained and binding of [^{3}H]-DHA was determined in membrane preparations. Compared with controls, this treatment increased the concentration of β-adrenergic receptors by 76 %, as shown in Fig. 8.13. There was no effect on the K_D which was 0.78 and 0.96 nM in control and treated fetuses, respectively. In the same groups of animals, there was no difference in the concentration of DHA binding sites in fetal heart tissue. Recent autoradiographic studies indicate that glucocorticoids preferentially increase β-receptors in alveoli (Table 8.6).

The stimulatory effect of glucocorticoids on adrenergic receptors has been confirmed in subsequent studies using cultured tissue (Giannopoulos and Sommers-Smith 1982; Maniscalco and Shapiro 1983; Roberts et al. 1985). Representative data are presented in Table 8.7. In these experiments, explants of fetal rat or rabbit lung were cultured in serum-free medium. Addition of dex-

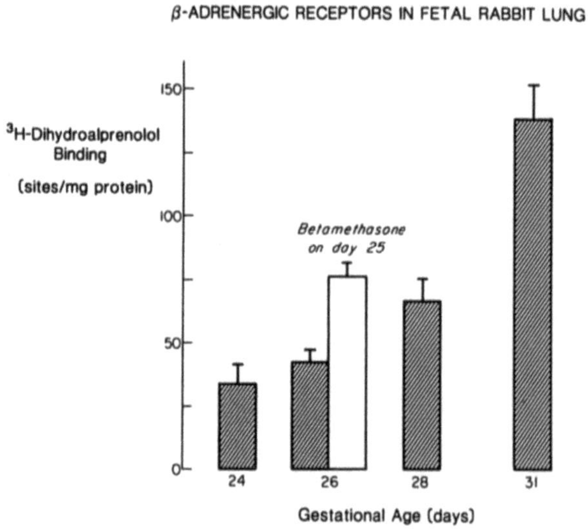

Fig. 8.13. Ontogeny of β-adrenergic receptor concentration in fetal rabbit lung and effect of betamethasone. Values are mean ± SE for binding capacity of untreated *(shaded)* and betamethasonetreated (0.17 mg/kg to mother at 25 days gestation, *open bar*) fetuses. Data of Cheng et al. (1980). From Ballard (1983), by permission

amethasone produced a 60–120% increase in receptor concentration within 24–48 h. An optimal response occurred with 100 nM steroid and the effect was greatly reduced in the presence of 50 μM cycloheximide. Glucocorticoids did not affect the K_D for $[^{125}I]$-HYP binding (Giannopoulos and Sommers-Smith 1982), but appeared to increase the K_D of DHA binding in rat lung (Maniscalco and Shapiro 1983). It is also noteworthy that this effect of glucocorticoid occurred in the absence of other exogenous hormones. By contrast, T_3 (10^{-7} M) did not alter the concentration of binding sites. These results indicate that glucocorticoids act directly in fetal lung tissue to increase receptor concentration. Insofar as they have been investigated, the properties of this effect are consistent with a glucocorticoid receptor-mediated process involving new synthesis of adrenergic receptor.

Table 8.7. Dexamethasone stimulation of β-adrenergic receptors in cultured lung. Lung of 25-day fetal rabbit and 19-day fetal rat were cultured in serum-free medium for 2-3 days with or without dexamethasone (1-10 μM). Beta-adrenergic binding was assayed with $[^{125}I]$HYP (rabbit) and $[^{3}H]$DHA (rat) as described by Giannopoulos and Sommers-Smith (1982) and Maniscalco and Shapiro (1983), respectively

	Binding sites (fmol/mg protein)		KD (nM)	
	Rabbit	Rat	Rabbit	Rat
Control	40.2 ± 2.9	63.2 ± 5.0	0.24 ± 0.03	0.43 ± 0.08
Dexamethasone	65.4 ± 2.1[a]	138.0 ± 8.8[a]	0.21 ± 0.03	0.85 ± 0.07[a]

[a] $p < 0.05$ vs. control

Glucocorticoids have also been shown to influence β-adrenergic receptors in other systems (reviewed recently by Davies and Lefkowitz 1984). Mano et al. (1979) found that 9 days treatment with hydrocortisone increased the concentration of receptors in rat lung by 70 %. Adrenalectomy decreased the concentration by about 30 %, and this change was prevented by administration of hydrocortisone. In human subjects, a single I.V. dose of methylprednisolone (2 mg/kg) did not affect β-adrenergic receptor concentration in lymphocytes isolated 16 h later. However, the same treatment did increase receptor number in asthmatic patients with a depressed number of receptors secondary to chronic terbutaline therapy (Hui et al. 1982). By contrast, Davies and Lefkowitz (1980) found an increase in both adrenergic receptor density and adenylate cyclase activity of human neutrophils 4 h after in vivo administration of cortisone, and Cotecchia and De Blasi (1984) report increased binding of DHA in lymphocytes exposed to hydrocortisone (time unspecified) in vitro.

The study of Fraser and Ventner (1980) is of particular interest with regard to the mechanism of the glucocorticoid effect. These workers used lines of both normal and SV-40 transformed human embryonic lung cells maintained in culture. These cells bind [^{125}I]-HYP with properties characteristic of β-adrenergic receptor. Exposure of these lung cells to hydrocortisone for 24 h produced a doubling in maximal HYP-binding with no change in receptor affinity. This response was dose-dependent with a half-maximal effect at approximately 0.3 μM; this relatively high value may reflect metabolism of cortisol to cortisone. The rate of receptor synthesis was examined by exposing the cells to an irreversible β-adrenergic antagonist which almost completely inactivates existing receptors. The appearance of new receptors was then determined by the development of HYP binding sites during further incubation. Pre-exposure of cells to hydrocortisone resulted in an approximate doubling of the rate of new receptor appearance.

In contrast with these findings in lung tissue and cultured lung cells, binding sites for HYP in rat liver increases after adrenalectomy in animals without replacement cortisone therapy (Wolfe et al. 1976). In 3 T 3-L_1 cells which are induced to differentiate into adipocytes, dexamethasone increases the number of β-adrenergic receptors and also promotes a switch in receptor subtype from β_1 to β_2 (Lai et al. 1982). Glucocorticoids may also influence the interaction between adrenergic receptor and the N-protein. Davies and Lefkowitz (1981) have utilized computer assisted techniques for estimating the relative amounts of low affinity and high affinity binding of agonists in isolated membranes. In experiments with neutrophils from 4 subjects, it was found that in vivo exposure to cortisone acetate (4 h) resulted in 80 % of the receptors in the high affinity state versus 66 % in the controls. A similar change in low and high affinity binding was observed after 4 h incubation of isolated neutrophils with hydrocortisone sodium succinate at approximately 3 μM. Although the properties and mechanism of this effect of glucocorticoids are not yet defined, these observations suggest a possible glucocorticoid-induced alteration of the N-protein. An increase in the proportion of high affinity state receptor should increase adenylate cyclase activity, and this effect was indeed observed after in vivo cortisone treatment. Studies are in progress with fetal lung to determine whether corticosteroids influence coupling of receptor to N-protein and cyclase as well as increasing receptor number. A combined effect would further increase the sensitivity of fetal lung to adrenergic stimulation.

Thyroid hormones are known to influence adrenergic receptors in myocardial cells of the rat (Williams et al. 1977; Tsai and Chen 1978; Scarpace and Abrass 1981). The possible role of these hormones in postnatal development of lung adrenergic receptor was investigated by Whitsett et al. (1980, 1982a). Rats were rendered hypothyroid by propylthiouracil (PTU) treatment both in utero and postnatally, and adrenergic binding by lung membranes was assayed during the first month postnatally. PTU treatment did not affect the concentration of receptors at 5 and 15 days of age compared with controls and hypothyroid pups treated with T_4. By 28 days, however, receptor concentration was low in hypothyroid animals but was increased after 3 days prior treatment with T_4. In adult animals, treatment with PTU did not alter receptor concentration, and, in a separate study, administration of T_3 did not affect receptor levels in lung while binding sites in the heart increased 60% (Scarpace and Abrass 1981). During fetal life, prenatal PTU treatment does not prevent the normal developmental increase in receptors (Whitsett et al. 1982a), and binding capacity is unaffected by treatment with either DIMIT in vivo (Cheng et al. 1980) or T_3 in cultured fetal lung (Giannopoulos and Sommers-Smith 1982). The specificity of the postnatal thyroid hormone influence observed by Whitsett et al. (1980), and its possible physiologic relevance, remain to be defined. It will be of interest, for example, to know whether such an effect is independent of endogenous corticosterone.

In many tissues, the concentration of adrenergic receptors is decreased by exposure to agonists (down regulation). Although it is likely that a similar form of regulation occurs in fetal lung, there is little information on this point.

8.2.3.3 Effect of Gender

The sex differences in lung maturation and responsiveness to corticosteroids (discussed in Chaps. 2, 3 and 5) prompted similar comparisons of the adrenergic system. Padbury et al. (1981) found slightly higher concentrations of adrenergic receptor (13–22%) in lungs of female versus male rabbits during the perinatal period. No difference was noted for the K_D of DHA binding. This finding has not been confirmed by subsequent studies (J. M. Roberts, personal communication; M. B. Jones, personal communication; Giannopoulos and Sommers-Smith 1982). The physiologic significance of a possibly small difference between sexes in adrenergic receptor number is not certain. In addition, Padbury et al. (1981; 1983a) found somewhat higher concentrations of adrenal epinephrine and PNMT in female versus male fetuses. They propose that the relative delay in development of the adrenal medulla may relate to the slower pulmonary maturation in the male.

8.2.4 Coupling to Adenylate Cyclase

The initial effect of the binding of β-adrenergic agonists by receptor is activation of the membrane-bound enzyme adenylate cyclase. This results in formation of intracellular cAMP which serves as a second messenger of adrenergic stimulation (Fig. 8.11). In many target tissues, cAMP has been shown to activate cAMP-dependent protein kinases, intracellular enzymes which catalyze phosphorylation of specific proteins.

As previously discussed in Sect. 8.1.1.2, β-adrenergic stimulation of adult Type II cells increases cAMP; derivatives of cAMP, but not of cGMP, mimic the effects of β-agonists on release of surfactant. As in other responsive systems, the maximal increase in cAMP occurs within minutes (see Fig. 8.5), preceding the biologic response. It has been proposed that phosphorylation of structural proteins (e.g., actin) within the cell cytoskeleton by cAMP-dependent protein kinases is part of the mechanism for surfactant release following adrenergic stimulation (Whitsett and Lessard 1984).

Involvement of cAMP with adrenergic stimulation of *fetal* lung is less well documented. Cyclase activity in fetal lung was first described by Barrett et al. (1974). They found a relatively high level of activity in lung homogenates from fetal rabbits compared with adult animals. Fluoride stimulated activity in lungs from late but not early third trimester fetuses, and there was an increasing response to epinephrine during the last week (from approximately 10–50 %). Subsequent studies have confirmed and extended these findings (Whitsett et al. 1981a, b, 1982a, 1983; J. M. Roberts, personal communication). In rat as well as rabbit, the basal concentration of adenylate cyclase activity in crude lung homogenate is high in fetal tissue compared with adult lung (Table 8.8). Addition of GTP or Gpp (NH) p, a nonhydrolyzable guanine nucleotide analog, enhanced cyclase activity in homogenates of both species. Although percent stimulation by isoproternol increases with age in both species the absolute stimulated level decreases in rat lung but does not change in the rabbit. There is a parallel rise in percent stimulation by NaF with development in the rat.

Whitsett et al. (1983a) found a different developmental pattern for cyclase activity using washed membrane preparations from rat lung. Basal activity with fetal and adult membranes were 53 and 37 pmol/mg/min, respectively, as compared with values of 130 and 25 using crude homogenate (Table 8.8). The high basal activity of fetal homogenates is apparently due in part to the presence of GTP and macromolecular GTP-like activity in cytosol of fetal and neonatal lung. These endogenous compounds, which are present in homogenates but not washed membranes, activate adenylate cyclase.

A distinctly different developmental pattern for adenylate cyclase has been reported by Nijjar (1979a, b) and Chaudhary and Nijjar (1984). In these studies basal activity increased several-fold in both homogenates and particulate preparations between birth and adulthood and was enhanced in the fetus by dexamethasone treatment. Stimulation by norepinephrine (30 μM) and by fluoride was maximal shortly after birth and not observed in adult tissue and GTP did not stimulate activity in membranes at any age. The level of cyclase activity was considerably lower than reported by other investigators, suggesting important differences in assay systems.

Production of cAMP has also been examined in intact lung cells in vitro (Palmer 1972). In 2 mm cubes of tissue in culture medium, β-adrenergic agonists increased cAMP content 10- to 15-fold within 6 min. Isoproterenol and epinephrine were maximally effective at ~0.1 and 10 μM, respectively,

Table 8.8. Adenylate cyclase activity in lung homogenate of rat and rabbit according to Whitsett et al. (1981a; 1981b). Adenylate cyclase activity was determined in crude homogenates in the absence of guanyl nucleotide and with or without isoproterenol (0.5 μM). Values are mean ± SD

	Basal activity (pmol/mg/min)		Stimulation by isoproterenol (%)	
	Rat	Rabbit	Rat	Rabbit
Fetal	130.1 ± 11.2	93.8 ± 12.8	21 ± 6	23 ± 14
Infant	101.0 ± 9.9	61.3 ± 3.0	29 ± 12	66 ± 10
Adult	25.4 ± 6.7	39.8 ± 18.5	71 ± 20	199 ± 38

and stimulation was reduced by propranolol. Basal rates of cAMP synthesis decreased somewhat between the perinatal period and adulthood, but not to the same extent as found for cyclase activity in homogenates (Table 8.8). At all pre- and postnatal ages studied, epinephrine stimulated cAMP to adult levels.

The high basal levels of cyclase activity in homogenates of fetal lung, and the meager response to catecholamine stimulation, implies that there is a developmental change in coupling of receptor and enzyme. However, the data of Palmer (1972) suggest that this change is observed only after cell disruption, which is consistent with the responsiveness of fetal lung to catecholamines in vivo. Further studies are needed to determine the type of developmental alterations occurring in homogenate and membrane preparations and whether these changes are reflected in cAMP generation upon catecholamine stimulation of intact lung cells.

A possible explanation for the decreased ability of agonists to stimulate adenylate cyclase in homogenates of fetal tissue is offered by recent studies of *β*-adrenergic binding (Roberts et al. 1985). In lung of fetal rabbit, agonist competition for ^{3}H-DHA binding to receptor indicates decreased formation of high affinity complex compared with adult tissue. This situation is apparently not due to defects in the N-protein, since reconstitution experiments with mutants of S-49 cells indicate normal function. Until this system is more fully investigated, one must be cautious in relating *β*-adrenergic receptor number with responsiveness to catecholamine.

The developmental changes observed for the adrenergic system of lung are not unique to this tissue. In a study of adenylate cyclase in hemolysates, enzyme activity was approximately twice as high in cells prepared from adult frogs compared with tadpoles. Catecholamines stimulated cAMP formation in frog hemolysate, but under the same conditions had no effect in tadpole hemolysate (Rosen and Rosen 1968). In a study with tissues from three human fetuses (12–13 week), cyclase activity was detected in homogenates of a variety of tissues. Activity in heart and liver homogenates was stimulated by epinephrine; however, there was no response to catecholamine with skeletal muscle and lung tissue (Menon et al. 1973). The adenylate cyclase system has been described in some detail during development of the rabbit heart (Schumacher et al. 1982). The basal activity of membrane preparations was somewhat greater in the fetus than the adult. The maximal response to isoproterenol was several-fold greater with adult tissue than with newborn or fetal heart; the concentration for half-maximal stimulation was lower for fetal vs. adult heart. In contrast with these developmental differences for stimulation of cyclase activity in membranes, newborn and adult hearts (isolated, perfused) did not differ in the dose-response relationship for isoproterenol induced contractility. In rat parotid gland, both adenylate cyclase activity and secretion are relatively insensitive to isoproterenol for the first two weeks postnatally, after which time responsiveness rapidly reaches adult levels. Receptor levels do not correlate with the increase in hormone sensitivity, but there is a temporal increase in the amount of N-protein as assayed by ADP-ribosylation in the presence of cholera toxin (Ludford and Talamo 1983). In 3T3-L1 cells prior to differentiation, adenylate cyclase is very sensitive to GTP and this response is increased little by β-agonist. However, after differentiation, the response to GTP decreases and adenylate cyclase requires β-adrenergic stimulation for expression (Lai et al. 1982). These examples indicate that responsiveness of adenylate cyclase to catecholamine stimulation in vitro changes during development in a number of tissues.

The sites of developmental modifications in hormone action are still unresolved. The list of possibilities includes changes in receptor concentration or structure, concentration and isoforms of N-protein, interaction between receptor and N-protein related to either the proteins per se or the membrane phospholipid environment, and changes in the adenylate cyclase system. With regard to the cyclase enzyme, a developmental increase in lung cytoplasmic activators has been reported (Nijjar 1979a; Nijjar et al. 1981). Finally, the relationship between responsiveness of the adenylate cyclase and functional response remains to be fully defined.

Subsequent steps in the cAMP system have been examined in rat lung by Whitsett et al. (1983b). Properties of both cAMP binding to regulatory subunits of cAMP-dependent protein kinase(s) and the kinase activity of catalytic subunits were similar to those in other systems. cAMP binding and cAMP-stimulated protein kinase activity were present in lung cytosol at all times in development (fetal to adult). A variety of protein substrates for cAMP-stimulated phosphorylation were found by radioautography and gel electrophoresis; the major proteins had molecular weights of 28,000, 44,000, 56,000, 97,000, 240,000 and 260,000 daltons. Ontogenic changes in certain of these protein substrates for protein kinase were observed. These findings suggest that some developmental changes in hormone effects in the lung may be mediated by the pattern of protein phosphorylation in response to cAMP.

8.3 Conclusions and Perspectives

Treatment with β-adrenergic agonists stimulates surfactant secretion and fluid reabsorption, two important processes in fetal lung maturation. The effect on surfactant release occurs rapidly, and is mediated through adrenergic receptor and accumulation of cAMP. Likewise, adrenergic stimulation of water reabsorption, as characterized in the fetal sheep, demonstrates the properties expected of a receptor-mediated event. The response is rapid, reversible, occurs with physiologic concentrations of catecholamines, and is inhibited by propranolol. Fluid reabsorption occurs, at least in part, as a result of increased active transport of sodium across alveolar epithelial cells in a lumenal to basal direction. The mechanism of catecholamine influence on this process is still largely unexplored and will no doubt be a fruitful area of research. Likewise, the intracellular mechanism of surfactant secretion, and its regulation by catecholamines, remains to be elucidated. There are other questions of obvious interest. Are the adrenergic effects on surfactant secretion and both ion and water transport separate or linked events in type II cells? Are there other effects of β-mimetics in the type II cell? Is increased secretion of surfactant a stimulus for increased synthesis? Are there effects of catecholamines on type I and other cell types in fetal lung?

The studies with administered β-adrenergic agonists generated the proposal that endogenous catecholamines are physiologically important in preparation for birth. According to this concept, a surge in circulating catecholamines during labor and birth prepares the lung for air breathing by stimulating both secretion of surfactant into alveolar spaces and reabsorption of water from these areas. This is an attractive hypothesis which is supported by several lines of evidence. First, adrenergic effects in fetal lung are mediated through receptor, indicating that physiologic rather than pharmacologic concentrations of catecholamine are sufficient to elicit responses. Secondly, the response to administered adrenergic agonist is rapid, which is consistent with a role for endogenous hormone during the relatively short time of labor and delivery. Third, endogenous catecholamines increase markedly during labor and delivery, and, in the fetal sheep there is a close association between circulating epinephrine concentrations and the rate of fluid reabsorption in the lung. Recent experimental approaches have involved either inhibiting catecholamine production by the fetal adrenal or blocking β-adrenergic receptors with an irreversible antagonist; both of these maneuvers reduce the amount of alveolar surfactant. Fourth, delivery of animals without exposure to labor, and presumably with a smaller increase in endogenous catecholamines, results in wetter lungs with less alveolar surfactant than in animals delivered after onset of labor. Finally, respiratory problems, including both RDS and retained lung fluid, are more common in infants delivered without labor than in those with labor. Despite this persuasive evidence, the relative contribution of endogenous catecholamines in preparing the lung for birth is not yet defined, and there are data suggesting differential adrenergic sensitivity for surfactant secretion vs. fluid clearance. Moreover, it is likely that other hormones and factors influence both surfactant secretion (e.g., prostaglandins) and fluid reabsorption (e.g., vasopressin) around the time of birth.

The possible influence of catecholamines in fetal lung earlier in gestation is largely unexplored. For example, do endogenous catecholamines influence the rate of surfactant secretion prior to onset of labor? Do they influence the rate of synthesis? Is the increase in receptor concentration during the third trimester reflected in increased sensitivity to endogenous hormone? The eventual answers to these and other questions, including the role of endogenous catecholamines at birth, probably await the development of experimental approaches which can specifically block the action of catecholamine in just the fetal lung.

The well documented effects of catecholamines in animals has suggested its potential usefulness as a clinical treatment. At present, however, benefit of prenatal β-adrenergic treatment for the premature human infant has not been established. There have been several clinical reports of decreased incidence of RDS with β-mimetic therapy, but multiple deficiencies in these studies preclude any firm conclusions. On the other hand, there are at least two reports that such therapy did not increase the L/S ratio of amniotic fluid. A critical aspect of this type of prophylactic treatment is the duration of exposure before birth. Based on results of the animal studies, a relatively brief exposure to β-agonist prior to birth should be sufficient to stimulate surfactant secretion and initiate fluid reabsorption. Longer exposures, such as frequently used clinically, may have adverse effects for the fetus. Alveolar surfactant may decrease, such as described in the rabbit, by depletion of intracellular stores and/or through down-regulation of the β-adrenergic receptor. On the other hand, chronic treatment with a β-mimetic might be a stimulus to the synthesis of phospholipids within type II cells. At present, the effect of catecholamines on surfactant synthesis is not well characterized, both as to mechanism and specificity for surfactant phospholipids. The possible use of adrenergic agonists for prevention of respiratory distress in the newborn is further complicated by the widespread use of these compounds as tocolytics. Currently, both the dose and duration of treatment are determined by the intensity of labor. Thus, until β-mimetics are replaced by other, more effective labor suppressants, adrenergic therapy cannot be tested in a standardized manner for its potential ability to improve the outcome for premature infants.

It is conceivable that therapy with catecholamines would be ineffective in infants delivered spontaneously after labor. In this circumstance, the rise in endogenous catecholamines with labor, fetal distress, and birth most likely are sufficient to optimally stimulate the fetal lung. A more likely application of adrenergic therapy, I believe, would be in both premature and term infants delivered by cesarean section before onset of labor. These infants have a higher incidence of respiratory distress, and presumably, they are exposed for only a relatively short period to elevated levels of endogenous catecholamines compared with infants delivered after labor. An alternative mode of therapy in this situation may be the methylxanthines, such as aminophylline. This drug stimulates surfactant secretion in animals, presumably via an increase in cAMP and stimulation of the same biochemical events as with β-adrenergic treatment. To date, however, there is insufficient data in both animals and humans on the action of aminophylline in the fetal lung. Before further clinical trials with either β-mimetics or aminophylline are undertaken, it will be helpful to generate more information in animal systems. In particular, studies of the dose and time effects of such therapy on both surfactant secretion and fluid absorption are needed. A useful experimental model in this regard might be the fetal lamb, where chronic measurements in utero and postnatal assessment after premature delivery is possible.

Beta-adrenergic receptor has been identified in fetal lung of every species examined. The increase in receptor concentration during development suggests that responsiveness of fetal lung to catecholamines is regulated in part at the level of membrane receptor. However, the developmental pattern of receptor concentration on type II cells is not yet known. There are also developmental changes in subsequent steps in the action of catecholamines. The basal levels of adenylate cyclase of lung membranes decrease with age, and the response to isoproterenol stimulation increases. Similar findings are recorded for other tissues, suggesting developmental alterations in the generation of cAMP may be a generalized biologic phenomenon. These observations have been made in membrane preparations, but appear not to hold true for studies with intact lung cells. If this difference is confirmed, it raises interesting questions regarding both the mechanism and physiologic significance of the developmental change. There is little information on the subsequent steps in the action of catecholamines in fetal type II cells. Future studies will need to explore cAMP-stimulated protein kinases, the proteins phosphorylated by these enzymes, and the relationship of such proteins to secretion and transport processes.

There are several levels of interaction between the β-adrenergic system and glucocorticoids in fetal lung. Glucocorticoid treatment increases the number of adrenergic binding sites and may also affect coupling between receptor and adenylate cyclase. The effect on receptor concentration is apparently mediated through glucocorticoid receptor with de novo synthesis of receptor protein. The mechanism of the glucocorticoid effect on coupling is still uncertain, but may involve modification or increased concentration of the N-protein. Both of these glucocorticoid effects enhance the sensitivity of the fetal lung to catecholamines. Thus, glucocorticoid treatment can be viewed as increasing both the synthesis of surfactant and the capacity for secretion in response to β-adrenergic agonists. Glucocorticoids also induce PNMT in fetal adrenal medulla. This increases concentrations of epinephrine and norepinephrine, which are available to act within the lung. Each of these effects of glucocorticoids represents accelerated maturation of normal developmental events, and as such, may be considered as physiologically relevant effects in preparing the fetus for birth. The role of endogenous corticosteroids in the normal developmental pattern for adrenergic receptor concentration and function has not been established. By analogy with the role of endogenous corticoids in other aspects of lung development (Chap. 4), it is likely that adrenergic receptor is also influenced by endogenous glucocorticoids. Additional studies involving both ablation procedures and maneuvers to precociously increase circulating corticoids will need to be performed.

References

Adams FH, Yanagisawa M, Kuzela D, Martinek H (1971) The disappearance of fetal lung fluid following birth. J Pediatr 78:837

Adamson TM, Boyd RDH, Platt HS, Strang LB (1969) Composition of alveolar liquid in the foetal lamb. J Physiol 204:159

Aeberhard EE, Scott ML, Barrett CT, Kaplan SA (1984) Effects of cyclic AMP analogues and

phosphodiesterase inhibitors on phospholipid biosynthesis in fetal type II pneumocytes. Biochim Biophys Acta 803:29
Aherne W, Dawkins MJR (1964) The removal of fluid from pulmonary airways after birth in the rabbit and the effect on this of prematurity and prenatal hypoxia. Biologia Neonat 7:214
Artal R, Hobel CJ, Lam R, Oddie TH, Fisher DA (1979) Free metanephrine in human amniotic fluid as an index of fetal sympathetic nervous system maturation. Am J Obstet Gynecol 133:452
Artal R, Platt LD, Kammula RK, Strassner HT, Gratacos J, Golde SH (1982) Sympathoadrenal activity in infants of diabetic mothers. Am J Obstet Gynecol 142:436
Avery ME (1961) Mechanics of respiration, in Normal and Abnormal Respiration in Children, 37th Ross Conference on Pediatric Research, p 15
Ballard PL, Kittermann JA, Bland RD, Clyman RI, Gluckman PD, Platzker CG, Kaplan SL, Grumbach MM (1982) Ontogeny and regulation of corticosteroid binding globulin capacity in plasma of fetal and newborn lambs. Endocrinology 110:359
Ballard PL (1983) Mode of action of glucocorticoids on lung maturation. In: The Cells of the Alveolar Unit. Curr Prob Clin Biochem 13:35
Barnes PJ, Basbaum CB, Nadel JA, Roberts JM (1982) Localization of β-adrenoreceptors in mammalian lung by light microscopic autoradiography. Nature 299:444
Barnes PJ, Jacobs MM, Roberts JM (1984) Glucocorticoids preferentially increase fetal alveolar beta-receptors: Autoradiographic evidence. Pediatr Res 18:1191
Barrett CT, Sevanian A, Kaplan SA (1974) Adenylate cyclase activity in immature rabbit lung. Pediatr Res 8:244
Barrett CT, Sevanian A, Lavin N, Kaplan SA (1976) Role of adenosine 3′, 5′-monophosphate in maturation of fetal lungs. Pediatr Res 10:621
Barrett CT, Sevanian A, Phelps DL, Gilden C, Kaplan SA (1978) Effects of cortisol and aminophylline upon survival, pulmonary mechanics, and secreted phosphatidyl choline of prematurely delivered rabbits. Pediatr Res 12:38
Bergman B, Hedner T (1978) Antepartum administration of terbutaline and the incidence of hyaline membrane disease in preterm infants. Acta Obstet Gynecol Scand 57:217
Bergman B, Hedner T, Lundborg P (1980) Pressure-volume relationship and fluid content in fetal rabbit lung after β-receptor-stimulating drugs. Pediatr Res 14:1067
Bergmann B (1981) Beta-mimetics and the preterm neonatal lung. An experimental and clinical study. Acta Physiol Scand Suppl 47:1
Bistoletti P, Nylund L, Lagercrantz H, Hjemdahl P, Strom H (1983) Fetal scalp catecholamines during labor. Am J Obstet Gynecol 147:785
Bland RD, Bressack MA, McMillan DD (1979) Labor decreases the lung water content of newborn rabbits. Am J Obstet Gynecol 134:364
Bland RD, McMillan DD, Bressack MA, Dong L (1980) Clearance of liquid from lungs of newborn rabbits. J Appl Physiol: Respirat Environ Exercise Physiol 49:171
Bland RD, Hansen TN, Haberkern CM, Bressack MA, Hazinski TA, Raj JU, Goldberg RB (1982) Lung fluid balance in lambs before and after birth. J Appl Physiol Respirat Environ Exercise Physiol 53:992
Bland RD, Boyd CAR (1984a) Birth activates cation exchange in rabbit lung epithelial cells. Fed Proc 43:1033 (abstract)
Bland RD, Boyd CAR (1984b) Effects of labor and air-breathing on cation exchange in lung epithelial cells of baby bunnies. Pediatr Res 18:386A (abstract)
Bland RD, Boyd CAR (1984c) Ion transport in rabbit lung epithelial cells. Clin Res 32:60A (abstract)
Boog G, Brahim MB, Gandar R (1975) Beta-mimetic drugs and possible prevention of respiratory distress syndrome. Br J Obstet Gynaecol 82:285
Brazy JE, Pupkin MJ (1979) Effects of maternal isoxsuprine administration on preterm infants. J Pediatr 94:444
Brazy JE, Eckerman CO, Gross SJ (1983) Follow-up of <1500 GM birth weight with antenatal isoxsuprine exposure. J Pediatr 102:611
Brown LA, Longmore WJ (1981) Adrenergic and cholinergic regulation of lung surfactant secretion in the isolated perfused rat lung and in the alveolar type II cell in culture. J Biol Chem 256:66
Brown MJ, Olver RE, Ramsden CA, Strang LB, Walters DV (1983) Effects of adrenaline and of

spontaneous labour on the secretion and absorption of lung liquid in the fetal lamb. J Physiol 344:137
Gastranova V, Jones GS, Miles PR (1983) Transmembrane potential of isolated rat alveolar type II cells. J Appl Physiol: Respirat Environ Exercise Physiol 54:1511
Cerione RA, Strulovici B, Benovic JL, Lefkowitz RJ, Caron MG (1983) Pure β-adrenergic receptor: the single polypeptide confers catecholamine responsiveness to adenylate cyclase. Nature 306:562
Chaudhary KC, Nijjar (1984) Effects of dexamethasone administration to pregnant rats on adenylate cyclase and cyclic AMP phosphodiesterase activities in the maternal and fetal lungs. Biol Neonate 45:188
Cheng JB, Goldfien A, Ballard PL, Roberts JM (1980) Glucocorticoids increase pulmonary β-adrenergic receptors in fetal rabbit. Endocrinology 107:1646
Comline RS, Silver M (1961) The release of adrenaline and noradrenaline from the adrenal glands of the foetal sheep. J Physiol 156:242
Comline RS, Silver IA, Silver M (1965) Factors responsible for the stimulation of the adrenal medulla during asphyxia in the foetal lamb. J Physiol 178:211
Comline RS, Silver M (1966) Development of activity in the adrenal medulla of the foetus and new-born animal. Br Med Bull 22:16
Conner MW, Reid LM (1984) Mapping of β-adrenergic receptors in rat lung: effect of isoproterenol. Exp Lung Res 6:91
Corbet AJS, Flax PK, Rudolph AJ (1976) Reduced surface tension in lungs of fetal rabbits injected with pilocarpine. J Appl Physiol 41:7
Corbet AJS, Flax PK, Rudolph AJ (1977) Role of autonomic nervous system controlling surface tension in fetal rabbit lungs. J Appl Physiol: Respirat Environ Exercise Physiol 43:1039
Corbet AJS, Flax P, Alstan C, Rudolph AJ (1978) Effects of aminophylline and dexamethasone on secretion of pulmonary surfactant in fetal rabbits. Pediatr Res 12:797
Corbet A (1981) Control of surfactant secretion in fetal and newborn rabbits. Prog Resp Res 15:78
Corbet A, Kolni H, Perreault T, Frink J, Rudolph J (1984) Development of sympathetic regulation of phospholipid secretion in fetal rabbit lung. Pediatr Res 18:136A (abstract)
Cotecchia S, De Blasi A (1984) Glucocorticoids increase β-adrenoreceptors on human intact lymphocytes in vitro. Life Sci 35:2359
Curet LB, Rao AV, Zachman RD, Morrison JC, Burkett G, Poole WK, Bauer C, Collaborative Group (1984) Association between ruptured membranes, tocolytic therapy, and respiratory distress syndrome. Am J Obstet Gynecol 148:263
Davies AO, Lefkowitz RJ (1980) Corticosteroid induced differential regulation of beta-adrenergic receptors in circulating human polymorphonuclear leukocytes and mononuclear leukocytes. J Clin Endocrinol Metab 51:599
Davies AO, Lefkowitz RJ (1981) Agonist-promoted high affinity state of the β-adrenergic receptor in human neutrophils: Modulation by corticosteroids. J Clin Endocrinol Metab 53:703
Davies AO, Lefkowitz RT (1984) Regulation of β-adrenergic receptors by steroid hormones. Ann Rev Physiol 46:119
Divers WA, Babaknia A, Hopper BR, Wilkes MM, Yen SSC (1982) Fetal lung maturation: amniotic fluid catecholamines, phospholipids, and cortisol. Am J Obstet Gynecol 142:440
Dobbs LG, Mason RJ (1979) Pulmonary alveolar type II cells isolated from rats. J Clin Invest 63:378
Dobbs LG, Mason RJ, Williams MC, Benson BJ, Sueishi K (1982) Secretion of surfactant by primary cultures of alveolar type II cells isolated from rats. Biochem Biophys Acta 713:118
Dudenhausen JW, Kynast G, Lange-Lindberg AM, Saling E (1978) Influence of long-term betamimetic therapy on the lecithin content of amniotic fluid. Gynecol Obstet Invest 9:205
Ekelund L, Burgoyne R, Brymer D, Enhorning G (1981) Pulmonary surfactant release in fetal rabbits as affected by terbutaline and aminophyllin. Scand J Clin Lab Invest 41:237
Ekelund L, Burgoyne R, Enhorning G (1983) Pulmonary sufactant release in fetal rabbits: immediate and delayed response to terbutaline. Am J Obstet Gynecol 147:437
Eliot RJ, Lam R, Leake RD, Hobel CJ, Fisher DA (1980) Plasma catecholamine concentrations in infants at birth and during the first 48 hours of life. J Pediatr 96:311
Eliot RJ, Klein AH, Glatz TH, Nathanielsz PW, Fisher DA (1981) Plasma norepinephrine, epinephrine, and dopamine concentrations in maternal and fetal sheep during spontaneous parturition and in premature sheep during cortisol-induced parturition. Endocrinology 108:1678

Enhorning G, Chamberlain D, Contreras C, Burgoyne R, Robertson B (1977) Isoxsuprine-induced release of pulmonary surfactant in the rabbit fetus. Am J Obstet Gynecol 129:197

Enhorning G, Chamberlain D, Contreras C, Burgoyne R, Robertson B (1979) Isoxsuprine infusion to the pregnant rabbit and its effect on fetal lung surfactant. Biol Neonate 35:43

Falconer AD, Lake DM (1982) Circumstances influencing umbilical-cord plasma catecholamines at delivery. Br J Obstet Gynaecol 89:44

Faridy EE (1976) Effect of distension on release of surfactant in excised dog's lungs. Respir Physiol 27:99

Faure-Fremiet E, Dragoiu J (1923) Le developpement du poumon foetal chez le mouton. Arch Anat Micro 19:411

Fedrick J, Butler NR (1972) Letter: Hyaline-membrane disease. Lancet ii:768

Finkelstein JN, Gallo RL, Notter RH, Shapiro DL (1984) Membrane potential responses of type II cells during surfactant secretion. Pediatr Res 18:391A (abstract)

Fraser CM, Venter JC (1980) The synthesis of β-adrenergic receptors in cultured human lung cells: Induction by glucocorticoids. Biochem Biophys Res Commun 94:390

Gallo RL, Finkelstein JN, Notter RH (1984) Characterization of the plasma and mitochondrial membrane potentials of alveolar type II cells by the use of ionic probes. Biochim Biophys Acta 771:217

Gatto C, Seybold V, Kulik T, Lock J, Johnson D (1984) Anatomic distribution and quantitative developmental changes in guinea pig pulmonary beta receptors. Pediatr Res:138A (abstract)

Giannopoulos G (1980) Identification and ontogeny of β-adrenergic receptors in fetal rabbit lung. Biochem Biophys Res Commun 95:388

Giannopoulos G, Sommers-Smith SK (1982) Hormonal regulation of β-adrenergic receptors in fetal rabbit lung in organ culture. Life Sci 31:795

Gilfillan AM, Rooney SA (1985) Arachadonic acid metabolites stimulate phosphatidylcholine secretion in primary cultures of type II pneumonocytes. Biochim Biophys Acta, 833:336

Gluck L, Motoyama EK, Smits HL, Kulovich MV (1967) The biochemical development of surface activity in mammalian lung. I. The surface-active phospholipids, the separation and distribution of surface-active lecithin in the lung of the developing rabbit fetus. Pediatr Res 1:237

Goldenberg VE, Buckingham S, Sommers SC (1969) Pilocarpine stimulation of granular pneumocyte secretion. Lab Invest 20:147

Goodman BE, Fleischer RS, Crandall ED (1982) Effects of metabolic inhibitors on dome formation by cultured alveolar epithelial cells. Fed Proc Am Soc Exp Biol 41:245 (abstract)

Gross I (1977) Nutritional and hormonal influences on lung phospholipid metabolism. Fed Proc, Fed Am Soc Exp Biol 36:2665

Gross I, Rooney SA (1977) Aminophylline stimulates the incorporation of choline into phospholipid in explants of fetal rat lung. Biochim Biophys Acta 488:263

Gross I, Wilson CM, Ingleson LD, Brehier A, Rooney SA (1980) Fetal lung in organ culture. III. Comparison of dexamethasone, thyroxine, and methylxanthines. J Appl Physiol: Respirat Environ Exercise Physiol 48:872

Hadjigeorgiou E, Kitsiou S, Psaroudakis A, Segos C, Nicolopoulos D, Kaskarelis D (1979) Antepartum aminophylline treatment for prevention of the respiratory distress syndrome in premature infants. Am J Obstet Gynecol 135:257

Hallman M (1977) Induction of surfactant phosphatidylglycerol in the lung of fetal and newborn rabbits by dibutyryl adenosine 3′:5′-monophosphate. Biochem Biophys Res Commun 77:1094

Handler JS, Perkins FM, Johnson JP (1980) Studies of renal cell function using cell culture techniques. Am J Physiol 238:Fl

Hastwell G (1977) Letter: Salbutamol and respiratory distress syndrome. Lancet ii:354

Hayden W, Olson EB, Zachman RD (1977) Effect of maternal isoxsuprine on fetal rabbit lung biochemical maturation. Am J Obstet Gynecol 129:691

Hildebran JN, Goerke J, Clements JA (1975) Air inflation releases phospholipids (PL) into the air-spaces of excised rat lungs. Fed Proc (abstract) 34:387

Hollingsworth M, Gilfillan AM (1984) The pharmacology of lung surfactant secretion. Pharmacol Rev 36:69

Hui KKP, Conolly ME, Tashkin DP (1982) Reversal of human lymphocyte β-adrenoceptor desensitization by glucocorticoids. Clin Pharmacol Ther 32:566

Humphreys PW, Normand ICS, Reynolds EOR, Strang LB (1967) Pulmonary lymph flow and the uptake of liquid from the lungs of the lamb at the start of breathing. J Physiol 193:1

Irestedt L, Lagercrantz H, Hjemdahl P, Hagnevik K, Belfrage P (1982) Fetal and maternal plasma catecholamine levels at elective cesarean section in general or epidural anesthesia versus vaginal delivery. Am J Obstet Gynecol 142:1004

Jones CT (1980) Circulating catecholamines in the fetus, their origin, actions and significance, In: Parvez H, Parvez S (eds), Biogenic Amines in Development, Elsevier/North-Holland Biomedical Press, pp 63–86

Jones GS, Miles PR, Lantz RC, Hinton DE, Castranova V (1982) Ionic content and regulation of cellular volume in rat alveolar type II cells. J Appl Physiol: Respirat Environ Exercise Physiol 53:258

Kanjanapone V, Hartig-Beecken I, Epstein MF (1980) Effect of isoxsuprine on fetal lung surfactant in rabbits. Pediatr Res 14:278

Karotkin EH, Kido M, Cashore WJ, Redding RA, Douglas WJ, Stern L, Oh W (1976) Acceleration of fetal lung maturation by aminophylline in pregnant rabbits. Pediatr Res 10:722

Kauppila A, Jouppila R, Moilanen K, Pakarinen A, Tuimala R (1981) Maternal, fetal and amniotic fluid ACTH, cortisol and prolactin in association with medical beta-adrenergic stimulation. Br J Obstet Gynaecol 88:1097

Kero P, Hirvonen T, Valimaki I (1973) Letter: Prenatal and postnatal isoxsuprine and respiratory distress syndrome Lancet 2:198

Kikkawa Y, Motoyama E, Gluck L (1968) Studies of the lungs of fetal and newborn rabbits: morphologic, biochemical and surface physical development. Am J Physiol 52:177

Kitterman JA, Ballard PL, Clements JA, Mescher EJ, Tooley WH (1979) Tracheal fluid in fetal lambs: spontaneous decrease prior to birth. J Appl Physiol: Respirat Environ Exercise Physiol 47:985

Lagercrantz H, Bistoletti P (1977) Catecholamine release in the newborn infant at birth. Pediatr Res 11:889

Lagercrantz H, Sjoquist B, Bremme K, Lunell N-O, Somell C (1980) Catecholamine metabolites in amniotic fluid as indicators of intrauterine stress. Am J Obstet Gynecol 136:1067

Lagercrantz H, Bistoletti P, Nylund L (1981) Sympathoadrenal activity in the foetus during delivery and at birth. In: Stern L, Salle B, Friis-Hansen B (eds), Intensive Care in the Newborn, Masson & Cie, New York, pp 1–12

Lai E, Rosen OM, Rubin CS (1982) Dexamethasone regulates the β-adrenergic receptor subtype expressed by 3T3-L1 preadipocytes and adipocytes. J Biol Chem 257:6691

Lawson EE, Brown ER, Torday JS, Madansky DL, Taeusch Jr HW (1978) The effect of epinephrine on tracheal fluid flow and surfactant efflux in fetal sheep. Am Rev Resp Dis 118:1023

Lefkowitz RJ, Stadel JM, Caron MG (1983) Adenylate cyclase-coupled beta-adrenergic receptors: Structure and mechanisms of activation and desensitization. Ann Rev Biochem 52:159

Lever JE (1979) Regulation of dome formation in differentiated epithelial cell cultures. J Supramol Struct 12:259

Ludford JM, Talamo BR (1983) Independent regulation of β-adrenergic receptor and nucleotide binding proteins of adenylate cyclase. J Biol Chem 258:4831

Maniscalco WM, Wilson CM, Gross I (1979) Influence on aminophylline and cyclic AMP on glycogen metabolism in fetal rat lung in organ culture. Pediatr Res 13:1319

Maniscalco WM, Shapiro DL (1983) Effects of dexamethasone on beta-adrenergic receptors in fetal lung explants. Pediatr Res 17:274

Mano K, Akbarzadeh A, Townley RG (1979) Effect of hydrocortisone on beta-adrenergic receptors in lung membranes. Life Sci 25:1925

Marino PA, Rooney SA (1980) Surfactant secretion in a newborn rabbit lung slice model. Biochim Biophys Acta 620:509

Marino PA, Rooney SA (1981) The effect of labor on surfactant secretion in newborn rabbit lung slices. Biochim Biophys Acta 664:389

Mason RJ, Williams MC, Widdicombe JH, Sanders MJ, Misfeldt DS, Berry Jr LC (1982) Transepithelial transport by pulmonary alveolar type II cells in primary culture. Proc Natl Acad Sci USA 79:6033

McDonald J V, Gonzales LK, Ballard PL, Roberts JM (1985) Role of β-adrenergic receptors and endogenous catecholamines in surfactant release but not lung water absorption in fetal rabbits. Pediatr Res 19:159A

Menon KMJ, Giese S, Jaffe RB (1973) Hormone- and fluroide-sensitive adenylate cyclases in human fetal tissues. Biochim Biophys Acta 304:203

Mescher EJ, Platzker CG, Ballard PL, Kitterman JA, Clements JA, Tooley WH (1975) Ontogeny of tracheal fluid, pulmonary surfactant, and plasma corticoids in the fetal lamb. J Appl Physiol 39:1017

Mescher EJ, Dobbs LG, Mason RJ (1983) Cholera toxin stimulates secretion of saturated phophatidylcholine and increases cellular cyclic AMP in isolated rat alveolar type II cells. Exp Lung Res 5:173

Mettler NR, Gray ME, Schuffman S, LeQuire VS (1981) β-adrenergic induced synthesis and secretion of phosphatidylcholine by isolated pulmonary alveolar type II cells. Lab Invest 45:575

Moore JR MB (1977) Regulation of intracellular cyclic GMP and cyclic AMP levels in mouse lung fragments by disopium cronoglycate, β-adrenergic agonists, cholinergic activators, and histamine. Res Commun Chem Path Pharmacol 17:639

Mortimer Jr EA (1981) Letter: Prevention of respiratory distress syndrome by antepartum aminophylline. Am J Obstet Gynecol 140:603

Motulsky HJ, Insel PA (1982) Adrenergic receptors in man. Direct identification, physiologic regulation, and clinical alterations. N Engl J Med 307:18

Newnham JP, Marshall CL, Padbury JF, Lam RW, Hobel CJ, Fisher DA (1984) Fetal catecholamine release with preterm delivery. Am J Obstet Gynecol 149:888

Nijjar MS (1979a) Regulation of rat lung adenylate cyclase by cytoplasmic factor(s) during development. Biochim Biophys Acta 584:43

Nijjar MS (1979b) Role of cyclic AMP and related enzymes in rat lung growth and development. Biochim Biophys Acta 586:464

Nijjar MS, Au AWY, Chaudhary KC (1981) Partial purification and properties of the cytoplasmic factors modulating adenylate cyclase activity in rat lung plasma membranes. Biochim Biophys Acta 677:153

Niles RM, Makarski JS (1979) Regulation of phosphatidylcholine metabolism by cyclic AMP in a model alveolar type 2 cell line. J Biol Chem 254:4324

Nylund L, Lagercrantz H, Lunell NO (1979) Catecholamines in fetal blood during birth in man. J Dev Physiol 1:427

Olsen DB (1972) Neurohumoral-hormonal secretory stimulation of pulmonary surfactant in the rat. Physiologist 15:230 (abstract)

Olver RE, Strang LB (1974) Ion fluxes across the pulmonary epithelium and secretion of lung liquid in the foetal lamb. J Physiol 471:327

Olver RE (1981) Of labour and the lungs. Arch Dis Child 56:659

Olver RE, Ramsden CA, Strang LB (1981) Adrenaline induced changes in net lung liquid volume flow across the pulmonary epithelium of the fetal lamb: evidence for active sodium transport. J Physiol (London) 319:55P (abstract)

Oyarzun MJ, Clements JA (1977) Ventilatory and cholinergic control of pulmonary surfactant in the rabbit. J Appl Physiol: Respirat Environ Exercise Physiol 43:39

Oyarzun MJ, Clements JA (1978) Control of lung surfactant by ventilation, adrenergic mediators, and prostaglandins in the rabbit. Am Rev Resp Dis 117:879

Padbury JF, Hobel CJ, Lam RW, Fisher DA (1981) Sex differences in lung and adrenal neurosympathetic development in rabbits. Am J Obstet Gynecol 141:199

Padbury JF, Roberman B, Oddie TH, Hobel CJ, Fisher DA (1982) Fetal catecholamine release in response to labor and delivery. Obstet Gynecol 60:607

Padbury JF, Hobel CJ, Gonzales FA (1983a) Ontogenesis and sex differences in rabbit fetal adrenal phenylethanolamine N-methyltransferase. Biol Neonate 43:205

Padbury JF, Lam RW, Hobel CJ, Fisher DA (1983b) Identification and partial purification of phenylethanolamine N-methyl transferase in the developing ovine lung. Pediatr Res 17:362

Padbury JF, Jacobs HC, Lam RW, Conaway D, Jobe AH, Fisher DA (1984) Adrenal epinephrine and regulation of pulmonary surfactant selease in neonatal rabbits. Expt Lung Res 7:177

Palmer GC (1972) Cyclic 3′,5′-adenosine monophosphate response in the rabbit lung – adult properties and development. Biochem Pharmacol 21:2907

Rice WR, Osterhoudt KC, Whitsett JA (1984) Surfactant release from isolated type II epithelial cells: role of microfilaments (actin). Pediatr Res 18:144A (abstract)

Roberts JM (1981) Receptors and transfer of information into cells. Seminars in Perinatology 5:203

Roberts JM, Jacobs MM, Cheng JB, Barnes PJ, O'Brien AT, Ballard PL (1985) Fetal pulmonary

beta-adrenergic receptors: Characterization in human and in vitro modulation by glucocorticoids. Pediatr Pulmonol 1:S69
Robertson PA, Herron M, Katz M, Creasy RK (1981) Maternal morbidity associated with isoxsuprine and terbutaline tocolysis. Europ J Obstet Gynec Reprod Biol 11:371
Rooney SA, Gobran LI, Wai-Lee TS (1977) Stimulation of surfactant production by oxytocin-induced labor in the rabbit. J Clin Invest 60:754
Rosen OM, Rosen SM (1968) The effect of catecholamines on the adenyl cyclase of frog and tadpole hemolysates. Biochem Biophys Res Commun 31:82
Scarpace PJ, Abrass IB (1981) Thyroid hormone regulation of rat heart, lymphocyte, and lung β-adrenergic receptors. Endocrinology 108:1007
Schumacher WA, Sheppard JR, Mirkin BL (1982) Biological maturation and beta-adrenergic effectors: Pre- and postnatal development of the adenylate cyclase system in the rabbit heart. J Pharmacol Exper Therap 223:587
Sevanian A, Gilden C, Kaplan SA, Barrett CT (1979) Enhancement of fetal lung surfactant production by aminophylline. Pediatr Res 13:1336
Smith DM, Sidhu NK (1984) In vivo autoradiographic demonstration of β-adrenergic binding sites in adult rat type II alveolar epithelial cells. Life Sci 34:519
Sommers-Smith SK, Giannopoulos G (1983) Identification of beta-adrenergic receptors in pulmonary alveolar type II cells. Life Sci 33:2071
Stahlman MT, Gray ME, Lieu S, Chytil F (1974) The role of cyclic AMP in lamellar body synthesis and secretion. Pediatr Res 8:196
Stoner J, Manganiello DC, Vaughn M (1974) Guanosine cyclic 3′,5′-monophosphate and guanylate cyclase activity in guinea pig lung: Effects of acetylcholine and cholinesterase inhibitors. Mol Pharmacol 10:155
Taeusch W, Wyszogrodski I, Wang NS, Avery ME (1974) Pulmonary pressure-volume relationships in premature fetal and newborn rabbits. J Appl Physiol 37:809
Tordet C, Bertin R, Gardey C, Richard MO, Dameron F, Marin L (1981) Lung catecholamines and cyclic nucleotides during perinatal development in the rat. Possible relationships with biochemical and morphological differentiation. Pediatr Res 15:787
Tsai JS, Chen A (1978) L-triiodothyronine increases the level of β-adrenergic receptor in cultured myocardial cells. Nature 275:138
Usher RH, Allen AC, McLean FH (1971) Risk of respiratory distress syndrome related to gestational age, route of delivery, and maternal diabetes. Am J Obstet Gynecol 111:826
Wallace RL, Herrick CN (1981) Pulmonary maturity studies in the evaluation of premature labor. Am J Obstet Gynecol 140:512
Walters DV, Olver RE (1978) The role of catecholamines in lung liquid absorption at birth. Pediatr Res 12:239
Whitsett JA, Darovec-Beckerman C, Adams K, Pollinger J, Needleman H (1980) Thyroid dependent maturation of β-adrenergic receptors in the rat lung. Biochem Biophys Res Commun 97:913
Whitsett JA, Manton MA, Darovec-Beckerman C, Adams K, Moore JJ (1981a) β-adrenergic receptors in the developing rabbit lung. Am J Physiol 240:E351
Whitsett JA, Manton MA, Darovec-Beckerman C, Adams K, (1981b) Current concepts. II. β-adrenergic receptors and catecholamine sensitive adenylate cyclase in the developing rat lung. Life Sci 28:339
Whitsett JA, Darovec-Beckerman C, Pollinger J, Moore JJ (1982a) Ontogeny of β-adrenergic receptors in the rat lung: Effects of hypothyroidism. Pediatr Res 16:381
Whitsett JA, Machulskis A, Noguchi A, Burdsall JA (1982b) Ontogeny of α_1- and β-adrenergic receptors in rat lung. Life Sci 30:139
Whitsett JA, Darovec-Beckerman C, Rice WW (1983a) Ontogeny of adenylate cyclase activity in rat lung: guanine nucleotides and cytosolic factors. Pediatr Res 17:553
Whitsett JA, Matz S, Darovec-Beckerman C (1983b) cAMP-dependent protein kinase and protein phosphorylation in developing rat lung. Pediatr Res 17:959
Whitsett JA, Lessard J (1984) Appearance of c-AMP dependent actin phosphorylation in rat lung and type II epithelial cells. Pediatr Res 18:147A (abstract)
Williams LT, Lefkowitz LK, Watanabe AM, Hathaway DR, Besch Jr HR (1977) Thyroid hormone regulation of β-adrenergic receptor number. J Biol Chem 252:2787
Wolfe BB, Harden TK, Molinoff PB (1976) β-adrenergic receptors in rat liver: Effects of adrenalectomy. Proc Natl Acad Sci USA 73:1343

Woodman DD, Watson D, Hatch U (1978) Noradrenalin to adrenalin ratio in amniotic fluid as an index of fetal maturity. Ann Clin Biochem 15:157

Wyszogrodski I, Taeusch HW, Avery ME (1974) Isoxsuprine-induced alterations of pulmonary pressure-volume relationships in premature rabbits. Am J Obstet Gynecol 119:1107

Zuspan FP (1974) Measurement and significance of epinephrine and norepinephrine in amniotic fluid. In: Natelson S, Scommegna A, Epstein MB (eds), Amniotic Fluid, John Wiley and Sons, New York, pp 101–108

9 Other Hormones

In addition to the three classes of hormones already discussed, effects of various other hormones in fetal lung have been reported. In general, the action of these hormones is not well characterized and in some cases conflicting results have been obtained. There is also relatively little information regarding possible physiologic roles. This chapter summarizes information on six hormones which have been investigated in recent years.

9.1 Prolactin

9.1.1 Background

Prolactin (PRL) was first discovered in 1928 as a lactogenic activity in extracts of pituitary gland. Recently, this hormone has been purified and the amino acid sequence determined. Among its diverse effects in the adult, PRL is required along with insulin and glucocorticoid for normal differentiation of mammary tissue and expression of the casein gene (recently reviewed by Topper and Freeman 1980). Production of PRL by the pituitary is under predominantly inhibitory regulation by dopamine of hypothalamic origin. Release of PRL is influenced by changes in psychic state and by both thyrotropin-releasing hormone (TRH) and estrogens (Frantz 1978).

PRL is present in the fetus, but the source, regulation, and physiologic effects of the hormone during fetal life are not well defined. In both the ovine and human fetus, plasma concentrations of PRL are low at mid-gestation, and rise to high concentrations by term (Mueller et al. 1979; Aubert et al. 1975; Clements et al. 1977; Schindler 1982; Flückiger et al. 1982). The levels of PRL in amniotic fluid are particularly striking, becoming quite high during mid-gestation. Dopaminergic inhibition of PRL release is operative during the second trimester in the sheep fetus (Gluckman et al. 1979), indicating that the high prenatal concentration of PRL is not due to immaturity of this regulatory mechanism. The origin of PRL in amniotic fluid is uncertain, and could arise from the fetus, mother and/or placenta.

The developmental pattern and elevated concentrations of PRL have prompted speculation and investigation as to the role and effects of this hormone during fetal life. PRL has an important role in fluid and electrolyte homeostasis in many vertebrates, which led to the hypothesis that PRL might influence amniotic fluid volume and tissue water stores in the fetal and neonatal animal. Evidence has been presented in support of this proposal (Josimovich et al. 1977a; Coulter and Avery 1980; Coulter 1983).

A second proposed role for PRL is regulation of surfactant synthesis in the

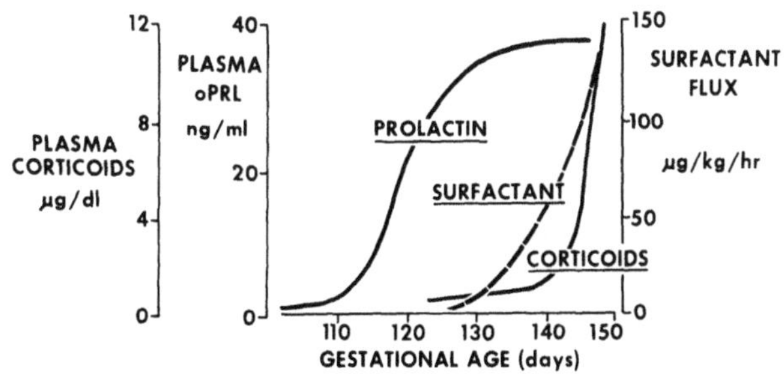

Fig. 9.1. Developmental pattern for plasma PRL, tracheal fluid surtactant and plasma corticoids in fetal sheep. From Ballard et al. (1978), by permission

developing lung. This idea originated from observations on the temporal pattern of PRL levels in the fetus as well as the role of this hormone in differentiation of the mammary gland. The developmental pattern for plasma PRL, plasma corticoids, and surfactant in tracheal fluid of the fetal sheep is shown in Fig. 9.1. PRL levels increase prior to the appearance of surfactant, whereas corticoids begin to rise later in gestation. A similar pattern occurs in the human with an increase in plasma PRL preceding the rise in amniotic fluid L/S ratio and plasma cortisol (Aubert et al. 1975; Winters et al. 1975; Gluckman et al. 1978; Hauth et al. 1978; Grosso et al. 1980).

9.1.2 Clinical Correlations

A possible role of fetal PRL in lung maturation is supported by studies examining the relationship between PRL concentrations in cord blood and occurrence of RDS. When regression lines of PRL vs. gestational age for infants with and without RDS were compared, the slopes were not different but the elevation of the line was significantly lower for infants who developed RDS (Gluckman et al. 1978). Data from this study by gestational age ranges are shown in Table 9.1. The mean concentration of PRL in cord plasma was significantly lower for infants developing RDS in the age range of 32–35.5 weeks. Similar results have been reported by Hauth et al. (1978), Smith et al. (1979), Grosso et al. (1980), and Dhanireddy et al. (1983), but not by Yuen et al. (1982). Concentrations of growth hormone, which decrease during the third

Table 9.1. Concentration of PRL in umbilical cord sera of infants with and without RDS. Data from Gluckman et al. (1978)

Gestational age (weeks)	Cord prolactin (ng/ml) mean ± SE				P
	No RDS	n	RDS	n	
28–31.5	75.5 ± 33.0	7	31.2 ± 9.4	7	NS
32–35.5	161.8 ± 18.9	23	101.7 ± 9.5	17	<0.025
36–40	135.6 ± 16.9	15	131.2 ± 17.5	8	NS

trimester, show no correlation with the occurrence of RDS (Gluckman et al. 1978). The possible influence of gender on PRL levels of cord blood are uncertain. No difference between the sexes has been observed (PL Ballard, unpublished data) and lower concentrations of PRL for male vs. female infants without RDS are reported (Dhanireddy et al. 1983). PRL levels in human amniotic fluid are quite variable and do not correlate with the L/S ratio (Hatjis et al. 1981).

The relationship between PRL and thyroxine levels has been investigated (Dhanireddy et al. 1983). A significant positive correlation between PRL and T_4 concentrations was found for infants with RDS, but not for healthy infants. This association might be related either to occurrence of RDS or to gestational age since the infants with RDS had a mean age 2 weeks less than the group of healthy infants. It is possible that TRH stimulates secretion of both thyroid hormones and PRL in the human fetus.

The cord blood studies indicate a slower developmental increase of serum PRL in less mature fetuses, at least during the first half of the third trimester. It is not known whether the association between PRL and RDS is causal or indirect. In a causal relationship, PRL could exert either a primary or permissive role in lung development. One possibility for an indirect association could involve estrogens. These hormones influence PRL during postnatal life, and fetal PRL concentrations are correlated with fetal estrogen (Aubert et al. 1974; Aubert et al. 1975; Kaplan et al. 1976). As discussed in the next section, estrogens influence pulmonary phospholipid synthesis in some systems. A similar argument could be made for TRH, which increases both PRL and thyroid hormones. Thus, it is conceivable that the association between PRL and RDS is secondary to the effect of estrogens or TRH on both PRL secretion and lung differentiation.

9.1.3 Effects in the Lung

The first study addressing the question of PRL effects on phospholipids in fetal lung was reported by Hamosh and Hamosh in 1977. Three litters of rabbit fetuses received in utero injections with PRL (1 mg) or diluent at 24 days gestation. Two days later, the fetuses were delivered by cesarean section for study. Treatment had no effect on fetal growth, lung weight, or DNA and protein content of lung tissue. As shown in Table 9.2, a substantial increase in

Table 9.2. Effect of prolactin on phospholipid content of fetal rabbit lung according to Hamosh and Hamosh (1977). Fetuses received 1 mg prolactin in utero on day 24 and lung lipids were analyzed 2 days later. Results are mean ± SEM

Treatment	Number of fetuses	Phospholipid	PC (μmol/g wet wt)	Dipalmitoyl PC
Prolactin	12	17.0 ± 0.85[a]	8.77 ± 0.81[a]	6.00 ± 0.35[a]
Control	13	12.16 ± 0.5	5.23 ± 0.44	2.30 ± 0.10

[a] $p < 0.001$ vs. control

phospholipid content of treated lungs was found. In particular, there was nearly a 3-fold increase in the concentration of saturated PC.

Subsequently, these experiments were repeated by Ballard et al. (1978) using the same protocol. In contrast to the results of Hamosh and Hamosh (1977), this study detected no influence of in utero PRL treatment on the content of either total phospholipid or saturated PC in fetal lung tissue (Table 9.3). A comparison of the lipid data in Tables 9.2 and 9.3 indicates close agreement for control fetuses, but different results after treatment. Surgery alone increased plasma corticoids and the rate of choline incorporation into PC, but PRL was not stimulatory. Plasma PRL immunoreactivity was elevated in treated animals, but not in control littermates, indicating that the hormone was absorbed. The reason for the discrepancy between these results and those of Hamosh and Hamosh (1977) has not been determined.

Most other in vivo studies of PRL administration have also been negative. Van Petten and Bridges (1979) examined pressure-volume characteristics after PRL treatment of rabbit fetuses using the protocol of Hamosh and Hamosh (1977). The deflation curves for PRL-injected fetuses at 26 days gestation were not different from control fetuses or those animals receiving diluent. Experiments carried out with older fetuses (28 days) gave similar results. Thus, this study failed to detect an effect of PRL on the content of alveolar surfactant as measured by deflation stability. In possible support of a role for PRL in lung maturation, Giussi et al (1981) found that administration of 2-bromo-α-ergocryptine to pregnant rabbits reduced the PC content of fetal lavage fluid; fetal weight was also decreased with treatment. Effects on PRL and other hormone levels in the fetus remain to be investigated.

In a study with fetal sheep, continuous infusions of ovine PRL at 1 mg/day did not influence the pattern of surfactant flux in tracheal fluid as determined by daily sampling (Fig. 9.2). This treatment did cause a marked increase in PRL concentrations of both fetal plasma and amniotic fluid, but did not influence levels of DHEA sulfate or corticoids in fetal plasma. Takahashi et al.

Table 9.3. Effect of PRL and surgery on choline incorporation, phospholipid and saturated PC content, and corticoids in the fetal rabbit according to Ballard et al. (1978) Rabbit fetuses were treated according to the protocol of Hamosh and Hamosh (Table 9.2). Mean ± SE values are shown with the number of determinations in parentheses

Determination	Unoperated control	Sham surgery control	Diluent injected	PRL injected
Choline incorporation into PC (pmol/mg protein/h)	33.2 ± 1.2 (47)	52.2 ± 5.1[a] (22)	45.6 ± 2.3[a] (21)	50.2 ± 3.1[a,b] (24)
Phospholipid, (μmol/g wet lung)	13.56 ± 0.52 (4)	14.62 ± 0.31 (3)	13.8 ± 0.59 (5)	13.74 ± 0.95 (5)
Saturated PC (μmol/g wet lung)	2.48 ± 0.16 (4)	2.30 ± 0.22 (3)	2.49 ± 0.14 (5)	2.23 ± 0.15 (5)
Plasma corticoids (μg/dl)	0.86 ± 0.06 (36)	1.15 ± 0.07[a] (20)	1.46 ± 0.12[a] (21)	1.35 ± 0.11[a,b] (26)

[a] $p < 0.05$ compared with unoperated control
[b] NS compared with diluent-injected and sham surgery control

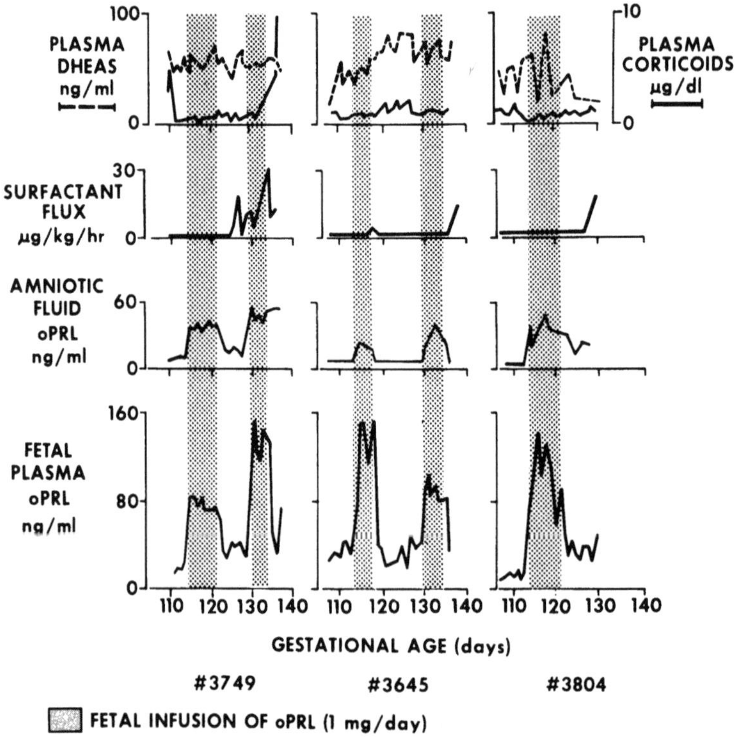

Fig. 9.2. Effect of PRL infusion to fetal sheep. Daily determinations of plasma DHEA sulfate, corticoids and PRL, amniotic fluid PRL, and surfactant in tracheal fluid were made in 3 fetuses which received oPRL at 1 mg/day during the *shaded times*. From Ballard et al. (1978), by permission

(1981) administered 2-bromo-α-ergocryptine (an inhibitor of PRL secretion) to fetal sheep for the last 2–3 weeks of gestation. This treatment reduced PRL to < 3 ng/ml but did not affect concentrations of cortisol or DHEA sulfate. All treated fetuses were healthy after spontaneous term delivery. Moreover, Kitterman et al. (1981a) found that endogenous fetal prolactin did not correlate with any of the physical or biochemical measurements made on lungs of third trimester fetal sheep. These findings in the sheep indicate 1) no stimulation of PRL administration alone on lung development, either directly or indirectly through an increase of endogenous cortisol, and 2) no association between endogenous PRL levels and lung maturity in late gestation.

Recently, Liggins and Schellenberg (1985) examined distensibility (V_{40}) of the ovine fetal lung (~ 128 days gestation) after hormone infusion in utero for 84 h. Administration of PRL (60 µg/h) plus cortisol (1 mg/h) was no more stimulatory of lung volume (0.66 ml/g) than cortisol alone (0.97 ml/g) compared with results in saline-infused fetuses (0.46 ml/g). However, the combination of cortisol with both PRL and T_3 (25 µg/h) produced a significant increase in distensibility (1.66 ml/g). Forthcoming data for phospholipids in these experiments will provide an assessment of surfactant levels. The apparent synergistic effect of the three hormones is discussed further in Chapter 10.

Conflicting results are described for studies of PRL with cultured lung tissue or cells. Cox and Torday (1981) exposed confluent cultures of fetal rabbit lung cells to various concentrations of ovine PRL for 48 h. One preparation of PRL (Sigma Chemical) influenced the amount of newly-synthesized PC which was saturated, but did not stimulate the overall rate of PC synthesis. By contrast, a second preparation of PRL (National Institutes of Health) did not affect either PC synthesis or percent saturation. The authors speculate that some component other than PRL in the commercial preparation affected remodeling of PC in this experimental system. Preliminary results on the effect of PRL in A-549 cells have been reported (Porreco et al. 1980). Cells were grown to confluence in medium containing 20% serum and exposed to PRL (2 ng/ml) for 12 h along with labeled precursor. Data from three experiments suggested that PRL stimulated the rate of incorporation of glycerol into PC and phosphatidylglycerol, but did not significantly increase the rate of choline incorporation into PC.

Additional studies on PRL have been carried out in organ culture. Mullon et al. (1983) used fetal rat lung obtained at day 18 of pregnancy and maintained in serum-free culture medium. Exposure of the cultures to PRL at a concentration of 2 μg/ml stimulated incorporation of both choline and glycerol into total phospholipids and PC and increased the tissue content of saturated PC 2-fold. In parallel experiments, however, little effect was noted with dexamethasone (1 μM). When dexamethasone and PRL were combined, there was nearly a 4-fold increase in the amount of saturated PC/mg DNA. This effect of PRL remains to be characterized with regard to dose and time.

Perhaps the strongest evidence for a direct effect of PRL on PC synthesis in fetal lung comes from the studies of Mendelson et al. (1981b). These experiments, which have also been discussed in Chapter 4, used organ culture of human fetal lung and treatment with various combinations of cortisol, insulin and PRL. As shown by the data of Table 9.4, none of the three hormones

Table 9.4. Effect of insulin, cortisol, and PRL on the rate of incorporation of choline into saturated PC of lung explants from a 22-week old human abortus according to Mendelson et al. (1981b). Explants of human fetal lung were incubated with the hormones indicated for 4 days and [^{3}H]choline was added the last 24 h of incubation. Values are the mean ± SE of determinations from three replicate cultures. I, insulin (2.5 μg/ml); F, cortisol (0.2 μg/ml); P, prolactin (2.5 μg/ml)

Treatment	Choline incorporated into saturated PC (nmol/24 h per mg protein)	Saturated PC: PC ratio
Control	5.9 ± 0.8	0.40
I	3.8 ± 0.3	0.36
F	6.2 ± 0.5	0.38
P	6.4 ± 1.0	0.40
I + F	14.2 ± 0.4	0.42
I + P	10.0 ± 0.7	0.42
F + P	17.9 ± 1.3	0.44
I + F + P	17.1 ± 1.0	0.45

alone stimulated saturated PC synthesis, but all combinations of the hormones were stimulatory. However, none of the treatment regimes appears to preferentially increase choline incorporation into saturated PC. In the presence of both insulin (2.5 μg/ml) and cortisol (0.2 μg/ml), PRL had an optimal effect at a concentration of 0.025 μg/ml with a decrease in stimulation at levels between 0.25 and 25 μg/ml.

In contrast with these data, recent studies with explants of rat, rabbit and human lung found little or no stimulatory effect of PRL alone or with corticosteroid; moreover, dexamethasone increased PC synthesis and content in the absence of PRL (Ballard et al. 1985; Gonzales and Ballard 1984). PRL obtained from both NIH and Sigma Chemical Co. was tested over a range of concentrations (0.001–8 μg/ml) and exposure time (1–6 days with human tissue), and with both choline and acetate as precursor. The reason for this puzzling discrepancy between studies is unknown.

9.1.4 Mechanism

The mechanism of a possible PRL effect on PC synthesis in fetal lung has not been investigated. Furthermore, conflicting results have been published regarding binding of PRL. Binding studies with [^{125}I]PRL and membrane preparations found little specific binding with fetal lung of the lamb (Chan et al. 1978), but substantial levels in lung of fetal Rhesus monkey (Josimovich et al. 1977b). Using an autoradiographic technique, Costlow and McGuire (1977) observed little PRL binding in lung of adult rat, whereas binding was present in various other tissues. Amit et al. (1984) also failed to detect PRL binding in adult rat lung, but report the presence of binding sites in fetal tissue. These workers also report the presence of PRL binding sites in membrane preparations from lungs of adult animals treated with PRL (Ben-Harari et al. 1983). It is apparent that further investigation of PRL binding in lung tissue and cells is desirable.

9.1.5 Conclusions

PRL is present at high concentrations during fetal life, but its physiologic role is uncertain. The developmental pattern for PRL (peak levels by the middle of the third trimester), and its well described effects in differentiation of mammary tissue, stimulated investigation of PRL action in fetal lung. Although the first study in this area indicated a marked effect of PRL administration on pulmonary phospholipids, subsequent work has not demonstrated any effects with PRL alone in either the rabbit or sheep. The reasons for the discrepancy with in vivo treatment in the rabbit are not known.

Experiments with cultured tissue have unfortunately not clarified the issue. Although one study with human lung found that PRL was required for expression of glucocorticoid stimulation, other studies with rat, rabbit, and human lung in culture find a response to glucocorticoid in the absence of serum and hormones, and little stimulatory effect of PRL. Thus, the bulk of the evidence indicates that glucocorticoids stimulate PC synthesis in cultured lung in the absence of exogenous PRL.

The recent observations of Liggins and Schellenberg (1985), however, support a role for PRL in hormone-induced lung maturation of the sheep. Based on their data, it may be hypothesized that sufficient levels of PRL are required to observe a synergistic response to glucocorticoid plus thyroid hormone (Chap. 10). In the second half of the third trimester, concentrations of endogenous PRL would be adequate to permit an effect of cortisol plus T_3. Earlier in gestation, when PRL levels are lower, administration of PRL plus the other two hormones would be necessary for a maximal response to treatment. This hypothesis of permissive action would explain the absence of response to infusion of PRL alone (Ballard et al. 1978). If this concept extends to other species, it might account for the variable results observed with PRL. Depending on the gestational age, the endogenous levels of PRL, T_3 and corticosteroid, and the amount of washout of endogenous hormones during culture studies, different responses to PRL and glucocorticoid would be observed. This hypothesis is also consistent with the observed relationship between plasma PRL levels and occurrence of RDS; the correlation is relatively weak and is only observed early in the third trimester. Hopefully, further characterization of glucocorticoid and PRL effects and investigation of differences in experimental design will clarify the influence of PRL.

Alternatively, the biologic link between PRL secretion and rate of lung maturation may involve other hormones such as estradiol or TRH which influence release of PRL. It has been suggested that PRL is adrenocorticotrophic in the fetus; however, in utero treatment of the sheep did not increase plasma levels of either cortisol or DHEA sulfate. PRL might also influence systems in the lung other than those related to surfactant (such as fluid reabsorption) which contribute to the occurrence of respiratory distress at birth.

9.2 Estradiol

9.2.1 Clinical Correlations

In human pregnancy, maternal estrogens increase throughout gestation, with the most pronounced rise occurring between 32 weeks and term. Unconjugated estriol concentrations in maternal and cord plasma and amniotic fluid at term are higher in pregnancies with labor and spontaneous delivery compared to cesarean section without labor (Goldkrand 1978). The continued rise in maternal estrogen concentrations has become an established index of fetal well-being. The relationship between estrogen levels and newborn survival has been recognized for many years, and there have been unsuccessful attempts to improve premature infant survival and weight gain by estrogen treatment after birth (Moncrieff 1936). In the 1960's, an association was noted between low urinary estrogen levels at birth and subsequent development of respiratory distress (Frank et al. 1965; Dickey and Robertson 1969). In a study with cord bloods, Conly et al. (1973) found lower concentrations of estriol in premature infants with RDS (as well as other types of respiratory distress) compared with normal premature infants. The temporal pattern of maternal estrogens, along with apparently lower fetal concentrations associated with respiratory distress, suggested a possible role of estrogen in lung maturation. This possibility has been examined in a series of studies since 1979.

9.2.2 Effects

Khosla and colleagues (Khosla and Rooney 1979; Khosla et al. 1980; Khosla et al. 1981; Khosla et al. 1983) tested the effect of administering 17β-estradiol to the pregnant rabbit. Treatment stimulated the rate of choline incorporation into PC by fetal lung slices and increased total phospholipid and PC content of lung tissue and lavage (Table 9.5). The most striking finding was the 4-fold increase in PC content of lung lavage. In addition, the PC/sphingomyelin ratio increased from 0.7 in controls to 2.0 in the treated fetuses. An effect on choline incorporation was observed with doses as low as 10 μg, plateauing at 25–75 μg/day. The effect of estradiol treatment on choline incorporation has been confirmed (Possmayer et al. 1981). In both studies, there was no effect of treatment on the percent of PC which was saturated.

Diethylstilbestrol was equally potent with 17β-estradiol in stimulating choline incorporation by lung slices after in vivo treatment. However, a similar response was also observed to maternal treatment with progesterone and testosterone. The anti-estrogen tamoxifen, which competitively binds to the estradiol receptor in other systems, was given in vivo both alone and with 17β-estradiol. At a dose of 0.22 mg/kg, tamoxifen did not affect the rate of choline incorporation nor did it block the effect of estradiol (0.44–1.1 μg/kg) on either choline incorporation or glycogen content in fetal lungs.

Both groups of investigators examined the effect of estradiol on activities of enzymes involved in phospholipid synthesis. These included enzymes of the de novo pathway for PC synthesis, enzymes for remodeling of PC, the de novo pathway for phosphatidylglycerol and phosphatidylinositol synthesis, and phosphatidic acid phosphatase. Of these enzymes, only the activity of CTP: cholinephosphate cytidylyltransferase was substantially increased after estradiol treatment (62–66%). Consistent with this finding, estradiol also reduced the tissue pool size of cholinephosphate and increased the pool of CDP-choline (Possmayer et al. 1981) Stimulation of cytidylyltransferase was observed

Table 9.5. Effects of maternal treatment with 17β-estradiol on fetal lung phospholipids. Pregnant rabbits received 50–75 μg 17β-estradiol or diluent (control) on day 25 (and 26) with choline incorporation assessed in lung slices on day 26 and lipid content on day 27. Data from Khosla und Rooney (1979) and Khosla et al. (1980)

	Control	Estradiol-treated	P
Choline incorporation into PC (cpm/min/mg)	47 ± 6	128 ± 8	<0.001
Lung tissue (mg P/g dry lung)	2.6 ± 0.1	4.3 ± 0.5	<0.02
total phospholipid	1.0 ± 0.04	1.6 ± 0.2	<0.005
PC			
Lung lavage (μg P/g dry lung)	11.3 ± 0.3	28.5 ± 4.6	<0.01
total phospholipid	2.6 ± 0.1	10.8 ± 0.8	<0.001
PC			

only in the absence of cofactor (phosphatidylglycerol), and this stimulation was markedly reduced by extraction of lipids from lung cytosol (Chu and Rooney 1985). These findings indicate that estrogen activates enzyme activity in a process mediated by cytosolic phospholipids, similar to effects observed with glucocorticoid and T_3.

Other effects of estradiol treatment have been described. Even at low doses, 24 h of treatment reduces both body and lung weight of the fetus. There is a dose-dependent loss of glycogen from fetal lung, but no effect on liver glycogen. Incorporation of labeled methionine and leucine into trichloroacetic acid-precipitable proteins was not altered by treatment, but thymidine incorporation into DNA was depressed. This latter finding is consistent with lower lung weight after treatment (Possmayer et al. 1981; Khosla et al. 1981). Two days after intra-amniotic injection of fetal rabbits, β-adrenergic binding capacity was 33% greater in lung membrane preparations from estradiol-treated versus saline-injected pups (Moawad et al. 1985).

On light microscopy, lungs of estradiol-treated fetuses demonstrated larger alveolar spaces with thinner septae on day 26 of gestation. In addition, blood vessels in the estrogen-treated group appeared more mature with larger lumens and thinner walls than in control specimens. At the electron microscopic level, treated lungs showed fewer undifferentiated epithelial cells, a greater percentage of type I cells, and increased occurrence of lamellar bodies within type II cells. All of these differences on morphologic analysis reached statistical significance (Khosla et al. 1981). These findings are consistent with an earlier observation that administration of the anti-estrogen ethamoxytriphetol to pregnant rabbits results in fetal pulmonary vessels with thicker walls and narrower lumens, an effect blocked by simultaneous administration of 17β-estradiol (Abdul-Karim and Prior 1969). The morphologic effects of estradiol treatment appear to represent accelerated differentation similar to that observed with glucocorticoid treatment. With both hormones, differentiation occurs concomitant with inhibition of lung growth.

Thursesson-Klein and co-workers (1985) recently described morphologic changes associated with estradiol treatment of fetal rats. Fetuses received estradiol phosphate (4 μg) or saline intraamniotically between days 15 and 20 and their lungs were studied by electron microscopy 48 h later. In a morphometric analysis of 11 animals, both the mean size and number of lamellar bodies per epithelial cell were increased with treatment, equivalent with 1–3 days accelerated development.

In contrast to the in vivo studies in rabbits and rats, estradiol treatment did not affect lung maturation in a study with fetal sheep (Rosenfeld et al. 1983). Fetal lambs received an infusion of 17β-estradiol at a rate of 100 μg/day for 2 weeks during the third trimester. This treatment produced a 400-fold increase in unconjugated estradiol of fetal plasma, approximating the levels reached at the onset of parturition. In samples of tracheal fluid, values for PC/total phospholipid ratio, L/S ratio, and PC content were similar for control and treated fetuses. At termination of the experiments (127 days), there were no differences between control and treated animals for total phospholipid, total PC, and percent saturation of PC in lung tissue. In addition, no differences in lung morphology by both light and electron microscopy were apparent. Thus, these investigators failed to detect any stimulatory effect of 17β-estradiol on the rate of lung maturation in the ovine fetus.

In organ cultures of fetal rat lung, 17β-estradiol at a concentration of 10 μM produced a modest stimulation of the rate of choline incorporation into PC and sphingomyelin. The rate of [^{3}H]acetate incorporation into all classes of phospholipids increased on exposure to estradiol. The relative distribution of radioactivity from acetate showed an increased percentage in phosphatidylglycerol and decreased percentage in phosphatidylinositol plus phosphatidylserine. Estradiol also increased the activity of cholinephosphate cytidylyltransferase, but neither this increase nor the enhancement of choline incorporation was blocked by tamoxifen, similar to the findings with in vivo treatment. A dose-response study found some stimulation with estradiol at 10 nM and the maximal effect at 10 μM, the highest concentration tested (Gross et al. 1979; Khosla et al. 1983). In cultures of fetal rabbit lung, 17β-estradiol (100 nM) did not affect the rate of choline incorporation (Gross et al. 1983).

9.2.3 Mechanism of Action

Although the effects of estradiol in fetal rabbit lung are partially characterized and confirmed, the mechanism of action remains uncertain. It is unlikely that estradiol is exerting its action through the classical estradiol receptor. Tamoxifen, an anti-estrogen acting through receptor, did not block the effects of estrogen both in vivo and in culture. The dose-response curve for estradiol obtained in organ culture is also inconsistent with receptor mediation. However, the dose-response question deserves further investigation, including analysis of estradiol metabolism in cultured tissue. For example, 30 min after injection of [^{3}H]estradiol to guinea pig fetuses, only one-third of the radioactivity found in lung tissue represented unmetabolized estradiol (Pasqualini et al. 1976). Adult human lung, like other tissues, supports the interconversion of estradiol and estrone (Milewich et al. 1982).

Fetal lung tissue contains binding sites for estradiol. In guinea pig lung, binding was detected in both cytosol and nuclear fractions, with a predominance of cytosol binding at term (Pasqualini et al. 1976; Pasqualini et al. 1977; Pasqualini et al. 1978). The identification of these binding sites as estradiol receptors, as characterized in other tissues, is not yet established. Subsequently, Mendelson et al. (1980, 1981a) examined estrogen binding in lung tissue of fetal rats and humans. A cytosolic estrogen binding protein was identified in both tissues by sucrose density centrifugation and charcoal-dextran analyses. The binding component sedimented at approximately 4S on sucrose gradients, and [^{3}H]estradiol was displaced by excess non-labeled estradiol but not by diethylstilbestrol. The complex of estradiol and cytosol binding protein did not bind to a nuclear fraction prepared from fetal rat lung. K_D values for binding were estimated at about 10 nM and 100 nM for rat and human lung, respectively.

These properties of estradiol binding in lung differ from the well described estrogen receptor of the uterus and other target tissues. Receptor sediments at 8S in low salt on sucrose gradients, binds estradiol with a high affinity ($K_D \leqq 1$ nM) and demonstrates a similarly high affinity for diethylstilbestrol.

The binding component found in lung tissue has some properties in common with α-fetoprotein. This protein could be present within lung cells or reflect plasma contamination of cytosol preparations. The identification and possible role of the estradiol binding protein of lung tissue remain uncertain.

Estradiol binding has also been detected in lung cytosol from adult rats (Morishige and Uetake 1978; Ben-Harari et al. 1983). Unlike the findings in fetal tissue, the binding component of adult cytosol sediments at approximately 8S on sucrose gradients, and binding was saturable with an apparent K_D of 0.1–1.0 nM. Binding capacity ranged between 5 and 10 fmol/mg protein at all postnatal ages examined (Morishige and Uetake 1978), but 100-fold higher concentrations were reported by Ben-Harari et al. (1983). Although further characterization is needed, this binding activity is consistent with the estradiol receptor. Specific binding of estradiol hemisuccinate in adult rat lung was also demonstrated by a histochemical approach (Pertschuk and Di Maio 1980). The fluorescent staining in this study was confined to the epithelial cells lining bronchi and bronchioles. Similar localization of binding sites is reported for lung of the guinea pig, rabbit, ferret and human.

Thus, both the binding studies and the data with lung explants argue against a direct effect of estradiol in fetal lung mediated by estradiol receptor. In view of this evidence, alternative mechanisms need to be considered. The clinical association between estrogen levels and respiratory distress in the newborn may reflect fetal adrenocortical function. The failure to observe effects after estradiol treatment of the sheep fetus might indicate that fetal effects are secondary to action in the mother. Estradiol treatment of the pregnant rabbit might stimulate maternal levels of other hormones which could pass to the fetus. It would be useful to determine maternal and fetal concentrations of cortisol, T_3, T_4, PRL, catecholamines, and insulin after estrogen treatment. Estradiol might increase blood flow in fetal lung analogous to the effect in the uterus; this could enhance *delivery* of hormones and/or substrates involved in surfactant synthesis without affecting circulating concentrations. Alternatively, metabolism of estradiol after maternal treatment could produce compounds which influence lung development. The mechanism of this postulated effect would presumably not involve estradiol receptor. Further insight into the mechanism of estradiol effects on lung maturation awaits additional studies both in culture and in vivo. At present, there is no evidence that endogenous estradiol has an important role in normal lung development.

9.3 Epidermal Growth Factor

Epidermal growth factor (EGF) was first identified as a protein from the mouse submaxillary gland which accelerated incisor eruption and eyelid opening in the newborn animal (Cohen 1963). Subsequently, this "tooth-lid" protein has been purified and its molecular weight determined to be 6045 daltons (Taylor et al. 1972). EGF has generalized effects on epithelial growth and keratinization in the mouse and other species. Mitogenic effects have been shown in many different cell types, including mammary epithelial cells, chondrocytes, corneal cells, vascular smooth muscle cells, prostatic cells, glial cells, fibroblasts, and epithelial cells of the uterus, vagina, ureter and ductus deferens. Stimulation of DNA synthesis in contact-inhibited fibroblasts occurs at EGF concentrations of 10–100 pM which are within the physiologic range for mouse serum (Jones 1966; Hollenberg and Cuatrecasas 1973; Armelin 1973; Baker and Cunningham 1978; Carpenter 1981). Under certain conditions, at least, EGF influences the expression of specific differentiated cell products independent of its effect on cell growth (Chen et al. 1977; Johnson et al. 1980). EGF has also been identified in human adult urine and newborn plasma; the amino acid sequence of the urine protein (also called urogastrone for its ability to inhibit gastric acid secretion) is similar to mouse EGF. Human and mouse EGF have similar effects, both in vivo and in culture systems (Starkey et al. 1975; Gregory 1975).

EGF acts in epithelial cells through a specific membrane receptor, which has been characterized and purified. Monoclonal antibodies to the receptor have been developed and used to identify chromosome 7 as the site of the structural gene in the human. Binding of the hormone is followed by phosphorylation and aggregation of receptor, with subsequent internalization and degradation in lysosomes (Carpenter and Cohen 1979; Fox and Das 1979; Waterfield et al. 1982; Kawamoto et al. 1983). The mechanism by which EGF-receptor interaction induces DNA synthesis is unknown. The stimulus may involve either a class of high affinity receptors, which remain on the cell surface after binding, or a second messenger produced after internalization.

The recognition of EGF as a normal growth hormone of the fetus, and its generalized action on epithelial cells, led to investigation of EGF in lung maturation. Catterton and colleagues (1979) administered purified mouse EGF (5 μg) in utero to rabbit fetuses at day 24 of gestation. This dose produces hyperplasia of esophageal epithelium in fetal rabbits without the increased mortality observed at the dose of 10 μg. Three days after the surgery, EGF-injected fetuses were compared with uninjected and saline-injected littermates. There was no effect of treatment on body or lung weight; however, treated lung showed greater distensibility at 35 cm H_2O and increased deflation stability at pressures of 0–15 cm H_2O. Each of the 8 fetuses receiving EGF showed evidence of enhanced morphologic maturity of alveolar epithelial cells, including an increase in the percentage of type II cells. It was also felt that treatment was associated with more attenuation of type I epithelial cells and more lamellar bodies per type II cell. Possible effects of EGF on lining cells of bronchioles, bronchi and trachea were not reported.

Sundell et al. (1980) infused mouse EGF in utero into fetal lambs of 124–131 days gestation. The administered doses ranged between 0.08–0.38 mg/day. On histologic examination, EGF treatment was associated with hyperplasia of the non-ciliated epithelial cells of the conducting airways and apparent accelerated differentiation of both type I and type II cells in aveoli. One group of treated and control fetuses were delivered and resuscitated at 128–131 days after inducing hypotension in the ewe the day before delivery. In this group, 6 treated lamps showed no evidence of developing hyaline membrane disease during the first 6 h of life; all 3 untreated lambs required oxygen and had pathologic evidence of membrane formation. EGF treatment also increased both thyroid and adrenal weight, but the authors state that plasma levels of cortisol, T_4 and TSH were not elevated. In a similar study, Thorburn et al. (1981) found thinning of pulmonary aveolar septae and a 3-fold increase in fetal cortisol within 24 h of EGF infusion. In the study of Liggins and Schellenberg (1985), EGF was infused into sheep fetuses at a lower dose (1 µg/h) for 84 h. EGF, both alone and in combination with cortisol (1 mg/h), did not increase lung distensibility (V_{40}).

EGF has also been tested in organ culture. The early study of Jones (1966) reported new growth of alveolar epithelial cells 48 h after addition of EGF to cultured lung of 4-week old rats. A preliminary study with fetal rat lung found a dose-dependent (half-maximal at 1 nM) stimulation of choline incorporation into PC by EGF (Gross and Dynia 1984).

The mechanism of EGF action in fetal lung presumably is receptor-mediated. There is specific binding of [^{125}]EGF by membrane preparations from fetal and maternal rabbit lung (Devaskar 1982) and by intact fibroblasts and type II cells of adult rat lung (Keller and Ladda 1981). The binding is saturable and dependent on both on both time and temperature. In dose response experiments with fetal membrane, the K_D was approximately 2 nM with a capacity of about 25 nmol/mg protein. The identification of binding sites, along with the response to EGF by lung in culture, suggests that EGF acts directly in fetal lung after treatment in vivo.

The physiologic importance of endogenous EGF in lung maturation is not known. Although high doses of EGF appeared to accelerate differentiation of alveolar epithelial cells in fetal lambs, there was also hyperplasia of epithelial cells in the conducting airways. The latter effect is not a normal occurrence, and would thus appear to be inconsistent with a physiologic role for EGF in normal pulmonary development. On the other hand, it is possible that lower doses of EGF might produce accelerated maturation along the normal pattern. There is no information at present on the concentrations of EGF within lung tissue during fetal life; in newborn mice, levels of endogenous EGF are relatively high in lung (and certain other tissues) compared with liver and heart (Lakshmanan et al. 1985).

Interrelationships between EGF and other hormones have not been extensively explored in fetal lung, but this possibility is suggested by other observations. In cultured pituitary cells (GH), EGF stimulates PRL synthesis, decreases growth hormone production, and blocks the induction of growth hormone by T_3 but not by dexamethasone (Johnson et al. 1980). In the newborn mouse, treatment with T_3 or T_4 for 6 days increases the concentrations of EGF in urine, eye and skin, but not in liver or submandibular gland. Similar treatment in the adult increased EGF in both skin and submandibular gland (Hoath et al. 1984; Perheentupa et al. 1984; Lakshmanan et al. 1985). The same dose of T_3 had little apparent effect on the timing of incisor eruption. Also, dexamethasone alone (50 ng/day) did not accelerate tooth eruption although the skin content of EGF was increased. When mice received both T_3 and dexamethasone, tooth eruption was accelerated. The mechanism of this synergistic interaction is not known, but it was found that combined therapy did not increase skin EGF greater than T_3 alone. There is no information on EGF concentrations in plasma and lung tissue (Hoath et al. 1983).

Effects of glucocorticoids on EGF receptor are also reported. Exposure of a fibroblastic cell line derived from mouse embryos to glucocorticoids increased the number of EGF receptors (Ivanovic and Weinstein 1981). The properties of this response were consistent with mediation through glucocorticoid receptor. Baker and Cunningham (1978) found that dexamethasone treatment of human fibroblasts increased both the affinity of EGF binding and the growth response to EGF. In a recent study in the rabbit, maternal betamethasone treatment for 2 days increased fetal lung EGF receptors about 3-fold (Sadiq and Devaskar 1984). These findings suggest the possibility that some effects of thyroid hormones and glucocorticoids on fetal lung development might be mediated through EGF.

9.4 Thyrotropin-Releasing Hormone

Administration of thyrotropin-releasing hormone (TRH), the hypothalamic peptide L-pyroglutamyl-L-histidyl-L-prolyl amide, to adults causes a prompt increase in plasma thyrotropin and a subsequent elevation of both plasma T_4 and T_3. In fetal lambs the pituitary-thryoid axis is responsive to TRF stimulation as early as 105 days gestation (Klein and Fisher 1980). In contrast to thyrotropin and the thyroid hormones, TRH readily crosses the placenta. Maternally-administered TRH increases fetal thyrotropin concentrations several-fold in both Rhesus monkeys and the human (Azukizawa et al. 1976; Roti et al. 1981). By 2 h after maternal treatment with 400 µg TRH, fetal plasma T_3 levels are increased about 3-fold. This rise is similar to the spontaneous increase occuring immediately after birth. TRH also stimulates prolactin release, and a response has been demonstrated in the fetal lamb at 88 days gestation (Thomsett et al. 1980). In cultured pituitary cell lines, at least, TRH regulated PRL through stimulation of gene transcription (Biswas et al. 1982; White and Bancroft 1983).

The ability of TRH to cross the placenta, and the responsiveness of the fetal pituitary-thyroid axis, suggests that maternal treatment with TRH might affect lung maturation. This hypothesis was addressed by a study in the rabbit (Rooney et al. 1979). Pregnant animals received intravenous TRH (20 µg/kg) as 4 injections over 2 days. Treatment did not affect either choline incorporation by lung slices or the phospholipid content or composition of lung tissue. In lung lavage, however, TRH treatment was associated with increased content of phospholipid and PC, and decreased amounts of phosphatidylethanolamine and sphingomyelin. The 2.5-fold increase in lavage PC is greater than usually observed with corticosteroid therapy. These findings are consistent with TRH stimulation of surfactant release but not synthesis. Effects of TRH on the fetal lung in vivo have not been further investigated in the rabbit. In preliminary studies with fetal sheep, infusion of TRH plus cortisol increased lung distensibility (V_{40}) more than cortisol alone (G. C. Liggins and J.-C. Schellenberg, personal communication).

There are several possible mechanisms for TRH action. TRH may stimulate T_3 and T_4 production in the fetal rabbit similar to the response in monkeys and humans. If this were the major mode of action in the rabbit, an increase in both PC synthesis as well as lavage content would be expected (see Chap. 7).

The action of TRH might also be mediated by PRL; however, the effect of PRL, when it has been observed, has been on the tissue content of PC. It is also possible that TRH acts directly in the lung. TRH is known to have effects in the central nervous system, acting as a neurotransmitter independent of the pituitary (Jackson 1982). TRH does not stimulate choline incorporation by fetal rabbit lung in organ culture (P.L. Ballard, unpublished observations), but its effect on surfactant release from isolated type II cells has not been examined.

There is an obvious need to examine the effects of TRH in more detail. Future studies should include assays of T_3 and T_4, as well as other fetal hormones, and explore interactions with glucocorticoids (see Chap. 10).

9.5 Fibroblast Pneumonocyte Factor

A series of studies since 1978 by Smith and colleagues (Smith 1978; Smith and Fletcher 1979; Tanswell and Smith 1979; Smith 1979; 1981 ab; Smith and Sabry 1983; Smith et al. 1983) describe a glucocorticoid inducible factor from pulmonary fibroblasts. This factor has been termed fibroblast-pneumonocyte factor (FPF) because of its observed effects on phospholipid synthesis by type II pneumonocytes and its proposed role as mediator of the glucocorticoid effect.

The existence of FPF was first suggested by the observation that epithelial cells derived from human fetal lung required the presence of fibroblasts for growth in culture (Tanswell and Smith, 1980). In these experiments, epithelial cells with characteristics of type II pneumonocytes were cloned from lung tissue of a 32-week gestation infant. Clones of cells were successfully grown from culture wells containing initially two cells each (presumably one fibroblast and one epithelial cell). After several weeks of further culture, a population of epithelial cells was isolated from the fibroblasts. These cells grew in culture medium containing 10% serum and were utilized as an assay system for FPF. This cell line resembled type II cells by virtue of their lamellar inclusions and phospholipid content (PC 76% with 35% saturated and 4% phosphatidylglycerol).

Figure 9.3 shows the effect of medium from fibroblasts cultured with cortisol on the rate of choline incorporation by the human epithelial cell line. The response to unheated medium is biphasic, but only stimulation is observed after heating the medium. The heating effect presumably represents inactivation of inhibitory substances in the culture medium. Although the fibroblast-derived medium used in these experiments contains 1 μM cortisol, addition of cortisol alone to the epithelial cells stimulated choline incorporation by only 50%. In a dose-response study, FPF activity was induced in fibroblasts at cortisol concentrations between 10 and 100 nM. By contrast, the response of the epithelial cells to cortisol was noted at 10-fold higher concentrations. Although it has been suggested that this divergence in the dose response curves might represent an amplification of the cortisol effect through generation of FPF, it is more likely that the decreased sensitivity of the epithelial cells reflects metabolism of cortisol to cortisone. Whereas fibroblasts demonstrate pri-

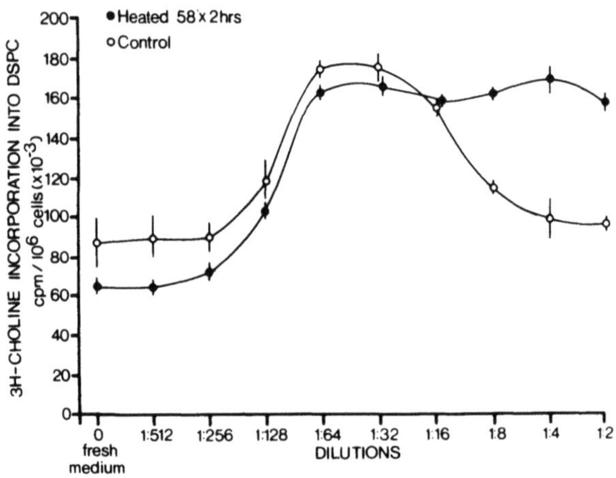

Fig. 9.3. Choline incorporation into saturated PC by fetal lung epithelial cells exposed to conditioned medium from cortisol-treated fibroblasts. All dilutions were made in 1 μM cortisol, and cells were exposed for 24 h to conditioned medium and [^{3}H]choline. From Smith (1978) by permission

marily reduction of cortisone to cortisol, intact human lung tissue (and presumably the epithelial cells) has primarily oxidative activity (discussed in Sect. 4.3.4).

FPF has been further characterized and purified from medium of cortisol-treated lung fibroblasts by both gel filtration and SDS-polyacrylamide gel electrophoresis. Pneumonocyte stimulating activity resides in a protein of molecular weigh ~ 8000 daltons which is soluble at acidic pH. FPF is stable to heating at 58 °C for 2 h (Fig. 9.3) and is inactivated by exposure to trypsin. Lung fibroblasts from a number of species (human, cat, rabbit, rat, monkey, chicken) show FPF activity, but no activity was observed in skin fibroblasts exposed to cortisol. FPF is not detected in medium of fibroblasts cultured in the absence of cortisol.

Production of FPF by primary cultures of lung fibroblasts varies markedly with gestational age (Fig. 9.4). In this experiment, fibroblasts were grown to confluence and exposed to 1 μM cortisol for 24 h. The medium was collected, heated (to inactivate the inhibitory factor), diluted, and added to cultures of human fetal lung epithelial cells. Under these conditions (and assuming equal densities of fibroblasts at each age), peak production of FPF occurred at 20 days gestation with a return to control levels shortly after birth. By comparison, the major increase in both free corticosterone and saturated PC synthesis in vivo occurs between 20 and 22 days (Chap. 4). This suggests that FPF responsiveness to glucocorticoid in vivo is decreasing during the period of surfactant accumulation. Alternatively, the decline in FPF production after 20 days could reflect age-dependent effects of in vitro culture conditions. With serial subculturing of fibroblasts, for example, the production of FPF in response to cortisol was found to decrease.

FPF has been tentatively identified in human amniotic fluid (Seybold and Smith 1980). Aliquots of fluid were tested for the ability to stimulate choline

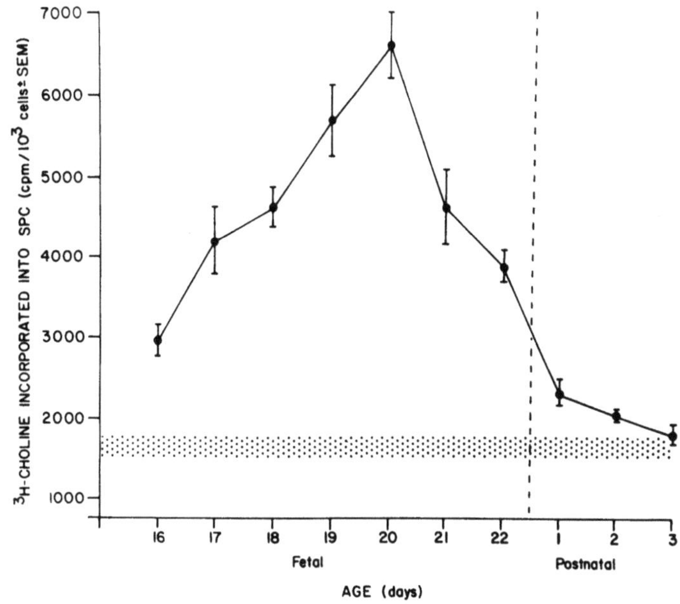

Fig. 9.4. Production of FPF by fibroblasts isolated from lungs of rats at various ages. Cells were grown to confluence and exposed to 1 μM cortisol for 24 h. The media was heat-treated and added to cultures of human lung epithelial cells for 24 h with addition of [^{3}H]choline for the last 6 h. The *shaded area* represents 1 ± SD below the mean for cells exposed to fresh medium containing cortisol. From Smith (1981b), by permission

incorporation by the cloned human lung epithelial cells. Stimulatory activity was detected in most samples of amniotic fluid from pregnancies of less than 36 weeks. This activity resembled FPF of fetal rat lung fibroblasts in molecular weight, heat stability, and solubility in acidic solution. The amount of stimulatory activity was compared with several variables. There was an inverse relationship with the number of epithelial cells in the tissue culture well after 24 h exposure to amniotic fluid, possibly indicating that stimulation of choline incorporation is inversely related to support of continued cell growth. There were also significant inverse correlations between activity and gestational age, L/S ratio, and cortisol concentration in the amniotic fluid. In addition, there was no apparent relationship to the occurrence of RDS. These observations do not support a physiologic role for FPF in human lung development, although it may be argued that the concentration of FPF in amniotic fluid does not necessarily represent intrapulmonary levels.

Probably the strongest evidence regarding a physiologic role for FPF was obtained in a recent study using monoclonal antibodies against FPF (Post et al. 1984). When the antibody was tested in culture systems, it decreased the stimulatory effect of FPF and cortisol on saturated PC synthesis in type II and organotypic cultures, respectively. In vivo effects of antibody were tested in chick embryos. As summarized in Table 9.6, treatment with antibody markedly decreased the synthetic rate and content of saturated, but not total, PC. This effect is consistent with retarded lung maturation in this species. It will

Table 9.6. Effects of antibodies against FPF on PC synthesis in the chick embryo (Post et al. 1984). Chicks were injected intraperitoneally at day 15 with saline or monoclonal antiboldy against FPF (278–415 µg protein). Lung phospholipids were assessed on day 20 (choline incorporation) and day 21 (PC content). Control data for unmanipulated embryos at day 14 and 19 are shown for comparison

	Day 20-21 of incubation			Uninjected embryos[a]	
	Saline	Antibody	P	Day 14	Day 19
Lung PC (% of total phospholipids)	45.3	42.1	NS	44.7	44.0
Lung saturated PC (% of PC)	46.5	32.9	<0.05	29.5	44.6
Choline into PC (dpm/mg protein/2 h)	9755	9056	NS	21	32
Choline into saturated PC (dpm/mg 2 h)	3005	1815	<0.01	4.4	12.9

[a] Control data from Hylka and Doneen (1982)

be of interest to carry out similar experiments in mammals, where it might be predicted that antibody would both retard normal development and block stimulatory effects of surgery on lung maturation.

Table 9.7 compares effects of FPF and glucocorticoids in fetal rat lung. Experiments have been carried out with in vivo injection of FPF, and in cell cultures of both mixed cell type (28% type II cells) and enriched for type II cells (50 %). Injection of FPF into rat fetuses increased the rate of choline incorporation into saturated PC, and altered lung phospholipid composition in a manner consistent with increased surfactant production. The effects of FPF on precursor distribution among phospholipids has been examined with type II cells isolated from organotypic cultures of fetal rat lung (Post and Smith 1984). Medium from cultures of cortisol-treated fibroblasts served as the source of FPF, and fresh medium (rather than conditioned medium from untreated fibroblasts) with added cortisol was used as control. Cells were incubated overnight with radiolabeled precursor in the presence of FPF or control medium, and lipids were analyzed by thin layer chromatography. Compared with the control condition, FPF increased the rate of choline, glycerol and palmitate into PC but did not affect the percent saturation of PC (40%). With [^{3}H]glycerol, incorporation was increased more into phosphatidylglycerol than into other phospholipids, suggesting a preferential effect of FPF on surfactant-associated lipids. The overall distribution of radioactivity from glycerol, however, was not changed by addition of FPF. Moreover, the distribution was characterized by a relatively low percentage of counts in PC (~ 32 %) and a high ratio for phosphatidylinositol versus phosphatidylglycerol (~ 11) compared with data from adult type II cells (58% and 0.2, respectively) (Dobbs et al. 1982). These differences suggest that considerably less of total phospholipid synthesis in both control and FPF-treated fetal cells is directed toward surfactant than in mature cells. Other studies with organotypic cultures have raised similar concerns regarding their suitability as model systems for development of type II cells (Gross et al. 1981; Batenburg et al. 1983). It is possible

Table 9.7. Comparison of FPF and glucocorticoid effects in fetal rat lung. Data are from Smith (1979) and Smith and Sabry (1983) unless otherwise noted (for glucocorticoid results)

Effect	System	Stimulation	
		FPF	Glucocorticoid
Choline incorporation into saturated PC			
– rate	In vivo	+60 %	+53 %[a] (Gross et al. 1984)
	Mixed cell culture	+130 %	+105 %
	Enriched type II cell culture	+67–114 %	Not tested
– synergy with T_3	Mixed cell culture	Not tested	Yes
	Enriched type II cell culture	Yes	Not tested
Intracellular cAMP			
– increased content (at 24 h)	Enriched type II cell culture	+64–228 %	Not tested
	Mixed cell culture	Not tested	+100 %
– synergy with T_3	Enriched type II cell culture	Yes	Not tested
Phospholipid composition (% of total tissue phospholipids)	in vivo	PC 42.6→49.2	–
		PG 0.5→ 1.1	–
Saturation of PC (%)	in vivo	25.7.→40.9	21.6→27.8[a] (Gross et al. 1984)

[a] Maternal injection with betamethasone (1 mg/kg)

that longer exposure to FPF and cortisol would increase surfactant synthesis in the fetal cells.

Exposure of cultured cells to FPF also increases the content of cAMP (Table 9.7). The stimulatory effect of FPF on both cAMP content and PC synthesis is enhanced by exposure of the epithelial cells to T_3. In these culture systems, T_3 alone does not stimulate choline incorporation nor production of FPF by fibroblasts. These observations have led to the proposal that FPF stimulates choline incorporation in type II cells through generation of intracellular cAMP. Furthermore, it is postulated that T_3 acts on the type II cells to increase responsiveness to FPF, possibly by inducing a putative FPF receptor. Under the circumstances where it has been tested, this hypothesis is supported by the similarity of responses to FPF and glucocorticoid.

The mechanism of glucocortoid action in FPF production has been recently examined (Floros et al. 1985). Accumulation of FPF in medium of cortisol-treated fibroblasts was inhibited by both actinomycin D and cycloheximide, inhibitors of RNA and protein synthesis, respectively. When poly A^+ mRNA was isolated from treated fibroblasts, the in vitro translation product from one fraction contained FPF activity on bioassay. These findings are consistent with glucocorticoid action at a transcriptional level in the induction of FPF.

The studies on FPF have extended the concepts of epithelial-mesenchymal interactions from the period of organogenesis to later in development when differentiated cellular function is expressed. As with many embryonic organs, bronchial branching during pulmonary organogenesis requires the presence of mensenchymal tissue (Wessells, 1970). The mesenchymal requirement is both organ and region, but not species, specific. Furthermore, cortisol stimulation of glycogen deposition within epithelial cells of mouse embryonic lung requires the presence of homologous mesenchyme (Alescio and Dani 1972).

FPF within the lung appears to represent an example of paracrine regulation during later differentiation. Morphologic studies, demonstrating close contact between the basal surface of most fetal type II cells and mesenchymal lipofibroblasts, support this proposal (Marin et al. 1982). The properties of FPF generation and action, in as far as they have been characterized, are consistent with a role in glucocorticoid action on lung maturation. There are preliminary reports of similar mesenchymal factors affecting expression of differentiated functions in duodenum and liver (Smith and Zinman 1982; Dow et al. 1983).

Several questions remain to be examined with regard to FPF. Are all glucocorticoid effects on surfactant synthesis mediated through FPF? In two epithelial cell lines isolated from human fetal lung, cortisol stimulated choline incorporation into saturated PC in the apparent absence of fibroblasts (Tanswell and Smith 1979; Smith 1978). Although the degree of stimulation (50–67%) is less than observed with FPF, the increase resembles that seen in vivo and in organ cultures. Also, glucocorticoids are reported to stimulate choline incorporation in isolated "pre-alveolar type II cells", a culture system nearly devoid of fibroblasts (Scott et al. 1983) and in isolated type II cells of adult rat (Post et al. 1980).

The characteristics of these cell populations, and their response to glucocorticoid, deserve further study. Areas of interest include other parameters of responsiveness (incorporation of other precursors into saturated PC and phosphatidylglycerol, cell content of these two phospholipids, effect on the content and size of lamellar bodies, relationship between response and cell growth, etc.), and further characterization of the glucocorticoid effect (specificity for glucocorticoid, dose-response relationships with non-metabolized corticosteroids, time course of effects, effect on intracellular cAMP, etc.). It will also be of interest to test FPF in other culture systems. For example, FPF should mimic the effects of glucocorticoids in organ culture, and the response to both glucocorticoids and FPF should be blocked by antibodies to FPF.

Does FPF have a physiologic role in lung maturation? The stimulatory effects of administered FPF in vivo do not necessarily indicate a physiologic role, but the data with antibody are persuasive. When a more sensitive assay is available for FPF, it will be of interest to determine concentrations in lung tissue and in freshly-isolated fibroblasts at various points in gestation and after both hormonal stimulation and ablation.

Do fibroblasts produce FPF in the absence of corticosteroid? Present data indicate that basal FPF activity cannot be detected in cultures of fibroblasts. If this is truly the case, and not merely a reflection of the relative insensitivity of the assay system, then corticosteroid regulation of FPF may represent a relatively unique system. In most glucocorticoid inducible systems, there is a basal level of activity even in the complete absence of hormone. This question may be resolved with development of a sensitive radioimmunoassay for FPF.

What is the mechanism of action of FPF within type II cells? The increase in cAMP concentrations after FPF treatment suggests that this cyclic nucleotide may be a secondary messenger. The relatively slow response time in generation of cAMP, however, indicates that the process is not merely activation of adenylate cyclase such as occurs with other hormones interacting with membrane receptors. The question of membrane receptors for FPF should be testable in the near future as the polypeptide is purified in greater quantities and becomes available for iodination and binding studies. It will be of interest to determine whether the stimulation of cAMP requires de novo protein synthesis by type II cells. If cAMP is the only mediator of FPF effects, then similar responses should be obtained to the two compounds. In studies both in vivo and with organ culture of lung, differences in the effects of glucocorticoids and cAMP/aminophylline have been apparent. Further understanding of the involvement of cAMP in the glucocorticoid response will be forthcoming when comparative studies with glucocorticoids and FPF, including determinations of cAMP levels, are carried out in mixed cell systems and isolated type II cells.

Does T_3 stimulate surfactant synthesis only by increasing type II cell responsiveness to FPF? This appears unlikely, since multiple differences in the effects of T_3 and glucocorticoids have been described. These findings are discussed in Chap. 10. It is possible that surfactant synthesis is stimulated by two separate mechanisms. One apparently involves de novo protein synthesis, and may be independent of cAMP; a secondary stimulatory pathway, which may not be specific for surfactant phospholipids, may be responsive to intracellular cAMP and thus to FPF.

9.6 Insulin

9.6.1 Diabetes and Lung Maturation

The infant of the pregnant woman with milder forms of diabetes is characterized by a number of abnormalities. These include macrosomia with organomegaly, placental hypertrophy, polyhydramnios, and an increased incidence of congenital abnormalities and intrauterine death. Biochemically, infants of diabetic mothers are hyperglycemic and hyperinsulinemic in utero and have an increased proportion of body fat (reviewed in Farrell et al. 1982). It is generally accepted that these complications are related to the hyperinsulinemic state in fetuses of diabetic women. The hyperglycemia in the diabetic mother increases glucose concentrations in the fetus with secondary β cell hyperplasia and fetal hyperinsulinemia. Evidence for fetal hyperinsulinemia includes increased pancreatic insulin in fetuses of diabetic women, increased rate of glucose disposal in newborn infants, and elevated levels of both insulin (gestational diabetes) and C-peptide (produced by cleavage of proinsulin to insulin) in cord serum (Pedersen et al. 1954; Steinke and Driscol 1965; Isles et al. 1968; Neufeld et al. 1978; Sosenko et al. 1979). A direct demonstration of hyperinsulinemia in infants of women with overt diabetes has not been possible because of the transplacental passage of maternal antibodies produced by insulin therapy.

It has been suspected for a number of years that infants of diabetic mothers have delayed lung development. An increased incidence of respiratory distress among these infants was suggested by various clinical observation; however, these studies have received criticism as to study design (reviewed by Frantz and Epstein 1978). The report by Robert et al. (1976) appears to have firmly established the increased risk for RDS, independent of other confounding factors, in infants of diabetic women. In this study, the occurrence of RDS due to maternal diabetes per se was found to be approximately 5 times higher than for non-diabetic pregnancies for the age range of 32.5–38.5 weeks. The risk factor for RDS in infants of diabetic women has undoubtedly decreased in recent years with improved management of maternal diabetes and better perinatal care.

A second line of evidence for retarded lung maturation in diabetes come from studies of phospholipids in amniotic fluid. Gluck and Kulovich (1973) first described the abnormal developmental pattern of L/S ratio in diabetic pregnancies. The increase in L/S ratio occurs later than normal in diabetes of class A–C, whereas more severe forms of diabetes are associated with a precocious rise. In addition, the L/S ratio appears to be a less reliable predictor of lung maturity in the diabetic pregnancy. Whereas there is a low incidence of false positives for L/S ratios in normal pregnancies, there are many reports of infants of diabetic women who develop RDS despite having a mature L/S ratio (greater than 2.0) (reviewed by Frantz and Epstein 1978). The developmental profiles for phosphatidylglycerol and phosphatidylinositol in amniotic fluid are also abnormal in the diabetic pregnancy (Kulovich and Gluck 1979). Thus, human diabetes is apparently associated with delayed appearance of surfactant in amniotic fluid and possibly an abnormality of surfactant function and/or alveolar structure. These observations have prompted a variety of experimental studies to investigate the effects of insulin (and glucose) on lung maturation. Both clinical and experimental aspects of this topic were recently reviewed by Bourbon and Farrell (1985).

9.6.2 In Vivo Models

Table 9.8 summarizes the various experimental approaches to inducing diabetes in animal models. The approaches include chemical pancreatectomy (alloxan or streptozotocin), direct fetal infusion with insulin (producing secondary fetal hypoglycemia), and infusion of glucose to the fetus with secondary hyperinsulinemia. Treatment with either of the drugs causes considerable maternal mortality early in pregnancy and produces several metabolic and growth effects. There is considerably less experience with the infusion of insulin or glucose to the fetus. The effects of these various maneuvers on lung function or phospholipid metabolism are described below.

9.6.2.1 Alloxan

Alloxan, which was first synthesized in 1838 from uric acid, has been used ex-

Table 9.8. Characteristics of diabetic animal models used in lung studies

Drug	Dose	Species	Serum glucose (% of control)		Serum insulin (% of control)		Fetal growth (% of control)				References
			Maternal	Fetal	Maternal	Fetal	Placenta	Body	Lung	Liver	
Alloxan	60–130 mg/kg (maternal)	Rabbit	240–290	210–571	31–44	100–365	100	76–90	71–85	76	Sosenko et al. 1980a; Bose et al. 1980; Neufeld et al. 1981; Neufeld & Melmed 1981
Strepto-zotocin	40–180 mg/kg (maternal)	Rat	400–1590	700–1100	17–44	100–500	124–159	75–87	68–100	71–80	Ulane et al. 1982; Singh & Feigelson 1983; Tsai et al. 1981, 1983; Tyden et al. 1980; Gewolb et al. 1982, 1984; Mulay & McNaughton 1983;
Insulin	19 U/day (fetal)	Monkey		43		7900		130			Susa et al. 1979;
	12 U/day (fetal)	Sheep		53		950		Intrauterine death			Rooney et al. 1983; Warburton et al. 1981
Glucose	14–16 mg/kg/min (fetal)	Sheep	100	200	100	300		Intrauterine death			Warburton 1983a, b

tensively as a chemical agent causing partial pancreatectomy and experimental diabetes (reviewed by Lukens 1948). Some of the effects of alloxan treatment are summarized in Table 9.8. There is hyperglycemia in mother and fetus, and maternal insulin is decreased. Both serum levels and pancreatic content of insulin in the fetus (28-day) were in the normal range in the study of Sosenko et al. (1980c), whereas Neufeld et al. (1981) found elevated fetal insulin.

The effects of alloxan-induced diabetes on lung maturation have been investigated in recent years by two groups (Sosenko et al. 1980a; Demottaz et al. 1980; Sosenko et al. 1980b; Sosenko et al. 1983; Bose et al. 1980). At 27.5–28 days gestation, lungs of alloxan-treated rabbit fetuses demonstrated less stability on deflation during pressure-volume studies and contained approximately 25% less air at the maximum inflating pressure used (35–40 cm H_2O). By 29.5 days of gestation, deflation stability was similar in control and treated fetuses, although maximal lung volume remained less in diabetic animals. Although these two findings are consistent with delayed lung maturation, there is disagreement as to the etiology of this effect. Bose et al. (1980) report that lavage fluid of treated fetuses contains 35% less saturated PC (per g dry lung) than control animals, although there was no difference in the content of total phospholipid. Furthermore, there was a close correlation between air retention on deflation studies and the percent saturated PC of lavage phospholipid. They postulate that delayed pulmonary maturation in this diabetic model results from diminished alveolar content of saturated PC. By contrast, Sosenko et al. (1980a) found no differences between treated and control fetuses for lung content of saturated PC, L/S ratio of lavage fluid, and lavage saturated PC content (per g dry lung). On surface balance studies, however, lavage fluid of diabetic fetuses contained 55% less activity than control animals. No difference in choline incorporation into PC and saturated PC was found for diabetic vs. control groups, consistent with the data on tissue and lavage content of PC (Demottaz et al. 1980).

The disparity between results for surface activity and saturated PC content of lavage fluid is unexpected, since data with fetal sheep show a close correlation between the two parameters (Kitterman et al. 1981b). To investigate the possibility that surfactant of alloxan-diabetic fetuses had abnormal function, Sosenko et al. (1983) tested for the presence of an inhibitor of surface activity (mixing experiments with lavage from control and diabetic animals), measured the cholesterol content of lavage fluid, and determined the fatty acid composition of surfactant PC. No differences were found between diabetic and control fetuses. Thus, the reason for the observed deficit in surfactant function of diabetic fetuses remains unknown. If this observation is confirmed, subsequent studies will need to focus upon other lipid components of surfactant and surfactant associated proteins.

In a morphologic study, several differences were noted between alloxan-diabetic fetuses and controls (Sosenko 1980b). Diabetic lungs were characterized by thicker alveolar septae, less potential air space, increased density of capillaries within the interstitium, and increased amount of glycogen and rough endoplasmic reticulum within type II cells. On biochemical assay, the protein/DNA ratio was similar in normal and diabetic fetuses, but diabetic lungs contained six times more glycogen per DNA. These findings are compatible with delayed maturation in the diabetic fetus. A surprising finding was the similar number and size of lamellar bodies in type II cells of the two groups.

Treatment with cortisol increased deflation stability and the amount of surface activity in 27.5 day diabetic fetuses, but did not affect saturated PC or the L/S ratio (Sosenko et al. 1980c). Although data for similar cortisol treatment of control animals is not available for comparison, the authors suggest that glucocorticoids may produce a specific reversal of delayed lung maturation found in alloxan-induced diabetes. Endogenous corticoids have been examined in the alloxan-diabetic rabbit (Guleff and Beck 1981). Diabetes did not affect maternal plasma concentrations of cortisol and corticosterone throughout gestation, although in vitro production was reduced at 28 days compared with controls. In diabetic fetuses at 28 days, both the plasma levels and adrenal production rate of corticoids were approximately one-third less than in control animals.

The precise effects of alloxan-induced diabetes on development of the fetal rabbit lung remain somewhat confusing. The uncertainty regarding content of lavage saturated PC is obviously a critical point and deserves further study. The absolute levels of saturated PC are quite different in the two studies, and the variability within both control and treated groups was considerable. A possible abnormality in surfactant of diabetic fetuses might relate to the clinical observations that RDS is more common with "mature" L/S ratio values in diabetic compared with non-diabetic pregnancies. An alteration in the pattern of morphologic development as described by Sosenko (1980b) might also relate to the clinical situation. However, delayed structural development in itself cannot explain the decreased surface activity per saturated PC content in lavage of the diabetic fetus.

9.6.2.2 Streptozotocin

The effect of streptozotocin-induced diabetes in the rat has been investigated by several groups. In general, there is little agreement among the studies. The rate of choline incorporation into saturated PC at 19 and 20 days gestation is reported to be increased (Tsai et al. 1981; Tsai et al. 1983) and decreased by about 40 % (Tyden et al. 1980) compared with controls. Gewolb et al. (1982, 1984) found a small decrease (approximately 10 %) in lung content of total phospholipid, PC, and saturated PC expressed per mg protein. This deficit in diabetic fetuses was observed on day 21 of gestation but not at earlier or later times. Mulay and McNaughton (1983) also found less saturated PC (approximately 30 % expressed per g wet lung) in diabetic fetuses at 21 days gestation, but there was no decrease in total PC. Comparable results for phospholipid content are reported by Singh and Feigelson (1983) who examined fetuses at 22 days gestation. A survey of 8 enzymes involved in pulmonary phospholipid synthesis has been carried out with diabetic and control fetuses at days 20–22 of gestations (Gewolb et al. 1984). The only difference noted was *increased* activity of cholinephosphate cytydylyltransferase activity in the diabetic lung at 22 days. By contrast, Mulay and McNaughton (1983) found *decreased* activity of this enzyme associated with diabetes.

Streptozotocin-induced diabetes alters glycogen accumulation and metabolism, but again there is disagreement between investigators. Lung glycogen was increased in diabetic fetuses (Mulay and McNaughton 1983; Gewolb et al. 1982) and newborn pups (Rhoades et al. 1979), whereas Singh and Feigelson (1983) report less glycogen during the last 4 days of gestation. The activity of enzymes of glycogen metabolism appear to parallel the changes in glycogen concentration in these studies. Gewolb and coworkers (1982) found no change in active glycogen synthase activity of diabetic lungs and less active glycogen phosphorylase activity, whereas Singh and Feigelson (1983) report decreased synthase activity and unaltered phosphorylase activity in the diabetic animal.

In adult rats, streptozotocin-induced diabetes was found to decrease lung content of PC and saturated PC and reduce specific activities of three enzymes involved in phospholipid synthesis (palmitoyl-CoA synthetase, phospholipase A_2, and lyso PC acyltransferase). Of interest, values for each of these parameters were restored to normal by T_3 administration (Das 1983).

Experimental diabetes also decreases glucose uptake (Stubbs and Stubbs 1978), oxidation (Morishige et al. 1977) and incorporation into phospholipids (Moxley and Longmore 1977) in perfused lung of adult animals, but similar studies have not been described for the fetus. Using slices of lung from newborn rats, Rhoades et al. (1979) found that diabetes decreased glucose oxidation but had no effect on incorporation into phospholipids. Thus, the effect of streptozotocin-induced diabetes on glucose metabolism in fetal lung, and possible relationship to PC synthesis, is largely unexplored.

In a brief description, Tyden et al. (1980) report delayed morphologic development in lungs of diabetic fetuses. On light microscopy, the lung of the diabetic fetus at day 20 showed increased amounts of interstitial tissue with delayed development of alveolar ducts. Lamellar bodies were seen within type II cells of both control and treated animals, but the extracellular content appeared to be decreased in the diabetic fetus. This latter observation is supported by a morphometric analysis which found a greatly reduced number of luminal lamellar bodies in diabetic lungs (Gewolb et al. 1984). In adult rats, streptozotocin-induced diabetes causes dilatation of the endoplasmic reticulum and golgi saccules (Plopper and Morishige 1978). These ultrastructural changes were felt to be similar to those observed in other cell types with suppressed secretion of intracellular products. Treatment with insulin reversed the dilatation of the endoplasmic reticulum. Of note, however, diabetes did not affect the number of lamellar bodies in type II cells.

Dixon and Jersild (1983) examined binding of lectins (concanavalin A and wheat germ agglutinin) to lung alveolar cells of rats with severe streptozotocin-induced diabetes. Both mothers and fetuses with diabetes demonstrated binding of concanavalin A, indicating accessible glucose residues on membrane proteins, whereas no binding occurred in normal animals unless terminal sialic acid residues were removed by treatment with neuraminidase. This finding supports the concept that diabetes, probably through the hyperglycemia, alters the composition of carbohydrates on the cell surface of many organs including fetal lung.

In the pregnant Rhesus monkey, streptozotocin treatment produces polyhydramnios, placental hypertrophy, fetal macrosomia, increased fetal insulin concentrations, and more intrauterine death. Epstein et al. (1976) examined fetal lung phospholipids in streptozotocin-treated fetuses delivered prematurely. Compared with control fetuses, fetuses of the glucose-intolerant monkeys had greater L/S ratio and increased rate of choline incorporation by fetal lung slices; however, lung content of PC was somewhat reduced. These findings suggest alterations in phospholipid metabolism of the fetus of streptozotocin-treated monkeys. Until such animals are studied in greater detail, it is uncertain whether streptozotocin treatment of the Rhesus monkey is an appropriate model for the human situation.

Thus, the literature presents a confusing picture of the effect of streptozotocin-induced diabetes on lung maturation. It is likely that this situation reflects, at least in part, variable severity of diabetes in the different investigations. As illustrated in Table 9.8, there is a considerable range in the values for maternal insulin and glucose and fetal glucose. Concentrations of fetal insulin were determined in only two studies and found to be similar to control (Gewolb et al. 1982) and elevated (Mulay and McNaughton 1983). Despite the finding of increased fetal insulin in the latter study, the animals appear to have been severely diabetic as judged by glucose concentrations and birthweight. Birthweight and organ weight of diabetic fetuses was decreased in each study; lower birth weight occurs throughout the third trimester at the doses of streptozotocin used (Gewolb et al. 1983). Thus, in addition to the variability of observed effects, the studies addressing lung maturation have utilized experimental models resembling *severe* diabetes in the human. Since the clinical correlation between increased incidence of RDS and diabetes involves milder forms of the disease, characterized by hyperinsulinemia, macrosomia, and organomegaly (Naeye 1965), the studies of both streptozotocin and alloxan-induced diabetes do not provide an appropriate model for the clinical situation.

It has been recognized for some time that lower doses of streptozotocin (e.g., 30 mg/kg) or alloxan (e.g., 67 mg/kg to pregnant rats) induce a milder form of diabetes (Solomon 1959; Lazarow et al. 1960; Pitkin et al. 1971; Pitkin and Van Orden 1974; Aerts and Van Assche 1977; Kervran et al. 1978; Eriksson et al. 1980; Kim et al. 1981). Under these conditions, the fetuses show several similarities with the human infant of the diabetic mother. The concentration of maternal glucose after such treatment is increased less than 100% compared with controls and some animals are normoglycemic with an abnormal glucose tolerance test. Similarly, the increase in fetal glucose is much less than described with the higher doses of streptozotocin (Table 9.8). When it has been assayed, fetal levels of insulin were substantially increased at the lower doses of streptozotocin (Pitkin and van Orden 1974; Kervran et al. 1978). Fetuses born near term have body weights equal to or slightly greater than control animals. For example, in the study of Kim et al. (1981) the frequencies of macrosomia (defined as greater than +2.5 S.D. of the fetal weight in the control population) in control and diabetic animals were 1/98 and 15/110 on day 20.5 and 1/155 and 14/148 on day 19.5 of gestation, respectively. In mildly diabetic animals delivering at term, the stillbirth rate is increased. In one study, diabetic fetuses had increased fat and DNA content, and decreased water content, per body weight, and these changes were reversed by maternal treatment with insulin (Pitkin et al. 1971). On morphologic examination, the fetal pancreas of mildly diabetic animals shows both islet and beta cell hypertrophy and increased release of insulin in response to glucose compared with controls. By contrast, fetuses of rats receiving higher doses of streptozotocin showed degranulation of pancreatic beta cells. In one study, macrosomic fetuses of diabetic rats, but not littermates of appropriate body weight, had a striking increase of amino acid influx after injection of the mother (Kim et al. 1981). Thus, exposure of rats and rabbits to lower doses of compounds which produce chemical pancreatectomy results in diabetic fetuses resembling the human infant of a diabetic mother. It will be of considerable interest to examine lung maturation in animals with mild diabetes, assessing individual fetuses and correlating data on phospholipid synthesis and content with body weight and concentrations of glucose and insulin.

An alternative model for the infant of the diabetic mother is the litter reduction procedure as originally described by Van Marthens et al. (1972). This technique involves removing all but one fetus from each uterine horn of the rabbit at 8 days of gestation. At 28 days, the remaining fetuses are macrosomic and hyperinsulinemic, consistent with the close association between fetal weight and plasma insulin concentration in undisturbed fetuses (Girard et al. 1976; Bassett and Fletcher 1982; Fletcher et al. 1982). In a preliminary study with this model, Levine (1985) found lower values for the L/S ratio in those fetuses with higher serum insulin levels (>24 μU/ml). Further studies seem appropriate to define other aspects of lung maturation (e.g., synthesis and content of saturated PC, morphology) and the concentrations of other endogenous hormones.

9.6.2.3 Fetal Infusion

Another approach to the study of diabetes has been infusion of either insulin or glucose to the fetus. One model in which lung phospholipid metabolism has been investigated is the hyperinsulinemic fetal Rhesus monkey. In this preparation, insulin is continuously infused into the fetus by implanted minipump for up to several weeks. This treatment produces macrosomia, selected organomegaly (liver, placenta, heart and spleen), extreme fetal hyperinsulinemia (2385 μU/ml vs. 30 in controls), but only mild hypoglycemia (Susa et al. 1979; Rooney et al. 1983).

Lung phospholipid synthesis and content were investigated in Rhesus monkeys at 144 days gestation after approximately 3 weeks' exposure to insulin infusion (Rooney et al. 1983). Compared with control fetuses, insulin treatment did not affect total phospholipid content, PC content and percent saturation, and the L/S ratio of lung lavage. Also, there was no effect on phospholipid content or rate of choline incorporation into saturated PC in lung tissue. These findings thus provide no evidence of retarded lung maturation in the presence of extremely high fetal insulin concentrations and hypoglycemia. It is possible that effects might be observed at other times in gestation.

Infusion of insulin has also been carried out in the fetal sheep (Warburton et al. 1981). As in the monkey, insulin infusion markedly elevated fetal insulin concentrations and produced fetal hypoglycemia. Treatment delayed the appearance of surfactant in tracheal fluid compared with control animals, but did not alter the rate of tracheal fluid production. In two of the treated animals, surfactant was detected in tracheal fluid on days when the infusion pump malfunctioned, and surfactant again was not detected on subsequent days when appropriate insulin infusion rates were resumed. These findings, in contrast with those in the monkey, suggest that primary hyperinsulinemia in the presence of hypoglycemia decreased production of surfactant. However, interpretation of these data are complicated by the intrauterine death of all the insulin-treated fetuses, apparently secondary to severe hypoglycemia, at about 135 days gestation. Prior to this time, however, blood gases did remain in the normal range.

In an attempt to more closely mimic human diabetes, Warburton (1983a) produced fetal hyperglycemia with secondary hyperinsulinemia by direct fetal infusion of glucose. Infusion of glucose for 18–33 days during the third trimester did not affect blood gases or production of tracheal fluid; however, intrauterine death eventually occurred in 5 of the 6 glucose-treated lambs. Surface active material, as determined on a surface balance, appeared in tracheal fluid in each of 5 control fetuses between 123 and 132 days, and increased as previously described. By contrast, surfactant was not detected in fluid from the glucose-treated fetuses between 130 and 140 days gestation (Fig. 9.5). Assay of phospholipids in tracheal fluid confirmed the delayed developmental appearance of saturated PC and phosphatidylglycerol.

An important advantage of this experimental approach is the daily monitoring of surfactant flux. The data clearly indicate that glucose treatment delays the initial appearance of surfactant in tracheal fluid, but no information is

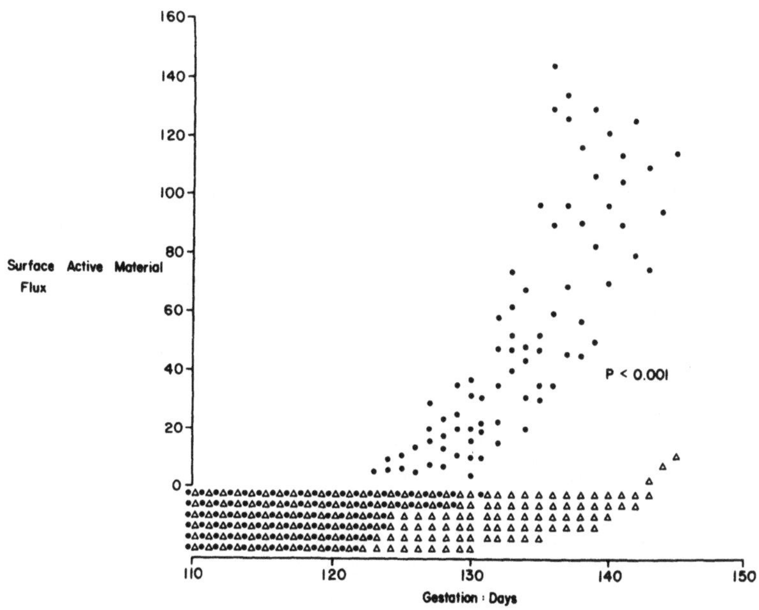

Fig. 9.5. Tracheal fluid surfactant in fetal lambs with *(open triangle)* and without *(solid circle)* glucose treatment. Daily measurements of surfactant flux were made using a surface balance. Glucose was infused into six fetuses at 14 mg/kg per min from 112 days as shown. From Warburton (1983a), by permission

available regarding late gestation because of fetal deterioration. The reversibility of the glucose effect, and the response to initiating glucose infusion after appearance of surfactant, were not examined. Thus, in the sheep, fetal hyperinsulinemia in the presence of either hypoglycemia or hyperglycemia reduces the flux of surfactant into tracheal fluid. These data suggest that hyperinsulinemia per se delays surfactant synthesis in this species.

This experimental model was further utilized by Warburton (1983b) to test the effect of hyperglycemia and secondary hyperinsulinemia on the response of the fetal lung to cortisol. Fetuses received in utero glucose infusions as described in the above experiments, and then were given intravenous cortisol (420 μg/h) between 128 and 130 days gestation. Whereas control fetuses receiving cortisol had increased flux of surfactant as expected, there was little response to cortisol in the glucose-infused animals. In addition, the saturated PC content of lung tissue was half the value in control fetuses, and lung volume at maximal inflation pressure was reduced. The concentrations of serum cortisol achieved with infusion were similar to term levels (8 μg/dl), suggesting that hyperglycemia with secondary hyperinsulinemia could potentially block the effect of endogenous cortisol in late gestation. The relationship between glucose, insulin and cortisol has not been defined and is undoubtedly complex. For example, it is unlikely that the inhibition of surfactant production by glucose infusion is secondary to blocking the action of endogenous cortisol, since the initial appearance of surfactant in the fetal lamb occurs in the absence of any increase in endogenous cortisol. The data do raise the possibility that diabetes would interfere with the response to exogenous glucocorticoids by the human fetus.

9.6.3 Studies in Culture

There are only a limited number of studies of insulin action in cultured lung tissue. The experimental systems include monolayer cell cultures from 28-day fetal rabbit lung (Smith et al. 1975), adult rat lung fibroblasts and an epithelial cell line (L-2) (Sharp et al. 1980), adult type II cells (Sugahara et al. 1984), fetal rabbit lung slices (Neufeld et al. 1979) and both fetal rat (Gross et al. 1980; Rooney et al. 1980) and human (Mendelson et al. 1981b) lung in organ culture. Insulin was tested at concentrations in the range of 1–100 μU/ml with monolayer cultures and 0.1–1 U/ml for slices and explants of lung. The higher doses of insulin with explant tissue presumably reflects restricted diffusion through the tissue blocks.

There is surprisingly little information regarding insulin effects on glucose metabolism. Addition of insulin for 24 h to explants of rat lung increased the rate of glucose oxidation to CO_2 and enhanced the glycogen content. In cultured rabbit cells, there was no evidence of increased glucose utilization based on depletion of glucose from the medium. Transport of 2-deoxy-D-glucose by adult type II cells in culture increased 68 % in the presence of insulin; this effect was half-maximal at an insulin concentration of 1.2 ng/ml, which is in the physiologic range for serum levels.

In most systems examined thus far, insulin by itself has no apparent effect on the rate of choline incorporation into saturated PC (Smith et al. 1975;

Gross et al. 1980; Sharp et al. 1980; Mendelson et al. 1981b; Carlson et al. 1984). In a preliminary report, Shapiro et al. (1984) describe-dependent increases with insulin for both choline incorporation into PC and glucose into fatty acid in type II cells from adult rat. Although insulin alone was inactive in explants of human lung, it enhanced the response to cortisol (Table 9.4). Neufeld et al. (1979) found a decrease in the incorporation of glucose into total lipids, PC, saturated PC and lyso PC after 90 min exposure to insulin. The effect of continued exposure to insulin on content of saturated PC is not known. In these experiments, insulin increased the total uptake of glucose but decreased oxidation to CO_2. The incorporation rate of acetate into saturated PC of lung explants was reduced somewhat (19 %) while rates of uptake into non-surfactant phospholipids were generally increased. Insulin also had little, if any, effect on the activity of enzymes involved in phospholipid synthesis, including cholinephosphate cytidylyltransferase. A morphologic analysis with explanted lung suggested that insulin delayed the appearance of type II cells and mature lamellar bodies (Gross et al. 1980). Thus, in the culture systems for fetal lung that have been used, insulin alone has not produced major effects on synthesis of surfactant phospholipid. The preliminary evidence for delayed morphologic maturation of type II cells deserves further study.

A more striking observation of insulin action relates to the interaction with glucocorticoids. Although insulin alone did not decrease choline incorporation by cultured rabbit cells, insulin blocked stimulation of this process by cortisol in a dose-dependent fashion. The same concentrations of insulin had no effect on the growth inhibitory effect of cortisol in these cultures (Smith et al. 1975). Insulin also blocked cortisol-stimulated increases in choline incorporation and FPF activity in cultures of mixed lung cells and fibroblasts, respectively, from fetal rat (Carlson et al. 1984). In organ cultures of rat lung, however, insulin did not inhibit stimulation of choline incorporation by dexamethasone. When the distribution of acetate incorporation into phospholipids was examined, insulin blocked the dexamethasone-induced increase into PC but not into phosphatidylglycerol. Insulin also decreased the stimulation of cholinephosphate cytidylyltransferase activity produced by dexamethasone (Rooney et al. 1980). Since glucocorticoid stimulation of enzyme activity is apparently mediated by increased content of phospholipid acting as cofactor, insulin may be blocking induced synthesis of acidic phospholipids. As noted, however, insulin did not block the effect of dexamethasone on increasing incorporation of radioactivity from acetate into phosphatidylglycerol. These observations suggest that insulin can antagonize at least some effects of glucocorticoids on fetal lung cells in culture, perhaps in part through effects on synthesis or secretion of FPF. The possible physiologic relevance of these observations is supported by the study in fetal sheep (Warburton 1983b).

Insulin also antagonizes responses to glucocorticoid in the liver. These include induction of argininosuccinate synthetase and argininosuccinate lysase in fetal liver explants (Raiha and Edkins 1977), tryptophane oxygenase in adult hepatocytes (Nakamura et al. 1980), tyrosine aminotransferase in cultured fetal hepatocytes (Ho et al. 1981) and phosphoenolpyruvate carboxykinase in Reuber H35 cells (Barnett and Wicks 1971). On the other hand, insulin enhances glucocorticoid responses in cultured adult hepatocytes

(Michalopoulos and Pitot 1975) and hepatoma cells (Gelehrter 1979), in explants of mammary gland (Bolander et al. 1981), and, in one report, in explants of human lung (see Table 9.4). In some of these instances, the positive influence of insulin on glucocorticoid response probably reflects better maintenance of cultured cells. In hepatoma cells, stimulation of tyrosine aminotransferase activity by insulin results from a generalized increase in protein synthesis and decreased rate of enzyme degradation.

There is limited information on the properties and mechanism of insulin inhibition of glucocorticoid action. In the cultures of fetal rabbit lung cells (Smith et al. 1975) the insulin effect was dose-dependent and occurred at physiologic concentrations. Inhibition of tyrosine aminotransferase induction in fetal hepatocytes by insulin was also dose-dependent from 1–1000 nM, but did not show saturability. The maximal effect of insulin required at least 12 h exposure. In this system, insulin did not affect dexamethasone binding either in vitro or by intact cells at 37 °C (Ho et al. 1981). The specificity of the insulin effect for glucocorticoid responsiveness in culture systems is complicated by the well recognized property of insulin to improve maintenance and growth of cultured cells.

9.6.4 Mechanism

The lung appears to be a target tissue for insulin. High affinity binding sites for ^{125}I-insulin have been described for plasma membrane preparations from lungs of adult (Morishige et al. 1977) and fetal rat (Neufeld et al. 1981; Ulane et al. 1982) and the fetal rabbit (Devaskar et al. 1982). The properties of the binding sites are similar in each system. In dose-response studies, curvilinear Scatchard plots are obtained which are consistent with either 2 classes of binding sites or negative cooperativity. Assuming the former situation, the apparent K_D for the first class of sites is 0.2–0.5 nM. There is a rapid degradation of iodinated insulin in these systems which is inhibited by bacitracin and by incubation at low temperature. Competition for labeled insulin binding to adult lung membranes showed insulin $\gg$ pro-insulin $\gg$ prolactin, glucagon, gastrin, growth hormone and ACTH. To the extent that it has been characterized, insulin binding in lung tissue resembles that described in other target tissues. The presence of insulin receptors on type II cells isolated from adult rat lung is also established (Bonnevie-Nielsen and Geppert 1982; Shapiro et al. 1984; Sugahara et al. 1984), and there are preliminary descriptions of high affinity insulin binding in human fetal lung (Sara et al. 1983).

The concentration of high affinity binding sites in plasma membrane preparations, based on membrane protein, is somewhat greater in fetal vs. adult lung (Neufeld et al. 1981; Devaskar et al. 1982). In both rat and rabbit lung the number of high affinity sites increases during the last week of fetal life without a change in the apparent K_D (Devaskar et al. 1982; Ulane et al. 1982). In an in vivo study with rat fetuses, Sodoyez-Goffaux et al. (1981) found that radio-labeled insulin was concentrated in lung tissue, although to a lesser extent than found for liver. The ontogenic pattern for insulin binding in lung is similar to that described for membrane preparations of fetal rat liver (Blazquez et al. 1976).

In rabbits, insulin binding by fetal lung membranes was decreased in hypothyroid pups and increased after betamethasone treatment (Devaskar et al. 1982), suggesting a possible role for these hormones in the normal developmental increase of insulin receptors. The possible effect of insulin on the concentration of its receptor is of particular importance with regard to the diabetic pregnancy. Whereas hyperinsulinemia results in "down regulation" of receptors in adult tissues, there is little evidence regarding effects in fetal lung. In a study with alloxan-induced diabetes in rabbits, Neufeld et al. (1981) observed no change in high affinity binding capacity of fetal lung membranes despite a 4-fold increase in insulin concentration of treated fetuses. Similarly, receptor levels were increased rather than decreased on monocytes in cord blood of human infants delivered of women with gestational diabetes (Neufeld et al. 1978).

The data on insulin binding are consistent with insulin acting directly on the lung during fetal life. Furthermore, type II cells as well as other pulmonary cell types are potential targets for insulin effects. Receptor levels may be influenced by the fetal hormonal milieu, although autoregulation of receptor by insulin is apparently not operative in the fetus. This latter observation, if confirmed, suggests that the fetus of a diabetic pregnancy may be subject to the situation of both hyperinsulinemia plus relatively high concentrations of insulin receptors. This combination of events could amplify effects of insulin in fetal tissues compared with the adult.

9.6.5 Conclusions and Speculations

Diabetes during pregnancy, particularly milder forms with inadequate insulin therapy, increases the occurrence of respiratory distress in premature infants. The types of abnormalities in lung development, and the mechanisms responsible, remain to be elucidated. The experimental models using chemically-induced diabetes have produced conflicting data regarding phospholipid metabolism in the fetal lung. A major shortcoming of this experimental approach is the severe form of diabetes which is usually induced. Under these circumstances the fetuses are runted and often do not show hyperinsulinemia. Thus, these experimental models are probably not relevant to the milder forms of diabetes observed in the human. Perhaps the most useful experimental approach has been infusion of insulin or glucose into the fetal lamb. The latter approach in particular is similar to the human situation. The results from these studies indicate that hyperinsulinemia in the fetus, in the presence of either hypo- or hyperglycemia, delays appearance of surfactant. These results, along with the data for adult lung, argue that abnormalities in fetal lung can result from insulin per se independent of changes in glucose concentration. However, studies of insulin in cultured lung tissue have not revealed any major effects on the rate of choline incorporation into PC, a measurement which appears to accurately reflect surfactant synthesis during both normal and hormone-stimulated conditions.

Possible mechanisms for the effects of diabetes in fetal lung remain entirely speculative. One possibility is that insulin acts directly on type II cells to alter glucose uptake, oxidation and metabolism. Surfactant synthesis could be affected by these metabolic alterations. If, for example, the surge in surfactant synthesis is causally related to glycogenolysis, increased glucose uptake in the diabetic fetus could delay this process. If insulin decreased glucose metabolism through the pentose shunt pathway, production of NADPH and synthesis of fatty acids would be reduced. A related hypothesis advanced by Stubbs and Stubbs (1978) proposes that hyperinsulinemia decreases glycerol production in lung cells, possibly through activation of pyruvate dehydrogenase; this would increase conversion of glucose to acetyl-CoA and reduce formation of dihydroxyacetone phosphate and glycerol-3-phosphate which are required for synthesis of PC. A direct effect of insulin is supported by the presence of insulin receptors on type II cells of adult lung and the morphologic changes observed with diabetes and insulin therapy.

Second, it has been proposed that diabetes affects fetal lung through changes in insulin receptor levels (Shapiro et al. 1984). According to this scheme, hyperinsulinemia produces down-regulation of insulin receptors in utero. At birth, the deficit in receptors would reduce the sensitivity of type II cells to circulating insulin and accordingly decrease surfactant synthesis immediately postnatally. Thus, this scheme proposes that the adverse effects of diabetes occur after birth rather than during fetal life. This scenario seems unlikely in view of the reported effects of hyperinsulinemia in the fetal lamb. Furthermore, down-regulation of insulin receptors during fetal life has not been established.

A third possible mechanism for diabetes to affect the lung involves changes in glycosylation of membrane proteins. This alteration probably results from the hyperglycemia either directly and/or through increased glucose uptake by lung cells, but conceivably could be induced by insulin. A change in membrane proteins could affect the secretion of lamellar bodies or the uptake and recycling of secreted surfactant. Diabetes might also alter the properties of surfactant apoproteins via glycosylation. A family of apoproteins is observed in surfactant preparations from several species, and the multiple forms represent variable amounts of glycosylation. If diabetes affected glycosylation of apoprotein, the surface activity or absorption of secreted surfactant could be reduced. This possibility is consistent with the experimental and clinical indications that lung stability is decreased despite apparently normal concentrations of saturated PC in alveolar spaces.

A fourth possibility is that diabetes affects lung function primarily through an influence on structural development. In human infants of diabetic women, there is both cell hypertrophy and hyperplasia in the lung. An altered growth pattern in the presence of excess insulin might affect the shape and size of alveoli or the volume of mesenchymal tissue. Either of these changes could reduce both maximal lung volume and lung compliance.

Fifth, it has been proposed that insulin interferes with the stimulatory influence of endogenous cortisol on lung maturation. This possibility is supported by the observations that insulin blocks cortisol stimulation of 1) choline incorporation by cultured cells, 2) surfactant flux in the fetal sheep preparation, 3) production of FPF activity by pulmonary fibroblasts and 4) surfactant apoprotein accumulation in cultured human lung. (Mendelson and Snyder 1985) Similar antagonism is observed for induction of several liver enzymes. By contrast, insulin potentiated cortisol stimulation of PC synthesis in human lung explants, raising the possibility that hyperinsulinemia could result in protein-deficient surfactant. This appealing hypothesis deserves further study. Possible interactions between insulin and other hormones also need investigations.

Sixth, diabetes may delay pulmonary differentiation in part as a direct consequence of the growth-promoting effects of insulin. In the lung, as in other developing tissues, the rate of cell division slows at the time that differentiation of specialized functions occurs. The presence of excess insulin and its effect on growth of the lung could delay enzyme induction during fetal development. The mode of this interaction is open to speculation, but presumably involves intracellular substrate levels or regulators of gene expression. If this mechanism is involved in insulin action, other growth promoting agents might be expected to also delay differentiation.

Finally, diabetes may influence lung development in part by indirect mechanisms. The failure to observe major effects of insulin on phospholipid synthesis in cultured tissue supports this possibility. The metabolic perturbations associated with diabetes may affect the supply of substrates (e.g., glucose, glycerol, fatty acids) available for PC synthesis by pulmonary cells. Hyperinsulinemia and/or hyperglycemia may increase availability, uptake, or utilization of myoinositol in the lung. Excessive myoinositol would favor synthesis of phosphatidylinositol over phosphatidylglycerol, delaying accumulation of phosphatidylglycerol in amniotic fluid, as noted in diabetic pregnancies. Alternatively, diabetes may alter the hormonal milieu. Several observations support a possible deficit of thyroid hormones in the diabetic animal. In adult animals, experimental diabetes is reported to decrease circulating T_3 levels (Table 7.4) and both phospholipid content and synthetic enzymes in the lung; the enzymatic and phospholipid deficits were restored by T_3 treatment (Das, 1983). In alloxan-diabetic rabbits, treatment with DIMIT reduced fetal glucose levels and increased lung phospholipid content (discussed in Sect. 7.1.2). It is also reported that T_3 levels in cord blood are lower in human infants of diabetic mothers compared to normal infants (Wilker et al. 1984). Thus, deficiencies in thyroid and other endogenous hormones may be partly responsible for the metabolic imbalances and clinical problems, including RDS, of infants of diabetic women.

References

Abdul-Karim RW, Prior JT (1969) The influence of estrogens on the lung vasculature of the premature rabbit neonate. J Reprod Med 2:140

Aerts L, Van Assche FA (1977) Rat foetal endocrine pancrease in experimental diabetes. J Endocrinol 73:339

Alescio T, Dani AM (1972) Hydrocortisone-increased glycogen deposition and its dependence on tissue interactions in mouse embryonic lung development in vitro. J Embryol Exp Morphol 27:155

Amit T, Barkey RJ, Gavish M, Youdim MBH (1984) Induction of prolactin (PRL) receptors by PRL in the rat lung and liver. Demonstration and characterization of soluble receptor. Endocrinology 114:545

Armelin HA (1973) Pituitary extracts and steroid hormones in the control of 3T3 cell growth. Proc Natl Acad Sci USA 70:2702

Aubert ML, Grumbach MM, Kaplan SL (1974) Heterologous radioimmunoassay for plasma human prolactin (hPRL): Values in normal subjects, puberty, pregnancy and in pituitary disorders. Acta Endocrinol 77:460

Aubert ML, Grumbach MM, Kaplan SL (1975) The ontogenesis of human fetal hormones. III. Prolactin. J Clin Invest 56:155

Azukizawa M, Murata Y, Ikenoue T, Martin CB Jr, Hershman JM (1976) Effect of thyrotropin-releasing hormone on secretion of thyrotropin, prolactin, thyroxine, and triiodothyronine in pregnant and fetal rhesus monkeys. J Clin Endocrinol Metab 43:1020

Baker JB, Cunningham DD (1978) Glucocorticoid-mediated alteration in growth factor binding and action. Analysis of the binding change. J Supramolec Struct 9:69

Ballard PL, Gluckman PD, Brehier A, Kitterman JA, Kaplan SL, Rudolph AM, Grumbach MM (1978) Failure to detect an effect of prolactin on pulmonary surfactant and adrenal steroids in fetal sheep and rabbits. J Clin Invest 62:879

Ballard PL, Gonzales LK, Gross I, Wilson CM (1985) Interaction of glucocorticoid, thyroid hormone and prolactin in stimulation of phosphatidylcholine synthesis in cultured fetal lung. Pediatr Res, 19:149A (abstract)

Barnett CA, Wicks WD (1971) Regulation of phosphoenolpyruvate carboxykinase and tryosine transaminase in hepatoma cell cultures. J Biol Chem 246:7201

Bassett JM, Fletcher JM (1982) Hormonal regulation of fetal metabolism and growth: The roles of pancreatic and adrenal hormones, In: The Biochemical Development of the Fetus and Neonate, Jones CT (ed), Elsevier Biomedical Press, Amsterdam, pp 393–423

Batenburg JJ, Funkhouser JD, Klazinga W, Van Golde LMG (1983) On the suitability of organotypic cultures of fetal rat lung type II cells for biochemical studies concerning development. Biochim Biophys Acta 750:60

Ben-Harari RR, Amit T, Youdim MBH (1983) Binding of oestradiol, progesterone and prolactin in rat lung. J Endocr 97:301

Biswas DK, Hanes SD, Brennessel BA (1982) Mechanism of induction of prolactin synthesis in GH cells. Proc Natl Acad Sci USA 79:66

Blazquez E, Rubalcava B, Montesano R, Orci L, Unger RH (1976) Development of insulin and glucagon binding and the adenylate cyclase response in liver membranes of prenatal, postnatal and adult rats: evidence of glucagon resistance. Endocrinology 98:1014

Bolander FF Jr, Nicholas KR, Van Wyk JJ, Topper JY (1981) Insulin is essential for accumulation of casein mRNA in mouse mammary epithelial cells. Proc Natl Acad Sci USA 78:5682

Bonnevie-Nielsen V, Geppert EF (1982) Presence of surface receptors for insulin and absence of glucagon receptors on rat alveolar type II cells. Am Rev Resp Dis 125:229 (abstract)

Bose CL, Manne DN, D'Ercole AJ, Lawson EE (1980) Delayed fetal pulmonary maturation in a rabbit model of the diabetic pregnancy. J Clin Invest 66:220

Bourbon JR, Farrell PM (1985) Fetal lung development in the diabetic pregnancy. Pediatr Res 19:253

Carlson KS, Smith BT, Post M (1984) Insulin acts on the fibroblast to inhibit glucocorticoid stimulation of lung maturation. J Appl Physiol Environ Exercise Physiol 57:1577

Carpenter G, Cohen S (1979) Epidermal growth factor. Ann Rev Biochem 48:193

Carpenter G (1981) Epidermal growth factor. In: Handbook of Experimental Pharmacology. Tissue Growth Factors, Baserga R (ed), Springer, Berlin, Heidelberg, New York, pp 89–132

Catterton WZ, Escobedo MB, Sexson WR, Gray ME, Sundell HW, Stahlman MT (1979) Effect of epidermal growth factor on lung maturation in fetal rabbits. Pediatr Res 13:104

Chan JSD, Robertson HA, Friesen HG (1978) Distribution of binding sites for ovine placental lactogen in the sheep. Endocrinology 102:632

Chen LB, Gudor RC, Sunn T-T, Chen AB, Mosesson MW (1977) Control of a cell surface major glycoprotein by epidermal growth factor. Science 197:776

Chu AJ, Rooney SA (1985) Stimulation of cholinephosphate cytidylyltransferase activity by estrogen in fetal rabbit lung is mediated by phospholipids. Biochim Biophys Acta, in press

Clements JA, Reyes, FI, Winter JSD, Faiman C (1977) Studies of human sexual development IV. Fetal pituitary and serum, and amniotic fluid concentrations of prolactin. J Clin Endocrinol Metab 44:408

Cohen S (1963) Isolation of a mouse submaxillary gland protein accelerating incisor eruption and eyelid opening in the newborn animal. J Biol Chem 237:1555

Conly PW, LeMaire WJ, Monkus EF, Cleveland WW (1973) Plasma estriol concentration in infants with the respiratory distress syndrome. J Pediatr 83:851
Costlow ME, McGuire WL (1977) Autoradiographic localization of the binding of ^{125}I-labelled prolactin to rat tissues in vitro. J Endocrinol 75:221
Coulter DM, Avery ME (1980) Paradoxical reduction in tissue hydration with weight gain in neonatal rabbit pups. Pediatr Res 14:1122
Coulter DM (1983) Prolactin: a hormonal regulator of the neonatal tissue water reservoir. Pediatr Res 17:665
Cox MA, Torday JS (1981) Pituitary oligopeptide regulation of phosphatidylcholine synthesis by fetal rabbit lung cells: Lack of effect with prolactin. Am Rev Respir Dis 123:181
Das DK (1983) Hormonal control of pulmonary surfactant synthesis. Arch Biochem Biophys 224:1
Demottaz V, Epstein MF, Frantz ID III (1980) Phospholipid synthesis in lung slices from fetuses of alloxan diabetic rabbits. Pediatr Res 14:47
Devaskar SU, Ganguli S, Devaskar UP, Sperling MA (1982) Glucocorticoids and hypothyroidism modulate development of fetal lung insulin receptors. Am J Physiol 242:E384
Devaskar UP (1982) Epidermal growth factor receptors in fetal and maternal rabbit lung. Biochem Biophys Res Commun 107:714
Dhanireddy R, Smith YF, Hamosh M, Mullon DK, Scanlon JW, Hamosh P (1983) Respiratory distress syndrome in the newborn: Relationship to serum prolactin, thyroxine, and sex. Biol Neonate 43:9
Dickey RP, Robertson AF (1969) Newborn estrogen excretion: Its relationship to sex, birth weight, maternal complications and idiopathic respiratory distress syndrome. Am J Obstet Gynecol 104:551
Dixon MT, Jersild RA, Jr (1983) Diabetic pregnancy: changes in lectin binding to the surface of rat lung alveolar epithelial cells. Am J Pathol 113:389
Dobbs LG, Mason RJ, Williams MC, Benson BJ, Sueishi K (1982) Secretion of surfactant by primary cultures of alveolar type II cells isolated from rats. Biochim Biophys Acta 713:118
Dow KE, Sabry K, Smith BT (1983) Evidence for epithelial-mesenchymal interactions mediating glucocorticoid effects in developing chick liver. Fibroblast-hepatocyte factor. Cell Tissue Res 231:83
Epstein MF, Farrell PM, Chez RA (1976) Fetal lung lecithin metabolism in the glucose-intolerant Rhesus monkey pregnancy. Pediatrics 57:722
Eriksson U, Andersson A, Efendic S, Elde R, Hellerstrom C (1980) Diabetes in pregancy: effects on the foetal and newborn rat with particular regard to body weight, serum insulin concentration and pancreatic contents of insulin, glucagon and somatostatin. Acta Endocrinologica 94:354
Farrell PM, Engle MJ, Frantz ID, Goldman AS, Kalkhoff R, Kemnitz JW, Perelman R, Stern JS, Susa JB (1982) Complications of pregnancy and fetal development. Diabetes 31 (Suppl):89
Fletcher JM, Falconer J, Bassett JM (1982) The relationship of body and placental weight to plasma levels of insulin and other hormones during development in fetal rabbit. Diabetologia 23:124
Floros J, Post M, Smith BT (1985) Glucocorticoids affect the synthesis of pulmonary fibroblast-pneumonocyte factor at a pretranslational level. J Biol Chem 260:2265
Flückiger E, del Pozo E, Werder Kvon (1982) Prolactin: Physiology, Pharmacology and Clinical Findings. Monographs on Endocrinology, Vol 23, Springer, Berlin, Heidelberg, New York
Fox CF, Das M (1979) Internalization and processing of the EGF receptor in the induction of DNA synthesis in cultured fibroblasts: The endocytic activation hypothesis. J Supramol Struct 10:199
Frank DJ, Yazitzis MP, Gebhard R (1965) Urinary estriol levels and respiratory distress in the premature infant. J Pediatr 67:677
Frantz AG (1978) Prolactin. N Engl J Med 298:201
Frantz ID, Epstein MF (1978) Fetal lung development in pregnancies complicated by diabetes. Seminars in Perinatology 2:347
Gelehrter TD (1979) Synergistic and antagonistic effects of glucocorticoids on insulin action. In: Glucocorticoid Hormone Action. Monographs on Endocrinology, Vol 12, Springer, Berlin Heidelberg, New York, pp 583–591

Gewolb IH, Barrett C, Wilson CM, Warhaw JB (1982) Delay in pulmonary glycogen degradation in fetuses of streptozotocin diabetic rats. Pediatr Res 16:869
Gewolb IH, Barrett C, Warshaw JB (1983) Placental growth and glycogen metabolism in streptozotocin diabetic rats. Pediatr Res 17:587
Gewolb IH, Rooney SA, Barrett C, Ingleson LD, Light D, Wilson CM, Walker Smith GJ, Gross I, Warshaw JB (1985) Delayed pulmonary maturation in the fetus of the streptozotocin-diabetic rat. Exp Lung Res 8:141
Girard JR, Rieutort M, Kervran A, Jost A (1976) Hormonal control of fetal growth with particular reference to insulin and growth hormones. In: Perinatal Medicine, Rooth G, Bratteby LE (eds). Almqvist and Wilksell International, Stockholm, pp 197–202
Giussi GA, Ballejo G, Bustos R, Caldeyro-Barcia R (1981) Effects of bromocriptine administration to pregnant rabbits upon fetal lung maturation. Pediatr Res 15:850
Gluck L, Kulovich MV (1973) Lecithin/sphingomyelin ratios in amniotic fluid in normal and abnormal pregnancy. Am J Obstet Gynecol 115:539
Gluckman PD, Ballard PL, Kaplan SL, Liggins GC, Grumbach MM (1978) Prolactin in umbilical cord blood and the respiratory distress syndrome. J Pediatr 93:1011
Gluckman PD, Marti-Henneberg C, Thomsett MJ, Kaplan SL, Rudolph AM, Grumbach MM (1979) Hormone ontogeny in the ovine fetus. VI. Dopaminergic regulation of prolactin secretion. Endocrinology 105:1173
Goldkrand JW (1978) Unconjugated estriol and cortisol in maternal and cord serum and amniotic fluid in normal and abnormal pregnancy. Obstet Gynecol 52:264
Gonzales LK, Ballard PL (1984) Glucocorticoid and thyroid hormone stimulation of phosphatidylcholine synthesis in cultured human fetal lung. Pediatr Res 18:310A (abstract)
Gregory H (1975) Isolation and structure of urogastrone and its relationship to epidermal growth factor. Nature 257:325
Gross I, Wilson CM, Ingleson LD, Brehier A, Rooney SA (1979) The influence of hormones on the biochemical development of fetal rat lung in organ culture I. Estrogen. Biochim Biophys Acta 575:375
Gross I, Walker Smith GH, Wilson CM, Maniscalco WM, Ingleson LD, Brehier A, Rooney SA (1980) The influence of hormones on the biochemical development of fetal rat lung in organ culture. II. Insulin. Pediatr Res 14:834
Gross I, Freedman RM, Wilson CM, Lindsey S (1981) Organotypic culture of fetal rat lung: evaluation and comparison with organ culture. Am Rev Resp Dis 123:313
Gross I, Ballard PL, Ballard RA, Jones CT, Wilson CM (1983) Corticosteroid stimulation of phosphatidylcholine synthesis in cultured fetal rabbit lung: evidence for de novo protein synthesis mediated by glucocorticoid receptors. Endocrinology 112:829
Gross I, Dynia DW (1984) Do EGF and glucocorticoids act at the same metabolic sites in fetal rat lung? Pediatr Res 18:392A (abstract)
Grosso DS, MacDonald CP, Thomasson JE, Christian CD (1980) Relationship of newborn serum prolactin levels to the respiratory distress syndrome and maternal hypertension. Am J Obstet Gynecol 137:569
Guleff PS, Beck RR (1981) Maternal and fetal adrenocortical function in the diabetic rabbit. Am J Physiol (Endocrinol Metab) 3:E217
Hamosh M, Hamosh P (1977) The effect of prolactin on the lecithin content of fetal rabbit lung. J Clin Invest 59:1002
Hatjis CG, Wu CH, Gabbe SF (1981) Amniotic fluid prolactin levels and lecithin/sphingomyelin ratios during the third trimester of human gestation. Am J Obstet Gynecol 139:435
Hauth JC, Parker CR Jr, MacDonald PC, Porter JC, Johnston JM (1978) A role of fetal prolactin in lung maturation. Obstet Gynecol 51:81
Ho KKW, Cake MH, Yeoh GCT, Oliver IT (1981) Insulin antagonism of glucocorticoid induction of tyrosine aminotransferase in cultured foetal hepatocytes. Eur J Biochem 118:137
Hoath SB, Lakshmanan J, Fisher DA (1983) Differential hormonal response of epidermal growth factor concentration in the developing mouse: Synergism of triiodothyronine and dexamethasone in epidermal maturation. Life Sci 32:2709
Hoath SB, Lakshmanan J, Fisher DA (1984) Thyroid hormone effects on skin and hepatic epidermal growth factor concentrations in neonatal and adult mice. Biol Neonate 45:49
Hollenberg MD, Cuatrecasas P (1973) Epidermal growth factor: Receptors in human fibroblasts and modulation of action by cholera toxin. Proc Natl Acad Sci USA 70:2964

Hylka VW, Doneen BA (1982) Lung phospholipids in the embryonic and immature chicken: Changes in lipid composition and biosynthesis during maturation of the surfactant system. J Exp Zool 220:71
Isles TE, Dickson M, Farquhar JW (1968) Glucose tolerance and plasma insulin in newborn infants of normal and diabetic mothers. Pediatr Res 2:198
Ivanovic V, Weinstein IB (1981) Glucocorticoids and benzo(a)pyrene have opposing effects on EGF receptor binding. Nature 293:404
Jackson IMD (1982) Thyrotropin-releasing hormone. N Engl J Med 306:145
Johnson LK, Baxter JD, Vlodavsky I, Gospodarowicz D (1980) Epidermal growth factor and expression of specific genes: effects on cultured rat pituitary cells are dissociable from the mitrogenic response. Proc Natl Acad Sci USA 77:394
Jones RO (1966) The in vitro effect of epithelial growth factor on rat organ cultures. Exp Cell Res 43:645
Josimovich JB, Merisko K, Boccella L (1977a) Amniotic prolactin control over amniotic and fetal extracellular fluid water and electrolytes in the Rhesus monkey. Endocrinology 100:564
Josimovich JB, Merisko K, Boccella L, Tobon H (1977b) Binding of prolactin by fetal Rhesus cell membrane fractions. Endocrinology 100:557
Kaplan SL, Grumbach MM, Aubert ML (1976) The ontogenesis of pituitary hormones and hypothalamic factors in the human fetus: Maturation of central nervous system regulation of anterior pituitary function. Recent Prog Horm Res 32:161
Kawamoto T, Sata JD, Le A, Polikoff J, Sato GH, Mendelsohn J (1983) Growth stimulation of A431 cells by epidermal growth factor: Identification of high-affinity receptors for epidermal growth factor by an anti-receptor monoclonal antibody. Proc Natl Acad Sci USA 80:1337
Keller GH, Ladda RL (1981) Correlation between phosphatidylcholine labelling and hormone receptor levels in alveolar type II epithelial cells: Effects of dexamethasone and epidermal growth factor. Arch Biochem Biophys 211:321
Kervran A, Guillaume M, Jost A (1978) The endocrine pancreas of the fetus from diabetic pregnant rat. Diabetologia 15:387
Khosla SS, Rooney SA (1979) Stimulation of fetal lung surfactant production by administration of 17β-estradiol to the maternal rabbit. Am J Obstet Gynecol 133:213
Khosla SS, Gobran LI, Rooney SA (1980) Stimulation of phosphatidylcholine synthesis by 17β-estradiol in fetal rabbit lung. Biochim Biophys Acta 617:282
Khosla SS, Walker Smith GJ, Parks PA, Rooney SA (1981) Effects of estrogen on fetal rabbit lung maturation: Morphological and biochemical studies. Pediatr Res 15:1274
Khosla SS, Brehier A, Eisenfeld AJ, Ingleson LD, Parks PA, Rooney SA (1983) Influence of sex hormones on lung maturation in the fetal rabbit. Biochim Biophys Acta 750:112
Kim YS, Yoon Y, Jatoi I, Kim Y (1981) Fetal macrosomia in diabetic multiparous animals. Diabetologia 20:213
Kitterman JA, Liggins GC, Campos GA, Clements JA, Forster CS, Lee CH, Creasy RK (1981a) Prepartum maturation of the lung in fetal sheep: relation to cortisol. J Appl Physiol: Respirat Environ Exercise Physiol 51:384
Kitterman JA, Liggins GC, Clements JA, Campos G, Lee CH, Ballard PL (1981b) Inhibitors of prostaglandin synthesis, tracheal fluid, and surfactant in fetal lambs. J Appl Physiol Respirat Environ Exercise Physiol 51:1562
Klein AH, Fisher DA (1980) Thyrotropin-releasing hormone-stimulated pituitary and thyroid gland responsiveness and 3,5,3'-triiodothyronine suppression in fetal and neonatal lambs. Endocrinology 106:697
Kulovich MV, Gluck L (1979) The lung profile II. Complicated pregnancy. Am J Obstet Gynecol 135:64
Lakshmanan J, Perheentupa J, Hoath SB, Kim H, Gruters A, Odell C, Fisher DA (1985) Epidermal growth factor in mouse ocular tissue: effects of thyroxine and exogenous epidermal growth factor. Pediatr Res 19:315
Lazarow A, Kim JN, Wells LJ (1960) Birthweight and fetal mortality in pregnant subdiabetic rats. Diabetes 9:114
Levine DH (1985) Hyperinsulinemia and decreased surfactant in fetal rabbits. Dev Pharmacol Ther 8:284
Liggins GC, Schellenberg J-C (1985) Aspects of fetal lung development. In: Physiological Development of Fetus and Newborn, Jones CT, Nathanielsz PW (eds). Academic Press, London, pp 179-189

Lukens FDW (1948) Alloxan diabetes. Physiol Rev 28:304
Marin L, Dameron F, Relier JP (1982) Changes in the cellular environment of differentiating type II pneumonocytes. Quantitative study in the perinatal rat lung. Biol Neonate 41:172
Mendelson CR, MacDonald PC, Johnston JM (1980) Estrogen binding in human fetal lung tissue cytosol. Endocrinology 106:368
Mendelson CR, Brown PK, MacDonald PC, Johnston JM (1981a) Characterization of a cytosolic estrogen-binding protein in lung tissue of fetal rats. Endocrinology 109:210
Mendelson CR, Johnston JM, MacDonald PC, Snyder JM (1981b) Multihormonal regulation of surfactant synthesis by human fetal lung in vitro. J Clin Endocrinol Metab 53:307
Mendelson CR, Snyder JM (1985) Insulin inhibits the synthesis of the major surfactant apoprotein in human fetal lung in vitro. Pediatr Res 19:159A (abstract)
Michalopoulos G, Pitot HC (1975) Primary culture of parenchymal liver cells on collagen membranes. Exp Cell Res 94:70
Milewich L, Hendricks TS, Romero LH (1982) Interconversion of estrone and estradiol-17β in lung slices of the adult human. J Steroid Biochem 17:669
Moawad AH, River LP, Lin C-C (1985) Estrogen increases β-adrenergic binding in the preterm fetal rabbit lung. Am J Obstet Gynecol 151:514
Moncrieff A (1936) The value of oestrin for premature babies. Arch Dis Child 11:9
Morishige WK, Uetake C-A, Greenwood FC, Akaka J (1977) Pulmonary insulin responsivity: In vivo effects of insulin on the diabetic rat lung and specific insulin binding to lung receptors in normal rats. Endocrinology 100:1710
Morishige WK, Uetake C-A (1978) Receptors for androgen and estrogen in the rat lung. Endocrinology 102:1827
Moxley MA, Longmore WJ (1977) Effect of experimental diabetes and insulin on lipid metabolism in the isolated perfused rat lung. Biochim Biophys Acta 488:218
Mueller PL, Gluckman PD, Kaplan SL, Rudolph AM, Grumbach MM (1979) Hormone ontogeny in the ovine fetus. V. Circulating prolactin in mid- and late gestation. Endocrinology 105:129
Mulay S, McNaughton L (1983) Fetal lung development in streptozotocin-induced experimental diabetes: cytidylyl transferase activity, disaturated phosphatidyl choline and glycogen levels. Life Sci 33:637
Mullon DK, Smith YF, Richardson LL, Hamosh M, Hamosh P (1983) Effect of prolactin on phospholipid synthesis in organ cultures of fetal rat lung. Biochim Biophys Acta 751:166
Naeye RL (1965) Infants of diabetic mothers: a quantitative, morphologic study. Pediatrics 35:980
Nakamura T, Shinno H, Ichihara A (1980) Insulin and glucagon as a new regulator system for tryptophan oxygenase activity demonstrated in primary cultured rat hepatocytes. J Biol Chem 255:7533
Neufeld ND, Kaplan SA, Lippe BM, Scott M (1978) Increased monocyte receptor binding of [^{125}I]insulin in infants of gestational diabetic mothers. J Clin Endocrinol Metab 47:590
Neufeld ND, Sevanian A, Barrett CT, Kaplan SA (1979) Inhibition of surfactant production by insulin in fetal rabbit lung slices. Pediatr Res 13:752
Neufeld ND, Corbo LM, Kaplan SA (1981) Plasma membrane insulin receptors in fetal rabbit lung. Pediatr Res 15:1058
Neufeld N, Melmed S (1981) 3,5-dimethyl-3′-isopropyl-L-thyronine therapy in diabetic pregnancy. J Clin Invest 68:1605
Pasqualini JR, Sumida C, Gelly C (1976) Cytosol and nuclear [^{3}H]oestradiol binding in the foetal tissues of guinea pig. Acta Endocrinol 83:811
Pasqualini JR, Sumida C, Gelly C, Nguyen BL (1977) A general view of the quantitative evaluation of cytosol and nuclear steroid hormone receptors in the fetal compartment of guinea-pig. J Steroid Biochem 8:445
Pasqualini JR, Sumida C, Gelly C, Nguyen BL, Tardy J (1978) Specific binding of estrogens in different fetal tissues of guinea pig during fetal development. Cancer Res 38:4246
Pedersen J, Bojsen-Moller B, Poulsen H (1954) Blood sugar in newborn infants of diabetic mothers. Acta Endocrinol 15:33
Perheentupa J, Lakshmanan J, Fisher DA (1984) Epidermal growth factor in neonatal mouse urine: maturative effect of thyroxine. Pediatr Res 18:1080
Pertschuk LP, DiMaio MFAC (1980) Histochemical demonstration of steroid hormone binding sites in the lung. J Steroid Biochem 13:1121

Pitkin RM, Plank CJ, Filer LJ Jr (1971) Fetal and placental composition in experimental maternal diabetes. Proc Soc Exp Biol Med 138:163

Pitkin RM, Van Orden DE (1974) Fetal effects of maternal streptozotocin-diabetes. Endocrinology 94:1247

Plopper CG, Morishige WK (1978) Alterations in granular (type II) pneumocyte ultrastructure by streptozotocin-induced diabetes in the rat. Lab Invest 38:143

Porreco RP, Merritt TA, Gluck L (1980) Effect of prolactin on phopholipid biosynthesis by alveolar cell carcinoma (A549) in monolayer tissue culture. Am J Obstet Gynecol 136:1071

Possmayer F, Casola PG, Chan F, MacDonald P, Ormseth MA, Wong T, Harding PGR, Tokmakjian S (1981) Hormonal induction of pulmonary maturation in the rabbit fetus. Effects of maternal treatment with estradiol-17β on the endogenous levels of cholinephosphate, CDP-choline and phosphatidylcholine. Biochim Biophys Acta 664:10

Post M, Battenburg JJ, vanGolde LMG (1980) Effects of cortisol and thyroxine on phosphatidylcholine and phosphatidylglycerol synthesis by adult rat lung alveolar type II cells in primary culture. Biochim Biophys Acta 618:308

Post M, Floros J, Smith BT (1984) Inhibition of lung maturation by monoclonal antibodies against fibroblast-pneumonocyte factor. Nature 308:284

Post M, Smith BT (1984) Effect of fibroblast-pneumonocyte factor on the synthesis of surfactant phospholipids in type II cells from fetal rat lung. Biochim Biophys Acta 793:297

Raiha NCR, Edkins E (1977) Insulin antagonism of dexamethasone-induced increase of argininosuccinate synthetase and arginosuccinate lyase activities in cultured fetal rat liver. Biol Neonate 31:266

Rhodes RA, Filler DA, Vannata B (1979) Influence of maternal diabetes on lipid metabolism in neonatal rat lung. Biochim Biophys Acta 572:132

Robert MF, Neff RK, Hubbell JP, Taeusch HW, Avery ME (1976) Association between maternal diabetes mellitus and the respiratory-distress syndrome in the newborn. N Engl J Med 294:357

Rooney SA, Marino PA, Gobran LI, Gross I, Warshaw JB (1979) Thyrotropin-releasing hormone increases the amount of surfactant in lung lavage from fetal rabbits. Pediatr Res 13:623

Rooney SA, Ingleson LD, Wilson CM, Gross I (1980) Insulin antagonism of dexamethasone-induced stimulation of cholinephosphate cytidylyltransferase in fetal rat lung in organ culture. Lung 158:151

Rooney SA, Chu AJ, Gross I, Marino PA, Schwartz R, Seghal P, Singer DB, Susa JB, Warshaw JB, Wilson CM (1983) Lung surfactant in the hyperinsulinemic fetal monkey. Lung 161:313

Rosenfeld C, Andujo O, Snyder J (1983) Failure to detect a stimulatory effect of estradiol 17-β on ovine fetal lung maturation. Pediatr Res 17:141A (abstract)

Roti E, Gnudi A, Braverman LE, Robuschi G, Emanuele R, Bandini P, Benassi L, Pagliani A, Emerson CH (1981) Human cord blood concentrations of thyrotropin, thyroglobulin, and iodothyronines after maternal administration of thyrotropin-releasing hormone. J Clin Endocrinol Metab 53:813

Sadiq HF, Davaskar UP (1984) Glucocorticoids increase pulmonary epidermal growth factor receptors in female and male fetal rabbit. Biochem Biophys Res Commun 119:408

Sara VR, Hall K, Misaki M, Fryklund L, Christensen N, Wetterberg L (1983) Ontogenesis of somatomedin and insulin receptors in the human fetus. J Clin Invest 71:1084

Schindler AE (1982) *Hormones in Human Amniotic Fluid. Monographs on Endocrinology*, Vol 21, Springer, Berlin, Heidelberg, New York

Scott JE, Possmayer F, Harding PGR (1983) Alveolar pre-type II cells from the fetal rat lung: Isolation and characterization. Biochem Biophys Acta 753:195

Seybold WD, Smith BT (1980) Human amniotic fluid contains fibroblast-pneumonocyte factor. Early Hum Devel 4:337

Shapiro DL, Livingston JN, Maniscalco WM, Finkelstein JN (1984) Insulin receptors and effects on type II pneumonocytes – an hypothesis for the etiology of decreased surfactant synthesis in infants of diabetic mothers. Pediatr Res 18:346A (abstract)

Sharp MJ, Borer RC Jr, Vadnay L, Douglas WHJ (1980) Choline incorporation into lecithin in response to insulin or dexamethasone in homogenous cell cultures of rat lung epithelial cells and fibroblasts. Pediatr Res 14:899

Singh M, Feigelson M (1983) Effects of maternal diabetes on the development of carbohydrate-metabolizing enzymes, glycogen deposition and surface active phospholipid levels in fetal rat lung. Biol Neonate 43:33

Smith BT, Giroud CJP, Robert M, Avery ME (1975) Insulin antagonism of cortisol action on lecithin synthesis by cultured fetal lung cells. J Pediatr 87:953
Smith BT (1978) Fibroblast-pneumonocyte factor: Intercellular mediator of glucocorticoid effect on fetal lung. In: *Intensive Care in the Newborn, II,* Stern L (ed), Masson, New York, pp 25–32
Smith BT (1979) Lung maturation in the fetal rat: acceleration by injection of fibroblast-pneumonocyte factor. Science 204:1094
Smith BT, Fletcher WA (1979) Pulmonary epithelial-mesenchymal interactions: beyond organogenesis. Hum Pathol 10:248
Smith BT (1981a) Lack of species specificity in production of fibroblast-pneumonocyte factor by perinatal lung fibroblasts. In: *Physiological and Biochemical Basis for Perinatal Medicine,* Monset-Kouchard M, Minkowski A (eds), S Karger, Basel, Switzerland, pp 54–58
Smith BT (1981b) Differentiation of the pneumonocyte: Optimization of production of fibroblast-pneumonocyte factor by rat fetal lung fibroblasts. In: *The Biology of Normal Human Growth,* Ritzen M (ed), Raven Press, New York, pp 157–173
Smith BT, Zinman HM (1982) Glucocorticoid induced maturation of duodenal epithelium *in vitro*: role of the mesenchyme. Pediatr Res 16:117 (abstract)
Smith BT, Post M, Stiles AD (1983) Paracrine regulation of lung growth and maturation: The substrate of normal functional development. In: *Abnormal Development of the Heart, Lungs and Kidneys: Approaches to Functional Teratology,* Kavlock RJ, Grabowski CT (eds), Alan R Liss, Inc, New York, pp 135–141
Smith BT, Sabry K (1983) Glucocorticoid-thyroid synergism in lung maturation: A mechanism involving epithelial-mesenchymal interaction. Proc Natl Acad Sci 80:1951
Smith YF, Mullon DK, Hamosh M, Scanlon JW, Hamosh P (1979) Serum prolactin and respiratory distress syndrome in the newborn. Pediatr Res 14:93
Sodoyez-Goffaux FR, Sodoyez JC, De Vos CJ (1981) Insulin receptors in the fetal rat lung. A transient characteristic of fetal cells? Pediatr Res 15:1303
Solomon F (1959) Embryomegaly and increased fetal mortality in pregnant rats with mild alloxan diabetes. Diabetes 8:45
Sosenko IR, Kitzmiller JL, Loo SW, Blix P, Rubenstein AH, Gabbay KH (1979) The infant of the diabetic mother: correlation of increased C-peptide levels with macrosomia and hypoglycemia. N Engl J Med 301:859
Sosenko IRS, Lawson EE, Demottaz V, Frantz ID III (1980a) Functional delay in lung maturation in fetuses of diabetic rabbits. J Appl Physiol: Respirat Environ Exercise Physiol 48:643
Sosenko IRS, Frantz ID III, Roberts RJ, Meyrick B (1980b) Morphologic disturbance of lung maturation in fetuses of alloxan diabetic rabbits. Am Rev Resp Dis 122:687
Sosenko IRS, Hartig-Beecken I, Frantz ID III (1980c) Cortisol reveseral of functional delay of lung maturation in fetuses of diabetic rabbits. J Appl Physiol: Respirat Environ Exercise Physiol 49:971
Sosenko IRS, Werthammer J, Cunningham MD, Frantz ID III (1983) Surfactant dysfunction in diabetic offspring: inhibitors and fatty acid lecithin content. J Appl Physiol: Respirat Environ Exercise Physiol 54:1097
Starkey RH, Cohen S, Orth DN (1975) Epidermal growth factor: Identification of a new hormone in human urine. Science 189:800
Steinke J, Driscoll SG (1965) The extractable insulin content of pancreas from fetuses and infants of diabetic and control mothers. Diabetes 14:573
Stubbs WA, Stubbs SM (1978) Hyperinsulinism, diabetes mellitus, and respiratory distress of the newborn: a common link? Lancet, Feb 11:308
Sugahara K, Friedenberg GR, Mason RJ (1984) Insulin binding and effects on glucose and transepithelial transport by alveolar type II cells. Am J Physiol 247:C472
Sundell HW, Gray ME, Serenius FS, Escobedo MB, Stahlman MT (1980) Effects of epidermal growth factor on lung maturation in fetal lambs. Am J Pathol 100:707
Susa JB, McCormick KL, Widness JA, Singer DB, Oh W, Adamsons K, Schwartz R (1979) Chronic hyperinsulinemia in the fetal Rhesus monkey. Effects on fetal growth and composition. Diabetes 28:1058
Takahashi K, Auletta F, Tseng H–Y, Scommegna A, Burd LI (1981) Lack of relationship between prolactin and adrenal steroidogenesis in the ovine fetus. Am J Obstet Gynecol 139:427
Tanswell AK, Smith BT (1979) Human fetal lung type II pneumonocytes in monolayer cell culture: The influence of oxidant stress, cortisol environment, and soluble fibroblast factors. Pediatr Res 13:1097

Tanswell AK, Smith BT (1980) Cultured pulmonary epithelial cells: clonal isolation of human fetal alveolar type II cells. In: *Birth Defects: Original Article Series,* Vol XVI, 1980 March of Dimes Birth Defects Foundation, pp 249–259

Taylor JM, Mitchell WM, Cohen S (1972) Epidermal growth factor. Physical and chemical properties. J Biol Chem 247:5928

Thomsett TJ, Marti-Henneberg C, Gluckman PD, Kaplan SL, Rudolph AM, Grumbach MM (1980) Hormone ontogeny in the ovine fetus VIII. The effect of thyrotropin releasing factor on prolactin and growth hormone in the neonate. Endocrinology 106:1074

Thorburn GD, Waters MJ, Young IR, Dolling M, Buntine D, Hopkins PS (1981) Epidermal growth factor: a critical factor in fetal maturation? In: *The Fetus and Independent Life,* Ciba Foundation Symposium 86, Pitman, London, pp 172–198

Thuresson-Klein A, Moawad AH, Hedqvist P (1985) Estrogen stimulates formation of lamellar bodies and release of surfactant in the fetal rat lung. Am J Obstet Gynecol 151:506

Topper YJ, Freeman CS (1980) Multiple hormone interactions in the developmental biology of the mammary gland. Physiol Rev 60:1049

Tsai MY, Josephson MW, Brown DM (1981) Fetal rat lung phosphatidylcholine synthesis in diabetic and normal pregnancies. A comparison of prenatal dexamethasone treatments. Biochim Biopys Acta 664:174

Tsai MY, Josephson MW, Donhowe J (1983) Delayed pulmonary phosphatidylglycerol synthesis and reversal by prenatal dexamethasone in fetal rats of streptozotocin-diabetic mothers. Exp Lung Res 4:315

Tyden O, Berne C, Eriksson U (1980) Lung maturation in fetuses of diabetic rats. Pediatr Res 14:1192

Ulane RE, Graeber JE, Hansen JW, Liccini L, Cornblath M (1982) Insulin receptors in the developing fetal lung. Life Sci 31:3017

Van Marthens E, Grauel L, Zamenhof S (1972) Enhancement of prenatal development by operative restriction of litter size in the rabbit. Life Sci 11:1031

van Petten GR, Bridges R (1979) The effects of prolactin on pulmonary maturation in the fetal rabbit. Am J Obstet Gynecol 134:711

Warburton D, Lew CD, Platzker ACG (1981) Primary hyperinsulinemia reduces surface active material flux in tracheal fluid of fetal lambs. Pediatr Res 15:1422

Warburton D (1983a) Chronic hyperglycemia reduces surface active material flux in tracheal fluid of fetal lambs. J Clin Invest 71:550

Warburton D (1983b) Chronic hyperglycemia with secondary hyperinsulinemia inhibits the maturational response of fetal lamb lungs to cortisol. J Clin Invest 72:433

Waterfield MD, Mayes ELV, Stroobant P, Bennet PLP, Young S, Goodfellow PN, Banting GS, Ozanne B (1982) A monoclonal antibody to the human epidermal growth factor receptor. J Cell Biochem 20:149

Wessells NK (1970) Mammalian lung development: interactions in formation and morphogenesis of tracheal buds. J Exper Zool 175:455

White BA, Bancroft FC (1983) Epidermal growth factor and thyrotropin-releasing hormone interact synergistically with calcium to regulate prolactin mRNA levels. J Biol Chem 258:4618

Wilker RE, Fleischman AR, Saenger P, Pan C, Surks MI (1984) Thyroid hormone levels in diabetic mothers and their neonates. Am J Perinatol 1:259

Winters AJ, Colston C, MacDonald PC, Porter JC (1975) Fetal plasma prolactin levels. J Clin Endocrinol Metab 41:626

Yuen BH, Phillips WDP, Cannon W, Sy L, Redford D, Burch P (1982) Prolactin, estradiol, and thyroid hormones in umbilical cord blood of neonates with and without hyaline membrane disease: A study of 405 neonates from midpregnancy to term. Am J Obstet Gynecol 142:698

10 Hormone Interactions

In this chapter I consider recent evidence regarding additive effects of combined hormone treatment in fetal lung. Although some in vivo effects have been reported, most of the data are from studies in cultured lung and relate to PC synthesis as assessed by incorporation of choline. The interaction of thyroid hormones and corticosteroids is partially characterized in three tissues; however, the specific biochemical effects of each hormone, resulting in additive stimulation, have not been determined. There is even less information about interaction of the other hormones discussed. The final section of the chapter considers the possible clinical application of combined hormone treatment.

10.1 Thyroid Hormones and Corticosteroids

10.1.1 In Vivo

One of the first indications that thyroid hormones and glucocorticoids had additive effects in vivo came from Hitchcock (1979). She carried out a morphologic study of fetal rat lung after intra-amniotic treatment with T_4 on day 19 of gestation. The greatest acceleration of structural development occurred with in utero administration of T_4 to otherwise unmanipulated animals. Major effects in type II cells included glycogen depletion and increased amounts of Golgi apparatus, rough endoplasmic reticulum, lamellar bodies, and secreted surfactant. In other experiments, adrenalectomy or metopirone treatment was used to reduce the levels of both basal and (surgical) stress-induced endogenous corticosteroids. In these situations, the morphologic effects of T_4 injection were much less pronounced. Replacement hydrocortisone therapy restored the stimulatory effect of T_4 injection. Although plasma concentrations of corticoids were not determined, these findings are consistent with complimentary and additive effects of exogenous T_4 and endogenous corticosteroids.

More recently, the effect of combined hormone therapy on PC synthesis has been examined in intact animals (Table 10.1). Gross et al. (1984) treated pregnant rats with T_3, betamethasone, or both hormones. Although there is only limited passage of T_3 across the placenta, fetal concentrations of T_3 were substantially increased with the high doses administered to the mother. T_3 therapy did not affect fetal corticosterone concentrations, but betamethasone caused a doubling of endogenous T_3. Fetal lungs were examined two days after treatment. Stimulation of choline incorporation into saturated PC was greater after combined hormone treatment than with betamethasone therapy alone. Comparable results were obtained for the activity of cholinephosphate

Table 10.1. Effects of in vivo combined hormone treatment on PC synthesis in the rat. Pregnant rats and fetuses received 7 mg/kg and 1 µg T_3, respectively. Choline incorporation was assessed in minces of lung at 20 days of gestation.

	Choline incorporation into saturated PC (% stimulation vs. control)		
	T_3	Corticosteroid	T_3 plus Corticosteroid
Maternal treatment (Gross et al. 1984)	20	53	79
Fetal treatment (Torday and Dow 1984)			
Male	−44	27	69
Female	−54	13	44

cytidylyltransferase assayed in the absence of cofactor. In contrast with these results, the tissue content of saturated PC (per mg protein) was similar for combined therapy vs. corticosteroid alone (0.93 vs. 1.0 µg P, respectively). The failure to observe any additive effect on PC content may reflect the relative insensitivity of this measurement compared with assessment of the rate of PC synthesis. Alternatively, this finding could reflect the failure of thyroid hormone to increase the percent saturation of PC (see Table 10.3), enhanced degradation of saturated PC in the presence of both hormones, or hormone effects on intracellular choline pool sizes in addition to synthetic rates.

In the study by Torday and Dow (1984), fetal rats were injected intraamniotically with T_3, dexamethasone, or both hormones. At all doses of T_3 employed (0.1–2 µg/fetus), choline incorporation was inhibited rather than stimulated, compared with saline-injected controls. There was a positive albeit limited response to dexamethasone treatment. Nevertheless, combined hormone therapy was substantially more effective than dexamethasone treatment alone in both male and female fetuses. Other parameters such as saturated PC content in lung tissue were not examined. The lack of response to T_3 in this study is perplexing in view of the stimulatory effects of thyroid hormone previously observed by others after both maternal and fetal treatment (discussed above and in Chap. 7). Differences in experimental approach compared with other in utero studies include using T_3 vs. T_4, a relatively long exposure (3 days), and measurement of PC synthesis vs. morphologic examination.

There is indirect evidence for additive hormone effects on PC synthesis from the study using DIMIT (Ballard et al. 1980). Treatment of the pregnant rabbit causes a dose-dependent increase of endogenous maternal and fetal corticoids. Under conditions in which there was a minimal effect on corticoids, and no induction of PAPase, DIMIT treatment increased both choline incorporation and lavage PC. In situations where DIMIT substantially increased endogenous corticoids and PAPase, greater responses were observed. Also, stimulation of choline incorporation with increasing dose of DIMIT did not plateau to the same extent as the rise in CBG capacity, a response induced by thyroid hormone but not corticosteroids. Finally, the magnitude of the effects on PC synthesis and lavage content with the highest dose of DIMIT were considerably greater than seen with an optimal dose of betamethasone. By contrast, glucocorticoid effects are generally greater than those of thyroid hormones both in vivo and in culture. It is likely that these results reflect, in part, combined effects of exogenous DIMIT and elevated endogenous corticosteroids.

In the fetal sheep, infusion of T_3 plus cortisol was no more effective than cortisol alone for increasing lung distensibility (Liggins and Schellenberg 1985); data are not yet available for saturated PC content of tissue. When PRL was infused along with cortisol and T_3, a greater increase in distensibility occurred than with cortisol. Treatment with cortisol and TRH, which stimulates production of both thyroid hormone, and PRL, was also very stimulatory; however, combinations of PRL and T_3 and PRL plus cortisol were not effective (Liggins and Schellenberg, personal communication). These results suggest that PRL has a permissive effect on the response to thyroid hormone plus glucocorticoid in lung of the fetal lamb at about 130 days gestation. It is conceivable that PRL administration would not be required to observe a synergistic effect with T_3 plus cortisol later in gestation when endogenous PRL levels are high. The synergistic response to cortisol and TRH supports the interpretation that the effect of PRL is a physiologic one. Further investigations into the nature of the inter-relationships between PRL, corticoids and thyroid hormones in vivo are needed.

10.1.2 In Cultured Lung

Additive or supra-additive effects of thyroid and adrenocortical hormones in explants of fetal lung are documented by several studies. Effects of combined therapy on PC synthesis are similar in organ culture of fetal rat (Gross and

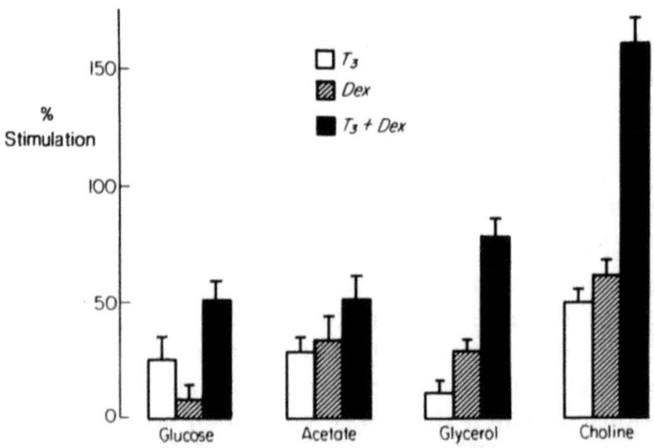

Fig. 10.1. Effect of T_3 and dexamethasone on incorporation of precursors into PC. Explants of 23-day fetal rabbit lung were cultured for 72 h in the absence of hormone (control) or with T_3 (2 nM), dexamethasone (Dex, 10 nM) or both hormones, and then exposed for 4 h to tritiated precursor. Data are mean ± SE (n = 3–5). From Ballard et al. (1984)

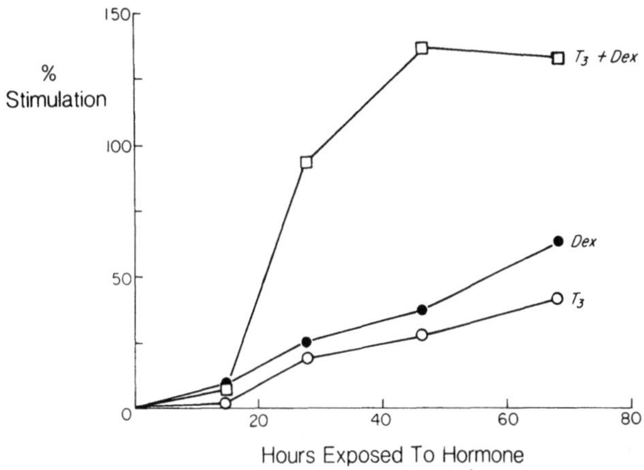

Fig. 10.2. Time-course of hormone stimulation in cultured fetal rabbit lung. Explants were cultured for 68 h without hormones or in the presence of T_3 (1 nM), dexamethasone (10 nM), or T_3 plus dexamethasone for the time intervals indicated. Choline incorporation into PC was assayed after 68 h of culture. Data from Ballard et al. (1984), by permission

Wilson 1982), rabbit (Ballard et al. 1984; Longmuir et al. 1982, 1985) and human (Gonzales and Ballard 1984). The effect of combined hormone treatment on precursor incorporation into PC of rabbit lung is illustrated in Fig. 10.1. An additive effect occurs with acetate and supra-additive stimulation is seen for incorporation of glycerol, glucose and choline. The greatest response occurs with choline incorporation. These data were obtained after exposure of the explants to optimal concentrations of hormones for 3 days, followed by a 4-h exposure to tritiated precursor at a concentration of 1 mM. Data for choline incorporation in cultured rat lung are comparable: the increase was 37 % with T_3, 100 % with dexamethasone, and 197 % with T_3 plus dexamethasone (Gross and Wilson, 1982). Assessment of choline incorporation has been used in further characterization of the synergistic effect.

Figure 10.2 shows the time course of response in explants of rabbit lung. In this experiment, lung from 23-day fetuses was cultured for 68 h and exposed to hormone for various times prior to assay of choline incorporation. After an initial lag period, the response to T_3 plus dexamethasone is considerably greater than with either hormone alone at each time point. The synergistic effect of both hormones is particularly striking at the earlier times of exposure to hormones. Comparable supra-additive responses were also observed after shorter periods of culture. When lung was cultured for only 24 h, the response with T_3 or Dex alone was minimal and inconsistent, whereas T_3 plus Dex was consistently stimulatory. After 48 h of culture, the percent stimulation with T_3, dexamethasone, and T_3 plus dexamethasone was 31, 37 and 116 %, respectively (Ballard et al. 1984). In this and other studies there was a close correlation between rate of choline incorporation and saturated PC content, indicating that the synthetic rate reflects accumulation of tissue saturated PC and lamellar body material (Longmuir et al. 1985).

T_3 and dexamethasone also produce supra-additive stimulation of choline

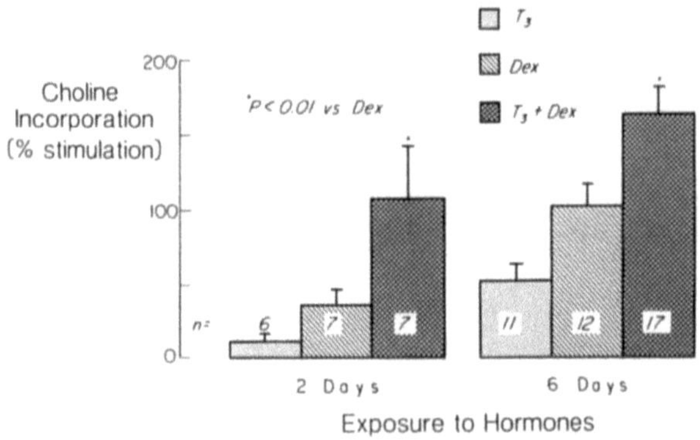

Fig. 10.3. Hormonal stimulation of PC synthesis in cultured human fetal lung. Explants were cultured for 6 days and exposed to T_3 (2 nM), dexamethasone (10 nM), or both hormones for the last 2 days or the entire 6 days. Data of Gonzales and Ballard (1984)

incorporation in cultures of human fetal lung (Gonzales and Ballard 1984). The maximal response occurs after 4–6 days exposure to hormone and the magnitude of the response is comparable to that in rabbit. Figure 10.3 shows the effect of individual and combined hormone treatment after exposure for 2 and 6 days. There is a synergistic response at the earlier time point and the effect is additive with longer exposure. Unlike the situation with rabbit tissue, T_3 does not stimulate incorporation of acetate into PC of human lung in either the absence or presence of dexamethasone (Gonzales and Ballard, unpublished data).

The effect of order of hormone addition has been examined in rabbit lung (Fig. 10.4). In these experiments, lung was cultured with either T_3 or dexamethasone alone for 48 h, and then the other hormone was added. The increase

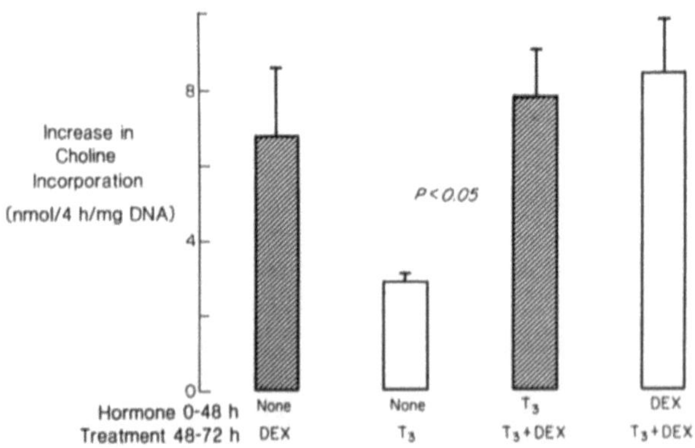

Fig. 10.4. Effect of order of hormone addition. Explants of fetal rabbit lung were exposed to dexamethasone (10 nM) and/or T_3 (2 nM) for the periods shown, and choline incorporation was measured after 72 h of culture. The data represent the increase in choline incorporation rate resulting from the hormone treatment between 48 and 72 h. Prior exposure of tissue to dexamethasone increases the response to T_3, but not vice versa. Data from Ballard et al. (1984)

in rate of choline incorporation with respect to cultures continuously exposed to only one hormone was determined. These results are compared with the stimulation observed by 24 h exposure to dexamethasone or T_3 without prior hormone treatment. The response to T_3 added during the last 24 h was greater in cultures pretreated with dexamethasone (+8.53 nmol/4 h/mg DNA) than in those cultures without prior glucocorticoid treatment (2.89 nmol). By contrast, prior exposure of tissue to T_3 did not enhance the rate of response to dexamethasone. These findings suggest that glucocorticoids increase the subsequent response to thyroid hormone, but not vice versa.

The synergistic interaction between thyroid and glucocorticoid hormones is apparently restricted to those effects which each hormone stimulates independently. T_3 alone stimulates choline incorporation in rat, rabbit and human tissue, and synergy with dexamethasone is seen. T_3 enhances acetate incorporation into PC in rabbit but not human tissue, and additive interaction shows the same pattern. T_3 does not increase the percent saturation of newly synthesized PC in either rat or rabbit lung, and the saturation with T_3 plus dexamethasone is no different from that for dexamethasone alone. With human lung, T_3 produces a small increase in the saturation of PC (Fig. 10.5). Dexamethasone causes a greater increase but there is no apparent additive effect. Finally, T_3 does not affect the distribution of radioactivity from acetate among phospholipids in rabbit, rat and human tissue, whereas dexamethasone does (see Table 7.7). In each of these tissues, treatment with T_3 plus dexamethasone is no more effective than dexamethasone alone in increasing radioactivity into PC and decreasing the percent in sphingomyelin.

There is little information regarding hormone interaction in monolayer cultures of lung cells. In an earlier study, Smith and Torday (1974) found that both cortisol and T_4 alone stimulated choline incorporation, but possible interactions were not tested. Smith and Sabry (1983) examined hormonal stimulation in monolayer cultures of fetal rat lung. In these mixed cell cultures, T_3 alone did not stimulate PC synthesis. However, when T_3 and dexamethasone

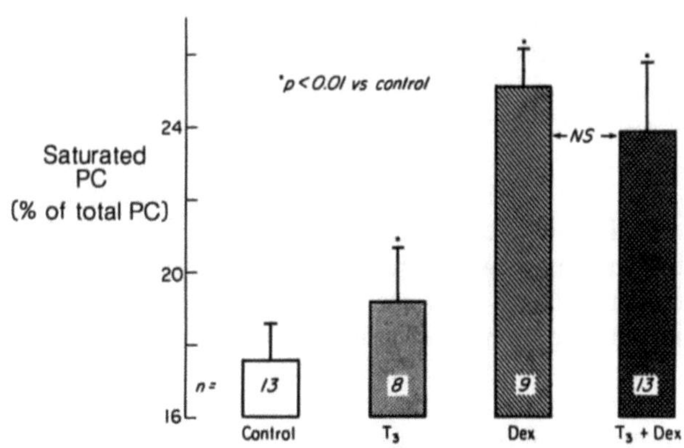

Fig. 10.5. Hormonal influence on saturation of PC in cultured human lung. Explants were cultured for 6 days and incorporation of choline into both saturated and unsaturated PC was determined. Data from Gonzales and Ballard (1984).

treatment was combined, the effect was greater than with glucocorticoid alone. This finding is an apparent exception to the concept discussed above that synergy occurs only for those parameters which are independently responsive to both hormones alone. It is not clear why dispersed rat lung cells show a different response to T_3 than the same tissue in organ culture.

Post et al. (1980) examined phospholipid synthesis in type II cells isolated from intact adult rats. Exposure of the cells to cortisol during 24 h of culture (in medium containing 10 % serum) stimulated incorporation of various precursors into PC, saturated PC and phosphatidylglycerol. Addition of T_4 or T_3, both in the presence and absence of cortisol, had no effect. Although these data argue against a role for thyroid hormones in surfactant synthesis in adult lung, additional experiments utilizing hypothyroid animals and serum-free culture conditions are needed.

The data from the organ culture studies indicate that neither hormone is necessary for a response to the other hormone. In particular, the order of addition experiments where tissue was incubated for 2 days without hormones, demonstrate a response to both T_3 and dexamethasone individually under conditions in which endogenous hormones should have been nearly completely removed. However, these experiments do not rule out possible effects of earlier in vivo exposure of tissue to both hormones. In fact, available data from in vivo thyroidectomy experiments (see Chap. 7) suggest that there is little glucocorticoid stimulation of surfactant synthesis in the absence of endogenous thyroid hormones.

The studies with cultured tissue have established the synergistic interaction of thyroid and adrenocortical hormones in PC synthesis. Since the actions of both hormones are receptor-mediated, it is likely that similar interactions occur in vivo with physiologic concentrations of endogenous T_3/T_4 and corticoids.

10.1.3 In Other Tissues

There are numerous observations of interactions between thyroid and corticosteroid hormones in other tissues. Table 10.2 lists several examples of hormonal effects on enzymes in 10 different tissues. Several of these enzymes have been studied in the adult animal and thus represent hormonal regulation of adaptive enzymes in differentiated tissue. The other entries represent precocious induction of enzymes in developing organs (reviewed by Henning 1981) and in this regard resemble the stimulation of PC synthesis in fetal lung. In these cases, the magnitude of enzyme induction frequently is dependent on the age when the effect is assayed, as well as the duration of hormone exposure (e. g., amylase activity in parotid). In several of the systems hormonal responsiveness is lost completely as differentiation proceeds.

The list of enzymes responding to both hormones includes examples where each appears to be the primary inducer. Corticosteroids have the major effect for induction of pancreatic amylase, pepsinogen, sucrase, maltase, α-lactalbumin, tyrosine aminotransferase, and for the inhibition of intestinal acid β-galactosidase. Thyroid hormones have a major role for the induction of esteroprotease, alkaline phosphatase, NaK-ATPase, NADPH cytochrome C reductase, α-glycerophosphate dehydrogenase, malic enzyme, glucokinase, α_{2u}-globulin and growth hormone. Differing results have been reported for the relative influence of the two hormones on parotid amylase. In the one instance where enzyme induction has been examined both in vivo and in culture (pancreatic amylase), the nature of the response to hormone treatment was similar in the adrenalectomized thyroidectomized animal in vivo and tissue cultured in serum (hormone)-free medium. This comparison supports the relevance of the in vitro results to the situation in vivo.

The data of Table 10.2 also provide some insight into circumstances where one hormone may be required for responsiveness to the other. An example from in vivo studies is induction of alkaline phosphatase in chick embryo intestine (Moog, 1961). There is a developmental increase in this enzyme which is precociously stimulated by cortisone treatment of the intact chick. Hypothyroidism induced by thiourea treatment delays the normal developmental pattern, and T_4 treatment restores the normal rate of enzyme accumulation; however, cortisone treatment has no effect on enzyme activity in the hypothyroid animal. These findings are consistent with a permissive role for thyroid hormones in glucocorticoid induction of alkaline phosphatase. In the case of pepsinogen induction, the experiments in adrenalectomized plus thyroidectomized animals suggest that each hormone is required for responsiveness to the other. In some of the in vivo studies, a permissive role for the one hormone cannot be ruled out since circulating levels of hormones were not determined after the various ablation procedures. These studies are also complicated by other interactions between thyroid and adrenocortical hormones: hypothyroidism in the developing rat greatly blunts the normal ontogenic rise in serum corticosterone concentrations, and high doses of replacement T_4 therapy (e.g., 10 µg/g body weight) increase levels of endogenous corticosterone. It is clear from these in vivo studies, however, that both thyroid hormones and corticosteroids of endogenous origin are involved in the timing of the normal developmental changes in a variety of enzymes.

The studies in organ and monolayer cultures provide an alternative approach to examining permissive action. As noted in Table 10.2, most investigations were carried out with tissue culture using serum-free medium. Among the enzymes listed, corticosteroids are required to observe an effect of thyroid hormone on tyrosine aminotransferase, and thyroid hormones play a permissive role for corticosteroid induction of α-glycerophosphate dehydrogenase, malic enzyme, and glucokinase. Although the studies with freshly isolated explants or cells have been carried out in serum-free medium, this experimental approach does not rule out the possibility that exposure of the tissue to hormone in vivo, prior to culturing, might influence in vitro responsiveness. In the pituitary cell lines, there is a relatively small effect of corticosteroids in the apparent absence of thyroid hormone. In this system, the kinetics of induction are quite different with the two hormones; induction by T_3 is optimal by about 48 h, whereas the glucocorticoid effect is first observed after this time interval. Induction in the presence of both hormones has a time course equivalent to that for T_3 alone (Samuels et al. 1979). The atypical kinetics for glucocorticoid induction of growth hormone in these cells has not been explained.

Table 10.2. Thyroid hormone-glucocorticoid interaction in other tissues

Tissue	Experimental system		Enzyme or protein induced	Hormone treatment (% stimulation) T_3/T_4	Corticosteroid	Both	References
Submandibular gland	Adult rat in vivo	Intact	Esteroprotease	214	–	225	Takuma & Kumegawa 1979
		Adx		182	69	353	
Pancreas	Suckling rat in vivo	Intact	Amylase	0	161	–	Kumegawa et al. 1980a
		Adx & Tx		0	22	114	
	Chick embryo	Organ culture (serum-free medium)	Amylase	0	202	403	Kumegawa et al. 1979b
			Chymotrypsinogen	0	161	329	
Parotid	Suckling rat in vivo	Intact	Amylase	190	275	484	Takeuchi et al. 1977
		Intact		200	52	183	Kumegawa et al. 1980b
		Adx & Tx		182	0	268	
Stomach	Suckling rat in vivo	Intact	Pepsinogen	0	118	180	Kumegawa et al. 1980c
		Adx & Tx		0	0	178	
Intestine	Suckling rat in vivo	Intact	Sucrase	0	1358	2530	Henning 1978
			Acid β-galactosidase	0	-78	-97	Leeper & Henning 1983
		Hpx	Alkaline phosphatase	562	328	1090	Yeh & Moog 1975
			Maltase	140	252	327	
			Sucrase	93	233	275	
	Chick embryo	Intact	Alkaline phosphatase	0	500	–	Moog 1961
		Hypo T		150	0	2600	
Kidney	Adult rat in vivo	Adx & Tx	Cortex Na K-ATPase	73	30	120	Klein et al. 1984
Mammary gland	Pregnant mice	Organ culture[b] (serum-free) medium)	α-lactalbumin	67	450	1500	Vonderhaar 1977
Skin	Adult human	Cultured fibroblasts	Acetate incorporation into cholesterol	58	0	471[a]	Amorosa et al. 1984
Liver	Fetal mouse	Organ culture (serum-free medium)	Tyrosine amino-transerase	0	97	193	Kumegawa et al. 1979a

	Fetal rat	Organ culture (serum-free medium)	NADPH cytochrome C reductase	74	20	167	Kriz et al. 1982
	Adult rat	Hepatocyte monolayers (serum-free medium)	α-glycerolphosphate dehydrogenase[a]	69	0	170	Wilson & McMurray 1981
	Adult rat Tx	Hepatocyte monolayers (serum-free medium)	Malic enzyme[a]	37	0	126	Wilson & McMurray 1981
			Glucokinase	81	0	289[c]	Spence & Pitot 1979
	Adult male rat	Hepatocyte monolayers (10% serum)	α_{2u}-globulin	110	57	302	Motwani et al. 1980
Pituitary	Rat tumor	GC cell line (in 10% Tx serum)	Growth hormone	1600	200	4400	Martial et al. 1977
		GH_1 cell line (serum-free medium)	Growth hormone	1200	250	4000	Samuels et al. 1979

Adx, adrenalectomized; Tx, thyroidectomized; Hypo T, hypothyroid; HPX, hypophysectomized
[a] Cultured in presence of insulin
[b] Cultured in presence of insulin and PRL
[c] T_3 continuously present with dexamethasone added from 36–60 h

The interaction of hormones in mammary tissue may be particularly relevant to fetal lung maturation. In organ culture, the minimal hormonal requirement for induction of the milk protein α-lactalbumin includes insulin, PRL, and corticosteroid. Addition of thyroid hormone to this system causes a several-fold increase in α-lactalbumin activity (Table 10.2). This response occurs at physiologic concentrations of hormone (T_3 and T_4 optimal at ~ 0.1 and 10 nM, respectively), requires 48–72 h for maximal response, and is inhibited by actinomycin D and cycloheximide. T_3 cannot substitute for any of the other hormones, and it does not affect production of casein (Vonderhaar 1975; Vonderhaar 1977; Bhattacharjee and Vonderhaar 1984). These properties are consistent with an effect of T_3, mediated by receptor, on synthesis and secretion of a specific milk protein during differentiation. The effect of T_3 and glucocorticoid individually, and the synergy with combined treatment, is dependent on the presence of PRL. A permissive role for PRL may also occur under certain circumstances in the developing lung (Chap. 9).

The mechanism of the hormone synergy in the various tissues is only partially understood. In the developing small intestine, enzyme induction is associated with both cytodifferentiation and cell migration. For example, there is a synergistic effect of thyroid and glucocorticoid hormones with regard to the depth of the crypts and the height of villi; hormones also cause a precocious increase in the rough endoplasmic reticulum and development of golgi complexes (Yeh and Moog 1975). For induction of sucrase, T_4 acts to enhance migration of sucrase containing enterocytes on intestinal villi. However, this mechanism apparently does not apply for other hormone responsive enzymes in the intestine such as acid β-galactosidose and neuraminidase which undergo a developmental *decrease* in activity.

It is likely that most, if not all, of the effects listed in Table 10.2 represent receptor-mediated hormonal events. In many of the systems it is known that relatively low concentrations of hormone are sufficient for enzyme induction. The multi-hormonal regulation of growth hormone in cultured pituitary cells is not due to effects of one hormone on receptor levels for the other. Cortisol had no effect on T_3 receptor, and conversely T_3 treatment did not alter either cytoplasmic or nuclear glucocorticoid receptors (Samuels et al. 1978; Samuels et al. 1977). For induction of both growth hormone in pituitary cells and α_{2u}-globulin in hepatocytes, T_3 and dexamethasone stimulate the synthesis of the specific mRNAs in a synergistic manner (Shapiro et al. 1978; Martial et al. 1977; Evans et al. 1982; Dobner et al. 1981; Kurtz et al. 1976).

Samuels et al. (1978) examined the question of whether multi-hormonal regulation was a general property for glucocorticoid-inducible enzymes in cells. In pituitary cells, where growth hormone is induced, there is no apparent effect of hormones on total cell protein synthesis as judged by both amino acid incorporation and gel electrophoretic patterns, and electrophoresis of in vitro translation products indicated hormonal stimulation primarily of pre-growth hormone. Glutamine synthetase, a glucocorticoid inducible enzyme in GH_1 cells, is not affected by T_3. Interaction of T_3 and dexamethasone was also examined in cultured Reuber H-35 hepatoma cells which contain T_3 receptors and are glucocorticoid-responsive for induction of tyrosine aminotransferase. T_3, both alone and in the presence of dexamethasone, did not influence the activity of this enzyme. These observations support the concept that multi-hormonal regulation is a selective process for specific inducible functions in target tissues.

Thus, for induction of growth hormone, the best characterized example of hormonal synergy, the evidence suggests that both thyroid hormones and glucocorticoids modulate synthesis by a pre-translational mechanism, presumably involving regulation of mRNA synthesis for the growth hormone genome. The experiments by Dobner et al. (1981) argue against the possibility that either hormone enhances gene expression by stimulating the processing of pre-growth hormone mRNA which was stored in the nucleus of unstimulated cells. However, it is unlikely that the growth hormone system is an appropriate model for multi-hormonal effects in fetal lung. As discussed below, there is considerable evidence that thyroid hormones and glucocorticoids regulate *different* proteins in the biosynthesis of PC. In fact, all of the examples of Table 10.2, except for acetate incorporation into cholesterol, represent induction of a specific enzyme and accordingly are probably not analogous to the synergistic stimulation of a biochemical pathway as presently described for the lung.

10.1.4 Mechanism in Lung

The biochemical sites of action of thyroid and adrenocortical hormones in lung cells are not yet fully defined. Accordingly, the details of the mechanism of interaction between the two hormones are not known. Nevertheless, partial characterization of the phospholipid response to hormone treatment allows some tentative conclusions regarding mechanisms and provides the opportunity for speculation.

Table 10.3 compares the effects of thyroid hormones and corticosteroids on several parameters in fetal lung. As is evident from discussion in previous chapters, there are several similarities between the effects of the two hormones. These include accelerated morphologic maturation in vivo, increased lavage PC, decreased tissue glycogen, increased choline incorporation into PC, and greater activity of cholinephosphate cytidylyltransferase. These results indicate that both hormones are affecting more than one pulmonary cell type (to produce the morphologic changes) and that both hormones influence synthesis of PC within type II cells which results in an accumulation of alveolar surfactant. Furthermore, the increase in cholinephosphate cytidylyltransferase activity probably means that both hormones are increasing the amount or availability of phospholipid cofactor. Stimulation of surfactant production, however, does not necessarily indicate that the hormones are acting directly in the type II cell.

Despite the similarities in overall effect, several important differences between thyroid hormone and glucocorticoid action are evident from recent studies (Table 10.3). The maximal effect on tissue content of saturated PC is greater for corticosteroid than T_3. Glucocorticoid treatment substantially increases the saturation of newly synthesized PC in three species, whereas thyroid hormone has little or no effect. Similarly, corticosteroids increase the distribution of radioactivity from acetate and glycerol into PC and

Table 10.3 Comparison of thyroid hormone and corticosteroid effects in fetal lung

Effect	System	Thyroid hormone	Cortico-steroid	References
Morphologic maturation	Rat in vivo	Yes	Yes	Hitchcock 1979
Increased lavage PC	Rabbit in vivo	Yes	Yes	Ballard et al. 1980
Decreased tissue glycogen	Rabbit and rat in vivo	Yes	Yes	Ballard et al. 1980 Gross et al. 1980
Increased rate of choline incorporation	Rat and rabbit, in vivo, and in culture; human in culture	Yes	Yes	Ballard et al. 1980 Brehier et al. 1977 Gross et al. 1980, 1983, 1984 Gonzales & Ballard 1984 Ballard et al. 1984 Gross & Wilson 1982
Increased activity of cholinephosphate cytidylytransferase	Rat in vivo and in culture	Yes	Yes	Gross et al. 1984
Increased tissue content of saturated PC	Rat in vivo	No	Yes	Gross et al. 1984
	Rat in culture	No	Yes	Ballard et al. 1984
	Rabbit in culture	+	++	Longmuir et al. 1985
Induction of PAPase	Rabbit in vivo	No	Yes	Ballard et al. 1980 Brehier et al. 1977
Increased saturation of tissue PC	Rat in vivo and in culture	No	Yes	Gross et al. 1980, 1984 Gross & Wilson 1982
	Rabbit in culture	No	No	Ballard et al. 1984 Gross et al. 1983 Longmuir et al. 1985
	Human in culture	+	+++	Gonzales & Ballard, 1984
↑ acetate cpm into PC	Rat, rabbit and human in culture	No	Yes	Gross et al. 1980 Gonzales & Ballard 1984 Ballard et al. 1984 Gross & Wilson 1982
↑ glycerol cpm into PG	Human in culture	No	Yes	Gonzales & Ballard 1984
Prior exposure enhances response to other hormone	Rabbit and human in culture	No	Yes	Ballard et al. 1984 Ballard unpubl. data
Sensitivity to actinomycin D and cycloheximide	Rabbit in culture	++	+	Ballard et al. 1984

"+ to +++" = degree of response

phosphatidylglycerol, respectively, while no such effect is detected with thyroid hormone treatment. These findings support the hypothesis that corticosteroids preferentially stimulate synthesis of surfactant, whereas thyroid hormones have a similar influence on most classes of phospholipids synthesized in lung cells. This interpretation implies that corticosteroids act preferentially in the choline incorporation pathway and perhaps in remodelling of newly-synthesized PC, whereas thyroid hormones may exert their influence at a biochemical site earlier in the pathways of phospholipid synthesis. Induction of PAPase by corticosteroids, but not by thyroid hormones, supports this possibility.

Both hormones act through their respective receptors. In view of their different effects on phospholipid biosynthesis, it is evident that the two hormones do not interact primarily through effects of one hormone on receptor concentration or affinity for the other. For example, Gross et al. (1984) found no effect of in vivo T_3 treatment on glucocorticoid binding both in vitro and in vivo. Also, the dose-response pattern for T_3 in cultured lung is equivalent in the absence and presence of dexamethasone (Ballard et al. 1984).

In rabbit tissue, at least, the effects of both hormones on PC synthesis are sensitive to inhibitors of RNA and protein synthesis. Thus, it appears that the mode of action of both hormones involves de novo protein synthesis. As indicated in Table 10.3, the sensitivity of hormone response to both actinomycin D and cycloheximide is greater for T_3 than dexamethasone. This finding is consistent with induction of different proteins by the two hormones.

Finally, there is a differential order of addition effect for T_3 and dexamethasone (see Fig. 10.4). Prior exposure of tissue to dexamethasone increased the rate of response to subsequent addition of T_3. By contrast, prior treatment with T_3 did not affect the rate of response to dexamethasone. Again, these findings are consistent with the two hormones acting at different biochemical sites in phospholipid synthesis.

A model for possible biochemical mechanisms of glucocorticoid and thyroid action in pulmonary surfactant production is presented in Fig. 10.6. One proposal for hormone interaction shown in this figure is that suggested by Smith and Sabry (1983). According to this scheme, glucocorticoids have their primary action in fibroblasts to induce synthesis of fibroblast pneumonocyte factor (FPF). This protein is secreted and influences type II cells through a putative membrane receptor. It is proposed that T_3 acts in part to increase the sensitivity of type II cells to FPF, possibly through increasing FPF receptor concentration, and that FPF stimulates synthesis of saturated PC through generation of cAMP and subsequent activation of protein kinases. With regard to thyroid hormone-glucocorticoid interaction, this model predicts that T_3 acts, at least in part, to amplify the effects of FPF. If this were a major action of T_3, then the responses observed with T_3 alone should resemble those seen after glucocorticoid stimulation of FPF production. The differences in responses noted in Table 10.3 argue against this possibility.

Alternatively (or additionally), thyroid hormones and corticosteroids may both act directly in type II cells as illustrated in Fig. 10.6. According to this proposal, each hormone acting through its receptor would induce different proteins. Thus, there would be stimulation of different enzymes involved in phospholipid biosynthesis resulting in an overall additive or synergistic effect on surfactant production. The possibility of a separate biochemical domain of the two hormones is supported by the observations that glucocorticoids, but not thyroid hormones, increase the concentration of β-adrenergic receptors in fetal lung (see Chap. 8).

A fuller understanding of the mechanism of the hormone interaction of course awaits more information on the details of each hormone effect. The enzymes possibly influenced by glucocorticoids and thyroid hormones have

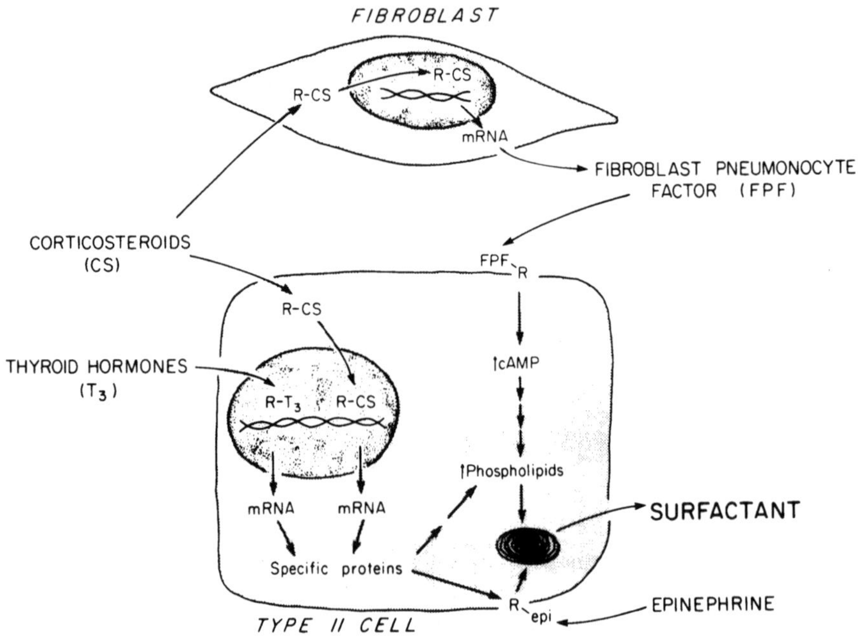

Fig. 10.6. Model of hormone action in lung cells. The different proposed pathways are discussed in the text. *R*, receptor. From Ballard and Gonzales (1984), with permission

been discussed in Chaps. 2 and 7, respectively. One possible scenario involves induction of PAPase, PC remodelling enzymes, fatty acid synthesis, and surfactant apoprotein by glucocorticoids, and induction of enzyme(s) involved in the choline pathway by thyroid hormone. The increased production of phospholipids would secondarily enhance the activity of cholinephosphate cytidylyltransferase through increased availability of cofactor. This indirect effect would further amplify the stimulation of surfactant synthesis by hormone treatment.

There may be additional indirect interactions between thyroid hormones and corticosteroids in vivo secondary to effects in tissues other than the lung. This might involve either production of substrates for phospholipid synthesis and/or effects on hormone synthesis or metabolism which would secondarily affect lung cells. One example is glucocorticoid stimulation of T_3 production from T_4 in fetal sheep. In this species, therefore, the response to increased corticoids includes effects secondary to elevated endogenous T_3. Corticosteroids may also influence T_3 production in the rat (Gross et al. 1984), but this effect apparently does not occur in the human (see Chap. 6). Nevertheless, it seems unlikely that indirect effects are a major part of in vivo thyroid and adrenocortical hormone action in lung in view of the responses seen in cultured tissue.

10.2 cAMP and Glucocorticoids

10.2.1 In Cultured Rat Lung

Studies of Gross and colleagues have examined the effect of cAMP and interactions with other hormones (Gross and Rooney 1977; Gross et al. 1980; Gross and Wilson 1982). Using organ culture of fetal rat lung, these workers have reported stimulation of choline incorporation by dibutyryl cAMP and methylxanthines. Comparable responses were observed with aminophylline, caffeine and theophylline. The response to theophylline is dose-dependent; most experiments were carried out at a concentration of 1 mM since higher doses were associated with cellular necrosis. It is presumed, but not demonstrated, that treatment of lung explants with methylxanthines increases the content of cAMP.

The data of Table 10.4 summarize effects of theophylline and dexamethasone, and combined treatment, in explants of rat lung. The two agents produce a similar stimulation for choline incorporation and tissue content of PC and saturated PC. In the presence of both compounds, the responses are greater than with dexamethasone alone. These findings are consistent with an additive effect of glucocorticoids and inhibitors of phosphodiesterase on both synthesis and accumulation of surfactant in cultured lung.

There were apparent differences in response when incorporation of acetate was examined. With dexamethasone treatment, the rate of [^{3}H]acetate incorporation into phospholipid *decreased* by 53 % during a 4 h exposure compared with control cultures. By contrast, exposure to aminophylline resulted in a 3-fold increase in incorporation (Gross et al. 1980). When the distribution of radioactivity from acetate was examined (Table 10.4), dexamethasone in-

Table 10.4. Effect of dexamethasone and theophylline on phospholipid synthesis in explants of rat lung according to Gross and Wilson (1982). Explants of 18-day fetal rat lung were cultured for 45 h without addition or with theophylline (1 mM), Dex (100 nM) or both agents

	Control	Theophylline	Dex	Theophylline plus Dex
Choline incorporation into PC (pmol/h/mg protein)	486 ± 26	1010 ± 113[a]	987 ± 76[a]	2260 ± 209[b]
Choline incorporation into saturated PC (pmol/h/mg protein)	120 ± 2	308 ± 24[a]	293 ± 9[a]	729 ± 43[b]
PC content (μg P/mg protein)	3.25 ± 0.17	4.30 ± 0.22[a]	4.39 ± 0.29[a]	5.11 ± 0.39[b]
Saturated PC content (μg P/mg protein)	0.80 ± 0.05	1.43 ± 0.11[a]	1.51 ± 0.05[a]	1.94 ± 0.19[b]
Radioactivity from acetate into:				
Saturated PC (%)	32.3 ± 2.5	34.1 ± 2.8	39.0 ± 3.2[a]	39.8 ± 2.4
Phosphatidylglycerol (%)	2.1 ± 0.3	6.1 ± 1.0[a]	6.1 ± 0.4[a]	7.0 ± 0.2

[a] $P < 0.05$; theophylline alone and Dex alone vs. control
[b] $P < 0.05$; theophylline plus Dex vs. Dex alone

creased the distribution of label into saturated PC whereas theophylline did not. Both agents increased the distribution into phosphatidylglycerol, but the response to combined treatment was not additive. Interpretation of these results is complicated by the decreased rate of incorporation with corticosteroid. In part, this may reflect hormonal effects on intracellular pool sizes and the fact that only tracer quantities of acetate were present.

These limited data suggest that glucocorticoids and methylxanthines have similar effects on PC synthesis in fetal lung. Further studies are required to document both the nature and the generality of the interactive effects.

10.2.2 In Other Tissues

There are several examples of coordinated modulation of enzymes by glucocorticoids and cAMP, or cAMP-generating hormones such as glucagon and epinephrine. These include glycerol phosphate dehydrogenase in brain cell cultures (Breen et al. 1978), argininosuccinate synthetase, argininosuccinase, and arginase in fetal rat liver (Hussen and Vaillant 1982), phosphoenolpyruvate carboxykinase (Barnett and Wicks 1971; Wicks et al. 1974) and albumin synthesis in cultured hepatoma cells (Brown and Papconstantinou 1979), and tyrosine aminotransferase in various populations of liver cells (Butcher et al. 1971; Barnett and Wicks 1971; Wicks et al. 1974; Ernest and Feigelson 1979; Gelehrter 1979; Ruiz-Bravo and Ernest 1982; Perry et al. 1983; Granner et al. 1979). In each of these systems, additive or synergistic effects of glucocorticoids and cAMP analogs occur. Where it has been examined, hormone regulation of liver enzymes in vivo is identical to that found in cultured cells.

The mechanism of hormone action has been studied most extensively for induction of tyrosine aminotransferase. Differences in hormone requirement are reported with various preparations of hepatocytes or hepatoma cells. In freshly-isolated liver cells, induction of tyrosine aminotransferase requires the presence of both glucocorticoid and cAMP or glucagon. In hepatoma tissue culture (HTC) cells, corticosteroid alone will induce the enzyme, but a response to cAMP is dependent on prior exposure to glucocorticoid. In other cell lines, cAMP is active in the absence of added corticosteroid. It is possible that these differences may reflect, in part, the presence or absence of serum (and endogenous hormones) in the culture systems.

The action of the two hormones on tyrosine aminotransferase involves increased levels of mRNA, enzyme protein, and enzyme activity. For both tyrosine aminotransferase and albumin, a synergistic response is seen for both mRNA and protein. It is well established that glucocorticoids act at the level of transcription for induction of liver enzymes, but the site of cAMP action remains uncertain. Differences in the response to glucocorticoids and cAMP have been noted. The time course of response to cAMP is faster than for corticosteroids, and prior exposure to dexamethasone produces a faster response to glucagon but not vice versa. Whereas stimulation by dexamethasone is abolished by actinomycin D, the initial response to dibutyryl cAMP is not inhibited. These and other observations imply that there are separate mechanisms of action for cyclic nucleotide and corticosteroid in the induction process.

It has been proposed that cAMP acts post-transcriptionally to increase the level of functional mRNA for inducible liver enzymes. To date, there is no evidence that glucocorticoids act at any of the known steps in cAMP synthesis, degradation, or activation of protein kinase. Thus, the details of the mechanism of synergy for liver proteins remains undefined. The possible relevance of the synergistic interaction in liver for the effects noted in fetal lung is only speculative at present. Nevertheless, the observations in liver cells establish a precedent for parallel and synergistic effects of corticosteroids and cAMP in other tissues such as lung. The response to corticosteroids plus other hormones which stimulate cAMP (e.g., β-adrenergic agonists) needs to be examined.

10.3 cAMP and T_3

Gross and Wilson (1982) also examined the effects of theophylline and T_3 in explants of rat lung (Table 10.5). T_3 alone increased the rate of choline incorporation into both PC and saturated PC, but not to the same extent as seen with dexamethasone (Table 10.4). The response to combined treatment was greater than with either compound alone, but again the response is less than found with the combination of theophylline and dexamethasone. Neither theophylline nor T_3 increased the distribution of radioactivity from acetate into saturated PC, and only theophylline enhanced incorporation into phosphatidylglycerol. The latter finding suggests that there are differences between cAMP and T_3 in biochemical sites of action for phospholipid synthesis. This implies that thyroid hormone does not affect surfactant synthesis via stimulation of cAMP. This conclusion is supported by the evidence discussed in Chap. 7 regarding receptor mediation of T_3 action.

Table 10.5. Effects of T_3 and theophylline on phospholipid synthesis in cultured rat lung according to Gross and Wilson (1982). Explants of 18-day fetal rat lung were cultured for 48 h without addition or with theophylline (1 mM), T_3 (100 nM) or both agents

	Control	Theophylline	T_3	Theophylline plus T_3
Choline incorporation into PC (pmol/h/mg protein)	483 ± 25	1076 ± 105[a]	664 ± 38[a]	1315 ± 114[b]
Choline incorporation into saturated PC (pmol/h/mg protein)	120 ± 2	296 ± 31[a]	162 ± 5[a]	338 ± 27[b]
Radioactivity from acetate into:				
Saturated PC (%)	32.3 ± 2.5	34.1 ± 2.8	29.8 ± 2.5	31.7 ± 1.1
Phosphatidylglycerol (%)	2.1 ± 0.3	6.1 ± 1.0[a]	2.0 ± 0.4	3.8 ± 1.0[b]

[a] $P < 0.05$; theophylline alone and T_3 alone vs. control
[b] $P < 0.05$; theophylline plus T_3 vs. T_3 alone

10.4 Multi-Hormonal Regulation: An Overview

Since the initial description of glucocorticoid effects on lung maturation, there has developed a growing list of hormones which influence the lung (Chap. 9). Thus, there is accumulating evidence that fetal lung is responsive to a variety of hormones and that several of these have a physiologic role during normal development. In this latter category, I include glucocorticoids, thyroid hormones and β-adrenergic agonists. Each of these hormones has effects directly in fetal lung, and there is considerable evidence supporting the involvement of the endogenous hormones.

A possible scenario for the effects and inter-relationships of these hormones is as follows. There is a basal developmental rate of lung maturation which is independent of the hormonal milieu. This basal rate is influenced by changes in the concentrations or availability of glucocorticoids, thyroid hormones, and catecholamines. In late gestation of normal pregnancies, or earlier in pregnancies complicated by stressful conditions such as premature onset of labor, increased hormone levels accelerate the rate of pulmonary maturation. An influence of T_3 and corticoids occurs in a variety of cell types but is most evident in type II cells. Here, cortisol and T_3 synergistically stimulate the rate of surfactant synthesis through effects at different biochemical sites, and thus cause a precocious accumulation of surfactant in potential airspaces. The rate and magnitude of hormonal stimulation is dependent on the concentrations of both T_3 and cortisol. Glucocorticoids acting independently of T_3 induce β-adrenergic receptors in alveolar cells, and thus increase the sensitivity to endogenous catecholamines. As the circulating levels of epinephrine and norepinephrine increase prior to delivery, the rate of surfactant release from type II cells is stimulated. Catecholamines also enhance reabsorption of lung water as an additional component of preparing the lung for air breathing. Thus, as a result of combined hormonal action, differentiation of the lung is accelerated prior to birth. Administration of exogenous hormones to the fetus mimics this normal regulatory process.

Other hormones may also be involved in regulating lung development. In the diabetic pregnancy, insulin may delay the maturational process, possibly by antagonizing glucocorticoid effects. The possible action of PRL is controversial, but conceivably this hormone may have a permissive action for response to corticoids and thyroid hormones. Similarly, the role of EGF of endogenous origin is uncertain. The effects observed for insulin, PRL, and EGF, and inter-relationships with glucocorticoids, have been discussed in Chap. 9. It seems likely that additional hormones will be identified in the future as influencing aspects of lung development. For example, surfactant secretion is probably under multi-hormonal control.

Objectives of future research will need to include further investigation into the mode of action of the various hormones in lung. Additional information on individual hormones will no doubt provide insight as to the mechanism of hormonal interactions. For example, 2-dimensional electrophoresis of lung proteins after different hormonal treatments may identify the domain of response for each agent. Studies with different cell types in the lung parenchyma can establish the sites of action of each hormone and possible paracrine interactions. With further understanding of basic mechanisms, it is possible that improved hormonal regimens can be devised for accelerating lung maturation in human fetuses.

10.5 Combined Hormone Therapy

Despite the efficacy of antenatal glucocorticoids for prevention of RDS, this therapy is not always effective. The major limitation is the in utero exposure time required for benefit to be observed. There is little, if any, benefit for infants delivered less than 24 h after initiation of maternal treatment, and optimal benefit is not achieved until 2–3 days after the first dose of corticosteroid (Chap. 5). Even with tocolytic therapy, many premature infants are delivered within 2 days after admission to the hospital and thus do not receive optimal treatment. Despite an optimal exposure to corticosteroid in utero, RDS still occurs in some infants. The reasons for treatment failure in many cases are not known, but a partial explanation may be a difference between sexes in glucocorticoid responsiveness (see Chap. 5). It is unlikely that treatment failure is related to the dose of administered corticosteroid, since higher dose regimens have not improved the efficacy nor shortened the interval required for optimal benefit.

Thus, there remains a substantial incidence of RDS among premature infants even in institutions where prenatal glucocorticoid therapy is used routinely. At the University of California, San Francisco, for example, the incidence of RDS among infants of 750–1750 g birthweight has remained around 40% during the interval between 1976 and 1983 (Ballard 1984). It is likely that a large proportion of these cases represents infants who were either not treated because delivery seemed imminent or received too brief an exposure time to betamethasone.

One approach to improving the efficacy of prophylactic treatment is combined hormonal therapy. The data in experimental systems regarding thyroid hormones and glucocorticoids suggest that this combination may be useful clinically. The faster response for PC synthesis by both hormones vs. dexamethasone alone suggests that clinical benefit might occur after shorter treatment intervals than currently seen with betamethasone therapy. The greater response with T_3 plus dexamethasone might also improve the clinical benefit for male infants and twins.

There are several possible approaches to treating the human fetus with thyroid hormone. Although maternal treatment with T_3 or T_4 will elevate fetal levels, high doses are required because of the restricted placental transfer. Alternatively, thyroid hormone could be administered intraamniotically as discussed in Chap. 7. This approach has the disadvantages of requiring an amniocentesis, producing variable concentrations of hormone in the fetus depending on fluid volume and absorption rate, and potentially allowing prolonged exposure of the fetus to elevated thyroid hormone levels if delivery is delayed.

A second therapeutic approach is maternal treatment with a non-iodinated synthetic thyroid hormone such as DIMIT, which readily crosses from mother to fetus. At appropriate treatment doses, DIMIT should produce the same effects in fetal lung as occur with the natural thyroid hormones. However, DIMIT is not yet available commercially, and toxicity testing will be required before application.

A third approach is stimulation of endogenous thyroid hormone production in the fetus. TRH readily crosses the placenta and elevates T_3 and T_4 concentrations of both fetal monkeys and humans at term. Treatment of women in labor at term with 400 µg TRH increased T_3 concentrations in cord blood by about 3-fold at 2 h and levels were elevated for up to 10 h (Roti et al. 1981). A similar response was observed in fetal Rhesus monkeys (Azukizawa et al. 1976). Jacobsen et al. (1977) administered TRH to preterm infants in the newborn period and found an increase in both TSH and T_3 comparable to that observed in term infants and adults. The levels of T_3 in cord plasma after maternal TRH treatment are also similar to the concentrations which normally occur immediately after birth. Based on the studies of T_3 action in organ culture, the increase in fetal T_3 levels with TRH stimulation would be sufficient to increase synthesis of surfactant. A possible added benefit of TRH therapy over administration of thyroid hormone would be the expected increase in fetal PRL levels. Although the role of PRL in lung maturation is not certain, initial experiments in fetal sheep suggest the possibility of a permissive action in the immature human fetus.

It appears likely that clinical trials of combined thyroid hormone and corticosteroid therapy will be carried out in the near future. At present, two approaches are being considered: 1) intraamniotic T_4 plus maternal dexamethasone, and 2) maternal treatment with both TRH and betamethasone. It is possible that such combined therapy will more closely mimic the normal hormonal influences on lung maturation in vivo than treatment with glucocorticoid alone. The potential risks of combined therapy, as well as possible benefits, need to be established before routine clinical use is considered.

References

Amorosa LF, Khachadurian AK, Harris JN, Schneider SH, Fung CH (1984) The effects of triiodothyronine, hydrocortisone and insulin on lipid synthesis by cultured fibroblasts preincubated in serum-free medium. Biochim Biophys Acta 792:192

Azukizawa M, Murata Y, Ikenoue T, Martin CB Jr, Hershman JM (1976) Effect of thyrotropin-releasing hormone on secretion of thyrotropin, prolactin, thyroxine, and triidothyronine in pregnant and fetal rhesus monkeys. J Clin Endocrinol Metab 43:1020

Ballard PL, Benson BJ, Brehier A, Carter JP, Kriz BM, Jorgensen EC (1980) Transplacental stimulation of lung development in the fetal rabbit by 3,5-dimethyl-3′-isopropyl-L-thyronine. J Clin Invest 65:1407

Ballard PL, Gonzales LK (1984) Mechanism of glucocorticoid and thyroid hormone action in fetal lung. In: Respiratory Distress Syndrome, Ravio K (ed), Academic Press, London, pp 67–86

Ballard PL (1984) Combined hormonal treatment and lung maturation. Seminars in Perinatology 8:283

Ballard PL, Hovey ML, Gonzales LK (1984) Thyroid hormone stimulation of phosphatidylcholine synthesis in cultured fetal rabbit lung. J Clin Invest 74:898

Barnett CA, Wicks WD (1971) Regulation of phosphoenolpyruvate carboxykinase and tyrosine transaminase in hepatoma cell cultures. J Biol Chem 246:7201

Bhattacharjee M, Vonderhaar BK (1984) Thyroid hormones enhance the synthesis and secretion of α-lactalbumin by mouse mammary tissue in vitro. Endocrinology 115:1070

Breen GAM, McGinnis JF, de Vellis J (1978) Modulation of the hydrocortisone induction of glycerol phosphate dehydrogenase by N^6, $O^{2'}$-dibutyryl cyclic AMP, norepinephrine, and isobutylmethylxanthine in rat brain cell cultures. J Biol Chem 253:2554

Brehier A, Benson BJ, Williams MC, Mason RJ, Ballard PL (1977) Corticosteroid induction of phosphatidic acid phosphatase in fetal rabbit lung. Biochem Biophys Res Commun 77:883

Brown PC, Papaconstantinou J (1979) Coordinated modulation of albumin synthesis and mRNA levels in cultured hepatoma cells by hydrocortisone and cyclic AMP analogs. J Biol Chem 254:9379

Butcher FR, Becker JE, Potter VR (1971) Induction of tyrosine aminotransferase by dibutyryl cyclic-AMP employing hepatoma cells in tissue culture. Exp Cell Res 66:321

Dobner PR, Kawasaki ES, Uy L-Y, Bancroft FC (1981) Thyroid or glucocorticoid hormone induces pre-growth-hormone mRNA and its probable nuclear precursor in rat pituitary cells. Proc Natl Acad Sci USA 78:2230

Ernest MJ, Feigelson PF (1979) Multihormonal control of tyrosine aminotransferase in isolated liver cells. In: Glucocorticoid Hormone Actin, Baxter JD, Rousseau GG (eds), Springer, Berlin, Heidelberg, New York, pp 219–241 Monographs on Endocrinology, Vol. 12

Evans RM, Birnberg NC, Rosenfeld MG (1982) Glucocorticoid and thyroid hormones transcriptionally regulate growth hormone gene expression. Biochemistry 79:7659

Gelehrter TD (1979) Synergistic and antagonistic effects of glucocorticoids on insulin action. In: Glucorticoid Hormone Action, Baxter JD, Rousseau GG (eds), Springer, Berlin, Heidelberg, New York, pp 583–591 Monographs on Endocrinology, Vol. 12

Gonzales LK, Ballard PL (1984) Glucocorticoid and thyroid hormone stimulation of phosphatidylcholine synthesis in cultured human fetal lung. Pediatr Res 18:310A (abstract)

Granner DK (1979) The role of glucocorticoid hormones as biological amplifiers. In: Glucocorticoid Hormone Action, Baxter JD, Rousseau GG (eds), Springer, Berlin, Heidelberg, New York, pp 593–611 Monographs on Endocrinology, Vol. 12

Gross I, Rooney SA (1977) Aminophylline stimulates the incorporation of choline into phospholipid in explants of fetal rat lung in organ culture. Biochim Biophys Acta 488:263

Gross I, Wilson CM, Ingleson LD, Brehier A, Rooney SA (1980) Fetal lung in organ culture. III. Comparison of dexamethasone, thyroxine, and methylxanthines. J Appl Physiol: Respirat Environ Exercise Physiol 48:872

Gross I, Wilson CM (1982) Fetal lung in organ culture IV. Supra-additive hormone interactions. J Appl Physiol: Respirat Environ Exercise Physiol 52:1420

Gross I, Ballard PL, Ballard RA, Jones CT, Wilson CM (1983) Corticosteroid stimulation of phosphatidylcholine synthesis in cultured fetal rabbit lung: evidence for de novo protein synthesis mediated by glucocorticoid receptors. Endocrinology 112:829

Gross I, Dynia DW, Wilson CM, Ingleson LD, Gewolb IH, Rooney SA (1984) Glucocorticoid-thyroid hormone interactions in fetal rat lung. Pediatr Res 18:191

Henning SJ (1978) Permissive role of thyroxine in the ontogeny of jejunal sucrase. Endocrinology 102:9

Henning SJ (1981) Postnatal development: coordination of feeding, digestion, and metabolism. Am J Physiol 241:G199

Hitchcock KR (1979) Hormones and the lung I. Thyroid hormones and glucocorticoids in lung development. Anat Rec 194:15

Husson A, Vaillant R (1982) Effects of glucocorticoids and glucagon on argininosuccinate synthetase, argininosuccinase, and arginase in fetal rat liver. Endocrinology 110:227

Jacobsen BB, Andersen H, Dige-Petersen H, Hummer L (1977) Pituitary-thyroid responsiveness to thyrotropin-releasing hormone in preterm and small for-gestational age newborns. Acta Paediatr Scand 66:541

Klein LE, Hsias P, Bartolomei M, Lo CS (1984) Regulation of rat renal ($Na^+ + K^+$)-adenosine triphosphatase activity by triiodothyronine and corticosterone. Endocrinology 115:1038

Kriz BM, Gates JA, Read FE, Fong BB (1982) Synergistic regulation of fetal rat liver nicotinamide adenine dinucleotide phosphate (reduced form) cytochrome c reductase activity: Effects of L-triiodothyronine and hydrocortisone. Endocrinology 110:2145

Kumegawa M, Takuma T, Hosoda S, Nakanishi M (1979a) Effects on induction of tyrosine aminotransferase in fetal mouse liver in vitro of prednisolone, insulin and thyroxine. Biochim Biophys Acta 587:20

Kumegawa M, Takuma T, Ikeda E, Nakanishi M, Hosoda S (1979b) Precocious differentiation of chick embryo pancreas in vitro. Roles of prednisolone, insulin and L-thyroxine. Biochim Biophys Acta 585:554

Kumegawa M, Maeda N, Yajima T, Takuma T, Ikeda E, Hanai H (1980a) Permissive role of L-thyroxine in induction of pancreatic amylase by cortisol in neonatal rats. J Endocrinol 86:497

Kumegawa M, Maeda N, Yajima T, Takuma T, Ikeda E, Minamide C (1980b) L-thyroxine, cortisol and diet affect the level of amylase in the parotid gland of developing rats. J Endocrinol 87:65

Kumegawa M, Yajima T, Maeda N, Takuma T, Hosoda S (1980c) Permissive role of L-thyroxine in the induction of stomach pepsinogen by cortisol in neonatal rats. J Endocrinol 87:431

Kurtz DT, Sippel AE, Feigelson P (1976) Effect of thyroid hormones on the level of the hepatic mRNA for α_{2u} globulin. Biochem 15:1031

Leeper LL, Henning SJ (1983) Hormonal control of postnatal development of ileal neuraminidase and acid β-galactosidase. Biol Neonate 44:28

Liggins GC, Schellenberg J-C (1985) Aspects of fetal lung development, In: Physiological Development of Fetus and Newborn, Jones CT, Nathanielsz PW (eds), Academic Press, London, pp 179–189

Longmuir KJ, Bleasdale JE, Quirk JG, Johnston JM (1982) Regulation of lamellar body acidic glycerophospholipid biosynthesis in fetal rabbit lung in organ culture. Biochim Biophys Acta 712:356

Longmuir KL, Resele-Tiden C, Sykes A (1985) The phospholipids of lamellar body material from fetal rabbit lung tissue in culture. Unusual phosphatidylcholine fatty acid profile. Biochim Biophys Acta 833:135

Martial JA, Seeburg PH, Guenzi D, Goodman HM, Baxter JD (1977) Regulation of growth hormone gene expression: Synergistic effects of thyroid and glucocorticoid hormones. Biochemistry 74:4293

Moog F (1961) The functional differentiation of the small intestine IX. The influence of thyroid function on cellular differentiation and accumulation of alkaline phosphatase in the duodenum of the chick embryo. Gen Comp Endocrinol 1:416

Motwani NM, Unakar NJ, Roy AK (1980) Multiple hormone requirement for the synthesis of α_{2u} globulin by monolayers of rat hepatocytes in long term primary culture. Endocrinology 107:1606

Partridge NC, Hoh CH, Weaver PK, Oliver IT (1975) Premature induction of glucokinase in the neonatal rat by thyroid hormone. Eur J Biochem 51:49

Perry ST, Rothrock R, Isham KR, Lee K-L, Kenney FT (1983) Development of tyrosine aminotransferase in perinatal rat liver: changes in functional messenger RNA and the role of inducing hormones. J Cell Biochem 21:47

Post M, Batenberg JJ, VanGolde LMG (1980) Effects of cortisol and thyroxine on phosphatidylcholine and phosphatidylglycerol synthesis by adult rat lung alveolar type II cells in primary cells. Biochim Biophys Acta 618:308

Roti E, Gnudi A, Braverman LE, Robuschi G, Emanuele R, Bandini P, Benassi L, Pagliani A, Emerson CH (1981) Human cord blood concentrations of thyrotropin, thyroglobulin, and iodothyronines after maternal administration of thyrotropin-releasing hormone. J Clin Endocrinol Metab 53:813

Ruiz-Bravo N, Ernest MJ (1982) Induction of tyrosine aminotransferase mRNA by glucocorticoids and cAMP in fetal rat liver. Proc Natl Acad Sci USA 79:365

Samuels HH, Horwitz ZD, Stanley F, Casanova J, Shapiro LE (1977) Thyroid hormone controls glucocorticoid action in cultured GH_1 cells. Nature 268:254

Samuels HH, Klein D, Stanley F, Casanova J (1978) Evidence for thyroid hormone-dependent and independent glucocorticoid actions in cultured cells. J Biol Chem 253:5895

Samuels HH, Stanley F, Shapiro LE (1979) Control of growth hormone synthesis in cultured GH_1 cells by 3,5,3′-triiodo-L-thyronine and glucocorticoid agonists and antagonists: Studies on the independent and synergistic regulation of the growth hormone response. Biochemistry 18:715

Shapiro LE, Samuels HH, Yaffe BM (1978) Thyroid and glucocorticoid hormones synergistically control growth hormone mRNA in cultured GH_1 cells. Proc Natl Acad Sci USA 75:45

Smith BT, Torday JS (1974) Factors affecting lecithin syntheis by fetal lung cells in culture. Pediatr Res 8:848

Smith BT, Sabry K (1983) Glucocorticoid-thyroid synergism in lung maturation: a mechanism involving epithelial-mesenchymal interaction. Proc Natl Acad Sci USA 80:1951

Spence JT, Pitot HC (1979) Hormonal regulation of glucokinase in primary cultures of adult rat hepatocytes. J Biol Chem 254:12 331
Takeuchi T, Ogawa M, Sugimura T (1977) Effects of various hormones and adrenalectomy on the levels of amylase in rat pancreas and parotid gland. Separtum Experienta 33:1531
Takuma T, Kumegawa M (1979) Synergistic effects of thyroxine and glucocorticoid in induction of trypsin-like esteroprotease in mouse submandibular gland. Biochim Biophys Acta 584:51
Torday JS, Dow KE (1984) Synergistic effect of triiodothyronine and dexamethasone on male and female fetal rat lung surfactant synthesis. Dev Pharmacol Ther 7:133
Vonderhaar BK (1975) A role of thyroid hormones in differentiation of mouse mammary gland in vitro. Biochem Biophys Res Commun 67:1219
Vonderhaar BK (1977) Studies on the mechanism by which thyroid hormones enhance α-lactalbumin activity in explants from mouse mammary glands. Endocrinology 100:1423
Wicks WD, Barnett CA, McKibbin JB (1974) Interaction between hormones and cyclic AMP in regulating specific hepatic enzyme synthesis. Fed Proc 33:1105
Wilson EJ, McMurray WC (1981) Regulation of malic enzyme and mitochondrial α-glycerophosphate dehydrogenase by thyroid hormones, insulin, and glucocorticoids in cultured hepatocytes. J Biol Chem 256:11 657
Yeh K-Y, Moog F (1975) Development of the small intestine in the hypophysectomized rat II. Influence of cortisone, thyroxine, growth hormone, and prolactin. Devel Biol 47:173

Subject Index

The abbreviation *re* is used to mean *in relation to.*

MIX
Papier aus verantwortungsvollen Quellen
Paper from responsible sources
FSC® C105338

If you have any concerns about our products,
you can contact us on
ProductSafety@springernature.com

In case Publisher is established outside the EU,
the EU authorized representative is:
Springer Nature Customer Service Center GmbH
Europaplatz 3, 69115 Heidelberg, Germany

Printed by Libri Plureos GmbH
in Hamburg, Germany